T0176539

Essentials of Dental Photography

Essentials of Dental Photography

Irfan Ahmad
Private Practice
Harrow, UK

WILEY Blackwell

Registered Offices
John Wiley & Sons, Inc., 111 River Street, Hoboken, NJ 07030, USA
John Wiley & Sons Ltd, The Atrium, Southern Gate, Chichester, West Sussex, PO19 8SQ, UK

Editorial Office
9600 Garsington Road, Oxford, OX4 2DQ, UK

For details of our global editorial offices, customer services, and more information about Wiley products visit us at
www.wiley.com.

Wiley also publishes its books in a variety of electronic formats and by print-on-demand. Some content that appears
in standard print versions of this book may not be available in other formats.

Library of Congress Cataloging-in-Publication Data
Names: Ahmad, Irfan, BDS, author.
Title: Essentials of dental photography / Irfan Ahmad
Description: Hoboken, NJ : John Wiley & Sons, 2020. | Includes
    bibliographical references and index.
Identifiers: LCCN 2019026632 (print) | ISBN 9781119312086 (paperback) |
    ISBN 9781119312130 (adobe pdf) | ISBN 9781119312147 (epub)
Subjects: MESH: Photography, Dental–methods | Photography,
    Dental–instrumentation | Image Processing, Computer-Assisted–methods
Classification: LCC RK51.5 (print) | LCC RK51.5 (ebook) | NLM WU 100 |
    DDC 617.60022/2–dc23
LC record available at https://lccn.loc.gov/2019026632
LC ebook record available at https://lccn.loc.gov/2019026633

Cover Design: Wiley
Cover Image: © Irfan Ahmad

Set in 10/12pt Warnock by SPi Global, Pondicherry, India
Printed and bound in Singapore by Markono Print Media Pte Ltd

10 9 8 7 6 5 4 3 2 1

For my intrepid wife Samar, and my loving children, Zayan and Zaina.

"And the swelling crescendo no longer retards" – Lou Reed

Contents

Foreword

Original French text

La photographie incarne an même titre que l'écriture, un instrument de prédilection, un outil efficace de formalisation de l'expérience apprécié pour son pouvoir de dénotation et son caractère d'empreinte fidèle et immédiate de la réalité.

C'est. vers la fin des années 1960 que la photographie, limitée à cette simple fonction documentaire ou support d'information va s'affranchir des antagonismes entre art et document à la faveur de la naissance de deux mouvements artistiques qui, sous la dénomination de «conceptuel» et «minimal» font suite aux propositions et travaux de M. Duchamp et Man-Ray et vont soutenir une démarche qui favorise son introduction et acceptation dans le monde de l'art.

Exempte d'intérêt esthétique, impersonnelle et dans le retrait expressif mais suivant un protocole de prise de vue immuable, rigoureux et systématique, cette démarche est en rupture avec la conception traditionnelle de la création et de la notion d'originalité.

Le travail d'Irfan Ahmad en s'interdisant toute incursion vers une attention esthétique, se situe parfaitement dans la ligne de cette mouvance qui va finalement servir et sublimer la finalité didactique qu'il s'était fixée: impressionnant.

Dr. Claude R. Rufenacht

English translation

Photography, like writing, embodies an instrument of predilection, an effective tool for formalising experience which is valued both for its capacity for denotation and its ability to offer a true and immediate account of reality.

It was towards the end of the 1960s that photography, limited to this simple documentary role of information carrier, freed itself from the opposition between art and documentation, thanks to the emergence of two art movements which, under the nomenclatures 'conceptual' and 'minimal', followed on from the proposals and works of Marcel Duchamp and Man Ray, sustained an approach that encouraged its introduction and acceptance in the art world.

Shorn of aesthetic interest, impersonal and utterly neutral, yet following an image-capturing protocol that is immutable, rigorous and systematic, this approach is at odds with the traditional art concept of creation and the notion of originality.

By excluding any hint of aesthetic sensibility, the work of Irfan Ahmad aligns perfectly with this movement to finally serve and sublimate the didactic purpose he set himself: impressive.

Dr. Claude R. Rufenacht

Preface

Photography represents an ineluctable modality of the visible (Joyce 1922). Recent technological advances in digital photography have allowed even the novice to take photographs that are so sharp they will cut your eye like a Buñuel film, with colours as tantalising as characters from a Fellini movie, nuances comparable to a Bergman drama, the depth of a Kubrick odyssey, and provocative as a Borowczyk tale. What was once reserved for the few, is now within reach of the many.

Nowadays, analogue or film photography is reserved for die-hard aficionados, an old school reliving their youths. In the twenty-first century, digital photography is the norm (Motta 2010), but comes in many guises, and requires novel approaches for creating superlative results. This is not unlike the demise of amalgam, and the rise of composite restorations, which requires a change in mindset, abandoning old techniques and learning new tricks. The world around us is analogue, everything is perpetual, days seamlessly fade into nights, time goes by without interruptions or delays. We have digitised the world for our convenience, utilisation and manipulation. Time is divided into second, minutes and hours, temperature into degrees of hot and cold, distance into lengths of miles or kilometres. In our digitised world, photography is no exception; light is expediently converted into binary or digital codes for producing visuals.

Today, dental photography is no longer an option, but an integral and indispensable tool for practising dentistry at every level and for every discipline. Furthermore, no matter how meticulously one articulates or writes clinical notes of an examination, a photograph will communicate the clinical scenario in a few seconds. Therefore, it is surprising that this subject does not form part of the undergraduate dental curriculum. Besides offering indisputable photodocumentation, pictures are probably the most powerful learning method for clinical dentistry and self-development. A series of images allow assessment, diagnosis, planning, delivery of treatment, and follow-up that no other medium can offer. Furthermore, photography is a vital communication tool between patients, fellow colleagues, specialists and technicians for discussing multi-disciplinary and for complex therapies. In addition, pre- and post-operative, as well as procedural images provide an invaluable record if a therapy fails to yield the desired results or satiate patients' expectations.

However, many clinicians are reticent about incorporating dental photography into their daily practice due to uncertainty about the choice of equipment, a steep learning curve and initial capital expenditure. These fallacious notions are fuelled by the plethora of dental literature on the subject, some scientifically based, some anecdotal, while others perversely complicate what is basically a simple procedure. It is the endeavour of this book to demystify many of these erroneous beliefs by proposing protocols for standardising photographs that are invaluable for intra- and inter-patient comparison. Once the essentials are mastered, a little experimentation will allow the operator to develop his or her own style for the intended use, and progress to the next level by modifying techniques for specific disciplines.

The dental team yearns for a book about photography that is reader-friendly, shows simple techniques, and gives pertinent advice for achieving repeatedly predictable results with a minimum of effort. Rather than endless descriptive text describing the theoretical aspects of photography, most of the discussion is focused on practical concepts. This is accompanied by copious illustrations and images, taking the reader by the hand and guiding him or her to learn about standardising images by showing simple set-ups and requisite equipment settings. Once assimilated, usually in a few days (preferably combined with a hands-on session), a routine photographic session should take no more than ten minutes. A small sacrifice, compared to the innumerable benefits that this medium offers. After obtaining predictable results, more advanced and special applications are presented for specific clinical and laboratory requirements.

The book is divided into three sections. The first deals with equipment and concepts, the second with photographic set-ups and the third with processing images. Each section is composed of modules that sequentially furnish the reader with the essentials, culminating in a complete manuscript that covers all aspects of the CPD (Capture, Processing and Display) triad of digital dental photography.

To summarise, this is a practical book, endeavouring to "show me" rather than "tell me", and informing the reader about what they *want* to know, rather than what they *need* to know.

Enjoy the journey into a world of infinite possibilities…

Irfan Ahmad

References

Joyce, J. (1922). *Ulysses*. Paris: Sylvia Beach.
Motta, R.J. (2010) The future of photography. Proceedings of the SPIE 7537: 753702.

Acknowledgments

The author would like to thank Fahad Al-Harbi for procuring the necessary photographic equipment for some of the pictures in Modules 5 & 6, and for arranging the model featured throughout the book, particularly in Module 6.

Section 1

Equipment and Concepts

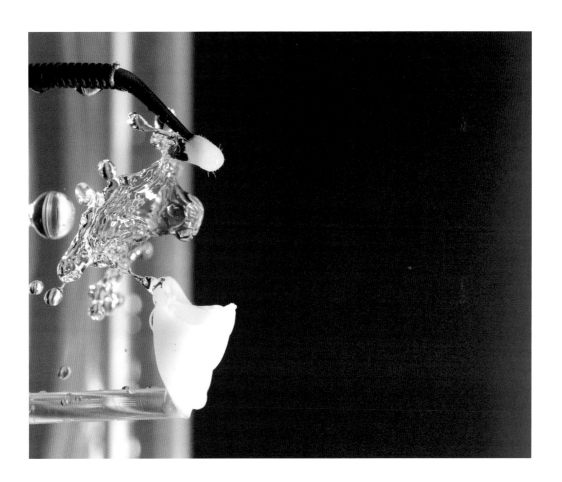

1

Photographic Equipment

The most frequently asked questions about dental photography are:

> 'Which equipment do I need?'
> 'What is the cost?'
> 'How long will it take to learn?'

The aim of this opening module is to provide answers to these questions.

Photography should be regarded as an integral part of daily clinical practice (Reddy et al. 2014), and photographic equipment as part of the dental armamentarium, no different to a dental handpiece. However, the common consensus is that a camera is an extraneous apparatus, exclusively reserved for specialists, or clinicians with a penchant for taking pictures. These are erroneous assumptions since photographic documenting is essential for diagnosis, treatment planning, treatment options, educating patients and ancillary staff, communicating with colleagues, recording treatment sequences, assessing and monitoring outcomes, marketing, and serves as irrefutable evidence if litigation ensues. Furthermore, it is important to emphasise that dental photography is not solely for specific treatments such as elective cosmetic procedures, but a requisite for recording pathological conditions of the oral mucosa or even the simplest treatment modalities such as tooth whitening.

The first thing to appreciate is that there are no 'quick fixes' and no 'deals', and fellow colleagues or companies who propagate these myths are misguided and misleading. A number of dental companies exploit photographic ignorance by offering 'quick fixes', with low-end cameras specifically adapted for dental photography, often sold at inflated prices for the gullible and uninitiated. However, most of these cameras are compromises, yielding inferior image quality, which is hopeless for precise diagnosis, treatment planning, follow-up and communication. If the objective is simply to produce bland and boring pictures, similar to passport or 'mug shots', then these devices fit the purpose. However, there is still a learning curve with these modified cameras, and it is questionable whether the toil is worthwhile for disappointing results. Alternately, the same time and effort can be channelled to learning correct techniques with appropriate equipment, which yield excellent and gratifying results.

Similar to learning a particular clinical technique such as crown preparation or implant surgical procedures, there is a learning curve for mastering dental photography that cannot be ignored. However, the time required to learn basic photographic techniques is reduced with proper advice and guidance. Taking pictures is probably easier than restoring a Class I cavity, but does require a degree of patience and perseverance. As mentioned in the Preface, once

Essentials of Dental Photography, First Edition. Irfan Ahmad.
© 2020 John Wiley & Sons Ltd. Published 2020 by John Wiley & Sons Ltd.

basic techniques are mastered in a few days (preferably combined with hands-on or online training course),[1] a routine photographic session should take no more than 10 minutes of clinical time; a small sacrifice compared to the innumerable benefits if offers.

Cameras

Before choosing a camera and the accompanying accessories, it is crucial to establish the basic requirements of dental photography. Dental photography is essentially divided into two types of picture: portraiture and macrophotography. Portraits are necessary for several disciplines and clinical scenarios such as orthodontics, prosthodontics, aesthetic/cosmetic dentistry, facial enhancement procedures, external traumas to the dentition, or accidents involving soft tissue bruising, lacerations and fractures of the facial skeleton. Macrophotography encompasses both intra-oral pictures of the oral environment consisting of the teeth and surrounding anatomy, and extra-oral pictures of the dento-facial composition and bench images of diagnostic casts or artificial prostheses/restorations. Therefore, it is essential to choose a camera and accessories that fulfil the requirements of both portraiture and macrophotography.

The market is awash with cameras offering countless functions, some superfluous, others essential, and deciphering which are useful or redundant is a challenging and annoying endeavour (Ahmad 2009a). Many camera features that are supposedly added to make life easier often end up as frustrating nuisances, and wading through never-ending cascading menus requires aptitude and endurance. This is probably the biggest turn-off for potential purchasers, who are bombarded with technical jargon, acronyms they do not understand and features they are unable to comprehend. Therefore, it is important to ignore manufacturers' hype and concentrate on salient specifications. The type of camera systems available is a minefield, such as point-and-shoot, compact, CCS (compact camera systems), EVIL (electronic viewfinder interchangeable lens), MILC (mirrorless interchangeable-lens compacts), rangefinders, dSLR (digital single lens reflex) and, of course, not forgetting the smartphone (cellphone) varieties (Figure 1.1).

Nowadays, no discussion on photography would be complete without mentioning smartphone cameras. In recent years the quality of smartphone cameras has increased exponentially, and these devices are capable of delivering images that were once only possible with dedicated digital cameras. In addition, many reputable camera manufacturers such as Leica˙, Hasselblad˙ and Carl Zeiss˙ are collaborating with phone companies to develop cameras and accessories for mobile hardware. The convenience, expediency and connectivity offered by smartphones and tablets is obviously the driving force for this rapidly evolving industry. Also, there has been a discussion in the dental literature about the suitability of cellphones or tablets for dental photography (Manauta and Salat 2012). The main purpose of smartphone cameras is that they are designed for social photography. Hence, to use these units for medical/dental purposes, the in-built cameras need to be calibrated and modified for macro use, which requires a degree of training. Whilst the disseminating convenience offered by mobile devices is unmatched, to achieve clinically useful images requires perseverance. Smartphones are ideal for random shots showing patients' particular oral problems, or sharing cursory images with dental technicians regarding oral rehabilitation, but to take this a step further, training is essential. Nevertheless, this technology is difficult to vilipend, because in the near future, mobile devices may evolve to be the standard for photodocumentation for many fields, including dentistry.

---

1 https://www.dentalphotomaster.com/online-training

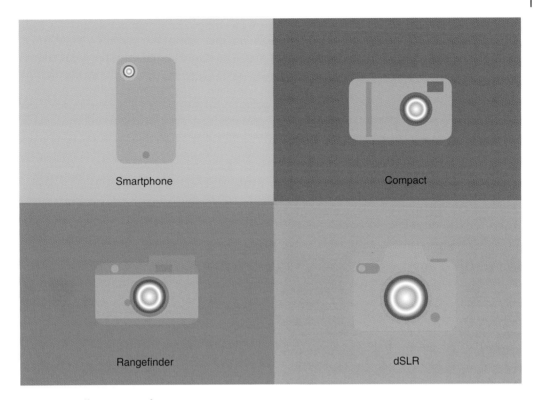

Figure 1.1 Different types of camera systems.

In order to satisfy the requirements of dental photography and produce images rich in detail, vibrancy, nuances of colour, texture, form, conveying emotions, feelings and unparalleled quality, the only choice at present is a dSLR.[2] Whilst other category of cameras can be tailored or adapted for dental use, the task is onerous, and probably not worth the frustration for the small cost saving that is often elusive. Having established that a dSLR is the ideal camera for dental applications, the next question is: which proprietary brand to choose?[3] The advice in this book concentrates on generic photographic equipment, which fulfils basic requirements for dental applications. Also, with technological advances, newer products are perpetually being introduced, which readily become obsolete in a short space of time. Furthermore, mid-range dSLRs from any major brands are almost identical in terms of features and the image quality they offer.

A dSLR consists of a body containing the mechanics and electronics, or brain, of the camera. A camera body usually comes as a kit with a lens and other basic accessories. However, most lens that form a kit are often unsuitable for dental applications, and, if possible, it is advisable to purchase the body alone, or exchange the accompanying lens for one that is more suited for dental use. The primary features to look for in a camera body are the physical size of the sensor, megapixel count, colour depth, numerical white balance input, external flash synchronisation via a hot-shoe with TTL (through-the-lens) metering, switchable manual focusing, sensor speed or ISO (International Standards Organisation) range, remote

---

2 http://www.dentalphotoapp.com/7.html
3 http://www.photomed.net

shutter release, tripod thread(s) and ease of sensor cleaning. The secondary features include exposure modes and metering, shutter speeds, sequential frames per second, colour space, dust and water spray sealing, anti-fingerprint and anti-scratch coating of the LCD (liquid crystal display) touch screen, RAW file formats, video capability, GPS (global positioning system), WiFi, storage media, interface for data transfer, built-in photo-editing software, build quality, size, weight and, of course, the price. Whilst there is no compromise of the mandatory primary features, the secondary features are desirable, but not necessary. Although the list of primary or secondary specifications may seem endless, there is no need to fret, since most dSLRs have these features as standard. But, like anything in this world, you get what you pay for; the higher the specifications, the higher the price. All major camera brands, such as Canon, Nikon, FujiFilm, Sony, Panasonic (Lumix), Pentax and Olympus, offer mid-range or semi-professional dSLRs suitable for dental requirements for around US$ 500 at current prices. Table 1.1 itemises the specifications for choosing a camera, and for those wishing to understand the relevance and importance of these features, an explanation of the major specifications is given below.

Sensors

The heart of a digital camera is the sensor, a solid-state device composed of tiny photosensitive diodes called pixels, (abbreviation of 'picture elements'). The pixels are stimulated by incoming light through-the-lens to create an electrical charge that is an analogue signal. The electrical signal is then converted by an analogue to digital converter (A–D converter) into a binary digital code, or data, for creating the image. The pixels are colour blind, only capable of registering black and white, or brightness and darkness (Figure 1.2), and require some types of filters to produce colour images using the additive red, green and blue (RGB) colour system. The additive RGB colour system represents the three primary colours RGB, which collectively produce white when mixed together. This is in contrast to the substrative colour system: cyan, magenta, yellow (CMY) – Figure 1.3. The colour filter system used by manufacturers for adding colour is either the mosaic Bayer pattern, or the Fovean X3˙ colour filters. The former uses a single layer with the imprinted Bayer pattern to add colour, whilst the latter has individual RGB filters stacked on top of each for capturing the corresponding RGB channels. In the Bayer system two green squares are included, representing greater sensitivity of the eyes to the colour green (Figures 1.4–1.8).

There are two types of sensors, CCD (charged couple device) and CMOS (complementary metal oxide semiconductors). CCD was the first type of sensor, offering superior image quality but with higher power consumption. The newer CMOS sensors are more efficient, better in low light conditions and offer high-speed capture. Furthermore, recent technical sophistication means that CMOS sensors are viable contenders to CCDs in terms of image quality. Most contemporary cameras use CMOS as the preferred type of sensor. Sensors are available in various physical sizes, some popular examples include medium format (up to 53.9 mm × 40.4 mm), full-frame (similar to 35 mm film – 36 mm × 24 mm), APS-H (Advanced Photographic System-type H – 28.7 mm × 17 mm), APS-C (Advanced Photographic System-type C – ranging from 23.6 mm × 15.7 mm to 22.2 mm × 14.8 mm), four thirds, micro-four thirds (17.3 mm × 13 mm), 1″ (13.2 mm × 8.8 mm), 1 : 2/3″ (8.6 mm × 6.6 mm), 1 : 1.7″ (7.6 mm × 5.7 mm) and 1 : 2.5″ (5.76 mm × 4.29 mm) – Figure 1.9. To complicate matters further, some sensors sizes are unique (or renamed) to a particular camera brand, e.g. the Nikon DX-format is equivalent to the APS-C format. The key issue is the physical size (or dimensions) of a sensor: the larger the sensor, the better the image quality, irrespective of the pixel count.

Table 1.1 Specifications of a digital single lens reflex (dSLR) camera for dental photography.

Specification	Must have	Wish list
Sensor size	minimum Advanced Photographic System-type-C (APS-C)	full-frame (36 mm × 24 mm), matching the focal length of lens
Pixel count in MP (megapixels)	minimum 18 MP (depending on physical size [dimensions] of sensor)	> 18 MP (depending on physical size [dimensions] of sensor)
No anti-alias filter	Desirable	Mandatory
ISO (International Standards Organisation) range	minimum 100–200: any maximum	
Sensor cleaning	Ease of manual sensor cleaning	Automatic, built-in sensor cleaning mechanism
Colour depth	8 bit/colour (channel)	16 bit/colour (channel)
Dynamic range (human eye = 24 f-stops)	minimum 6 f-stops	≥ 10 f-stops
White balance	Auto, or numerical input [5500 K]	
Focusing	Manual focus capability	
External flash connections	Hot-shoe, x-jack	Wireless/via smartphone
Remote shutter release	Wired hand/foot cable release	Wireless/via smartphone
Tripod screw thread	1/4–20 UNC (Unified National Coarse)	1/4–20 UNC or 3/8–16 UNC and a 1/4–20 UNC adapter
Exposure modes	Aperture priority and manual	
Metering modes	Centre-weighted, multi-zone, spot	
Shutter type	Focal plane	Built-in lens
Shutter drives	Single and multiple	
Shutter flash synchronisation speed	1/125 s or 1/250 s	Any shutter speed possible with built-in lens shutters
Colour space	sRGB, Adobe® RGB	
File format	Proprietary RAW or Adobe DNG (digital negative graphic), JPEG	
Storage	UHS I (30 MB/s writing speed) SD card	UHS II (100 MB/s writing speed) SD card or internal RAM storage
Data transfer	USB 3 or greater, audio in/out jacks, HDMI	WiFi
Video recording capability	HD 1080p (progressive) to 60 fps (frames per second)	> 4 K (similar quality to conventional cine film)
Location		GPS (global positioning system)
LCD (liquid crystal display)	Touch screen	Anti-fingerprint and anti-scratch coating
Camera protection		Dust and water spray sealing
Build quality, weight, size	Portable, light-weight, die-cast aluminium	Milled aluminium

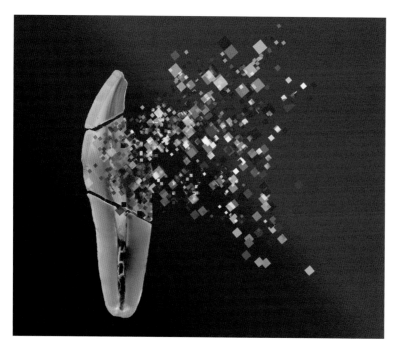

Figure 1.2 Pixels are only capable of registering lightness and darkness, i.e. black and white.

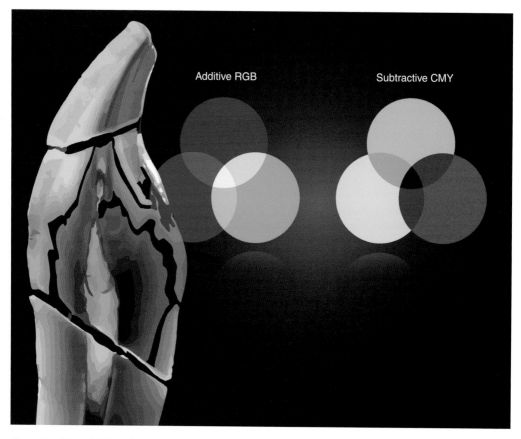

Figure 1.3 The additive red, green and blue (RGB) and subtractive cyan, magenta and yellow (CMY) colour systems.

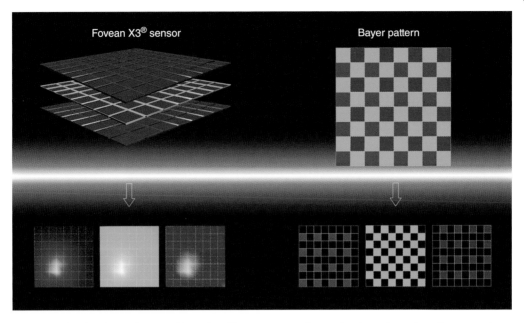

Figure 1.4 A colour image is created by colour filters corresponding to the three channels, red, green and blue, e.g. the Fovean X3 system or the mosaic Bayer pattern.

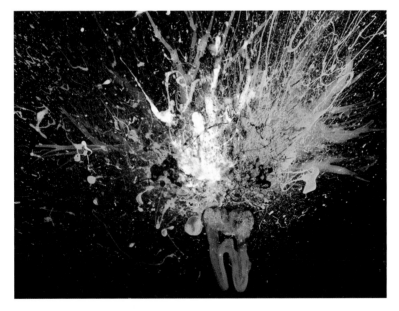

Figure 1.5 Red channel colouration.

Resolution

The resolution of an image is complex, depending on many variables, including the resolving power of the lens, sensor size, number and size of pixels, bit depth (range of colours), dynamic range (degree of contrast), signal to noise ratio (amount of 'noise' or graininess in an image), method of in-camera analogue to digital conversion, file format, subsequent post-capture editing with computer software, circle of confusion (distant from which an image is viewed) and the display media (monitor, projector, printing).

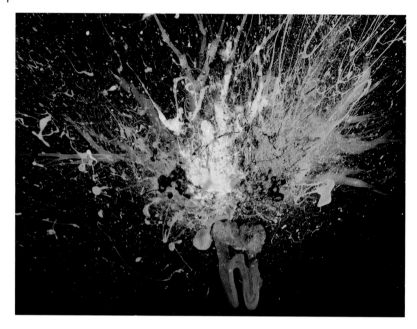

Figure 1.6 Green channel colouration.

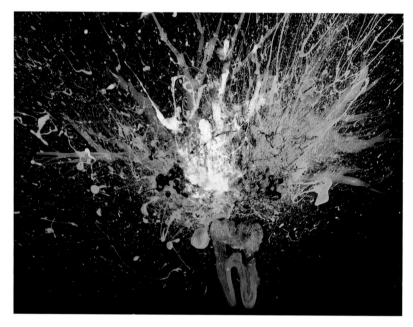

Figure 1.7 Blue channel colouration.

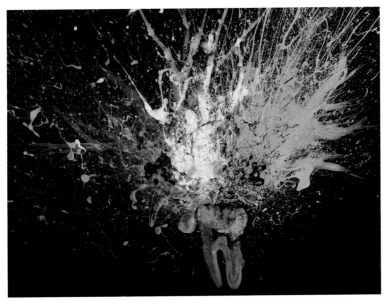

Figure 1.8 The final coloured image combining the three red, green and blue (RGB) channels.

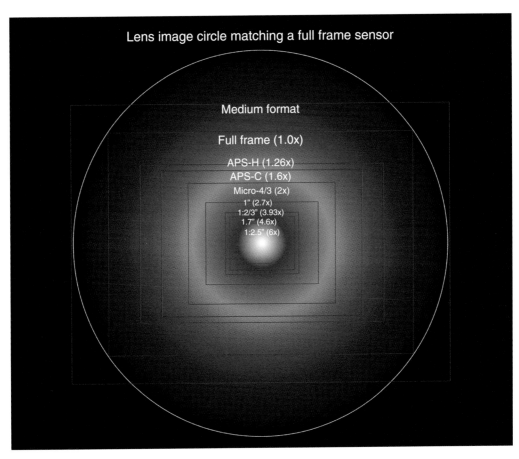

Figure 1.9 Comparison of digital camera sensor sizes, together with the corresponding crop factor in parenthesis.

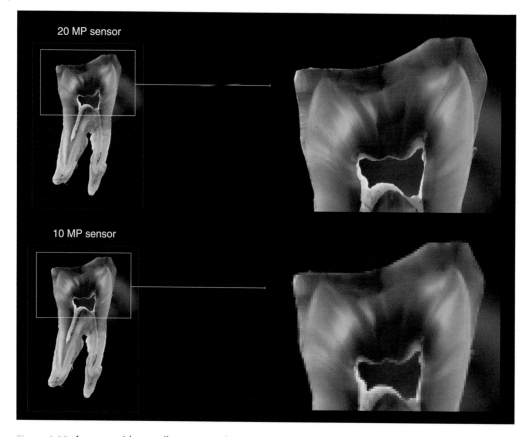

Figure 1.10 A sensor with a smaller megapixel count will result in deterioration in image quality when part of the image is magnified.

The resolution of the human eye varies from 324 megapixels (90° angle of vision) to 576 megapixels (120° angle of vision), which is far beyond any contemporary digital camera sensor.[4] However, one of the major misconceptions is relating pixel count to resolution, i.e. equating the number of pixels to image quality, often misleadingly perpetuated by camera manufacturers. The number of pixels determines the size of an image, not its ultimate resolution. However, a large pixel count is significant if the resolution is not to be compromised when part of an image is magnified or cropped. Hence, the resultant image quality depends on the number of megapixels (MP) and the physical size of the sensor (Figures 1.10 and 1.11). Understanding the significance of physical size of the sensor and its MP count are crucial when purchasing a camera. For example, a full-frame sensor with a pixel count of 20 MP yields a higher resolution than a smaller-sized sensor with the same or greater number of pixels. This is because the larger pixels found on large-sized sensors are capable of gathering more detail than the smaller pixels on small-sized sensors. Therefore, a small sensor with a large pixel count, often found in compact cameras, produces inferior quality images compared to a larger sensor with fewer pixels in a dSLR. Another factor to enquire about is the presence or absence of an anti-alias filter on the sensor. Newer cameras without anti-alias filters offer superior resolution and therefore better image quality. Further information about resolution can be found in Modules 3 and 8.

---

4 http://www.clarkvision.com/articles/eye-resolution.html

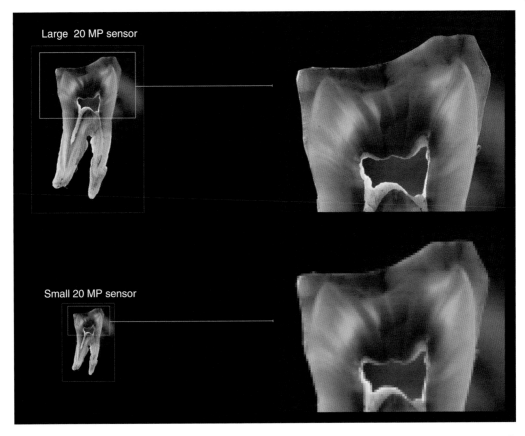

Figure 1.11 A large sensor will retain image quality when part of the image is magnified, compared to a small sensor with the same megapixel count.

Sensor Speed or ISO

The sensitivity of the sensor to light is represented by its ISO number. The ISO scale determines the intensity of light that is necessary for correct exposure; a lower ISO number requires more light, whilst a higher ISO number less light. Although higher ISO values have the benefit of taking pictures in low lighting conditions, the drawback is that the pictures are more grainy (with increased 'noise') and consequently with inferior resolution (Figure 1.12). As a general guide, an ISO value of 50–100 will produce insignificant noise but requires brighter illumination, whilst the ideal for dental use is between ISO 100 and ISO 200, and certainly should not exceed ISO 400.

Sensor Cleaning

Dust particles enter the camera at the junction where the lens is mounted onto the camera body, and also by the movement of the internal mirror (if any) within the camera. This is particularly significant when changing lenses or focusing screens, which should be performed in a dust-free environment, preferably with appropriate vacuum suction. The dust particles are a nuisance, adhering to the sensor surface and appearing as black or white specks on an image, especially noticeable with light backgrounds such as teeth (Figure 1.13). Although these

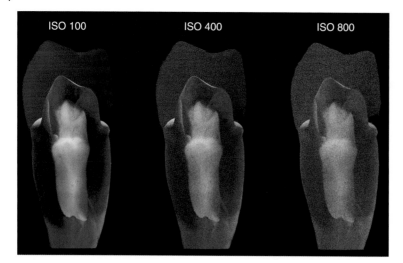

Figure 1.12 Increasing the ISO (International Standards Organisation) value has the advantage of taking pictures in low light, but at the expense of introducing graininess or noise that degrades image quality.

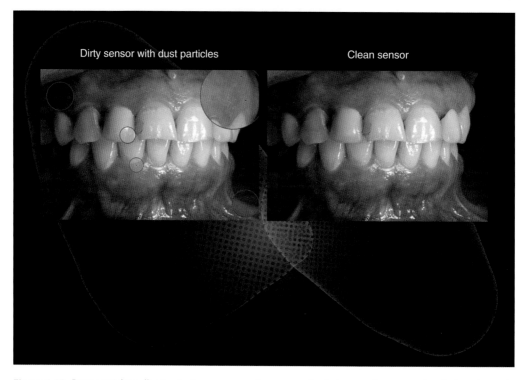

Figure 1.13 Dust particles adhering to the sensor surface are particularly conspicuous against light-coloured backgrounds.

blemishes can be erased with software during the editing stage, the process is tedious, time-consuming and best prevented at the outset. Sensors are difficult to access and clean manually, requiring a degree of dexterity to prevent inadvertent damage to the most delicate and expensive part of the camera body. Many proprietary sensor cleaning kits are available that

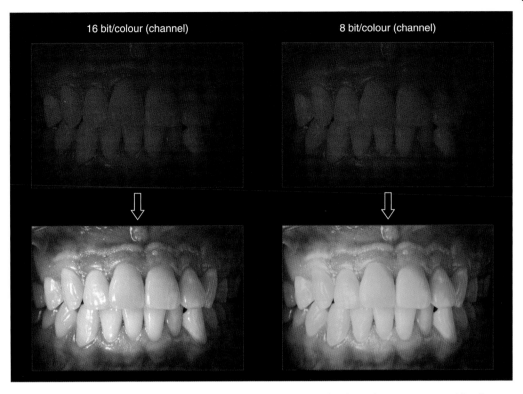

Figure 1.14 Bit/colour (channel) significance: A grossly underexposed 16 bit/colour image is capable of withstanding substantial exposure compensation without losing quality (left images), whereas an 8 bit/colour image is labile to degrade, often with resulting unwanted colour casts (right images, notice greenish colour cast after exposure compensation).

facilitate this process and provide invaluable and detailed instructions for mitigating irreversible damage to the sensors. In addition, many cameras have built-in sensor-cleaning mechanisms that minimise dust accumulation and facilitate its removal. Whichever mechanism a camera employs for sensor cleaning, it is important to enquire about ease of sensor cleaning, or built-in cleaning systems, when purchasing a camera body.

Colour (Bit) Depth

The colour, or bit depth, is a measure of the number of colours that can be captured by a sensor. It is expressed as bits/channel or bits/colour of the three photographic additive primary colours, red, green and blue. A camera with a colour depth of 8 bit/colour (channel) will have a total bit depth of 24, or 2^{24}, and is capable of producing 16.7 million colours, far more than the 10 million colours that the human eye can perceive.[5] High-end cameras have digital sensors with 16 bit/colour (channel) and are capable of discriminating 2^{48}, or 281 trillion colours. The advantage of having a larger bit depth is reducing degradation of image quality that occurs if substantial editing or manipulations are anticipated with post-capture software. Therefore, starting with a large bit depth at the outset compensates for this eventuality (Figure 1.14).

---

5 http://dmimaging.net/8-bit-vs-16-bit-images

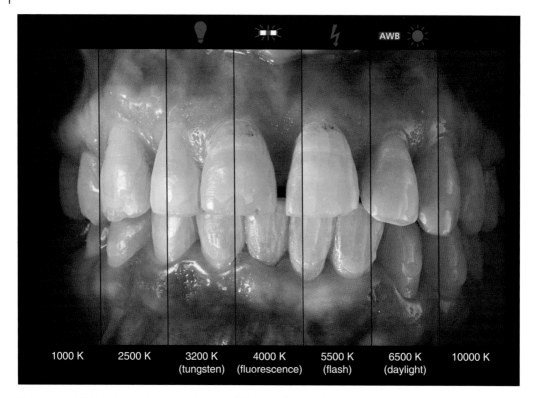

1000 K	2500 K	3200 K	4000 K	5500 K	6500 K	10000 K
		(tungsten)	(fluorescence)	(flash)	(daylight)	

Figure 1.15 White balance: An image showing different colour rendering by altering the white balance setting on the camera (AWB = automatic white balance).

White Balance

Unlike our brains, cameras do not possess colour adaptation, and have to be 'told' about the colour temperature of the illumination, a process known as setting or calibrating the white balance. Most cameras have pre-set automatic white balance (AWB) options that signify the quality, or colour temperature of the light, e.g. natural daylight of 6500 K, or indoor tungsten illumination of 3200 K. Photographic daylight is 5500 K because at this colour temperature all the three photographic primary colours (RGB) are present in equal proportions. This is an important issue for dental images because ensuring correct colour rendering is essentially from a dento-legal perspective. Therefore, the colour accuracy needs to be precise, without colour casts, for faithfully reproducing the actual colour of the soft and hard tissues. This allows distinguishing between health and pathological changes, as well as matching the shade of artificial restorations to natural teeth. Most dental photography uses artificial [flash] lighting, and it is important to ensure that the white balance on the camera is either set to AWB, or preferably input manually numerically to 5500 K (Figure 1.15).

Focusing

Almost every camera these days has auto-focus (AF) as standard, which is indispensable for the majority of photographic needs. However, for macrophotography, especially in the restricted confines of the oral cavity, AF often malfunctions. This is due to incessant patient or operator micro-movements, and extreme light thresholds of the highly reflective surfaces of teeth with the dark posterior regions of the mouth, which additively confuses the automatic focusing mechanism. Therefore, the ability to switch to manual focus (MF) is a prerequisite to compensate for the unique conditions of the oral environment. The usual method for ensuring sharply focused dental images is either using a mechanical focusing stage (discussed below), or moving hand-held cameras backwards and forwards until focusing is accomplished. Another advantage of MF is that it allows pre-set magnifications (e.g. 1 : 1 or 1 : 2) for consistent scaling of images that is useful for comparisons, whereas with AF, the magnification perpetually changes according to the distance of the subject from the lens.

External Flash

There are two types of external flash lighting necessary for dental applications: compact flashes and studio flashes or strobes. Compact flashes are mainly used for macrophotography and require a hot-shoe contact, usually found on top of the camera, to access the electronics of the camera for TTL metering for ensuring correct exposure. Once an initial contact with the camera is established via the hot-shoe, additional compact flashes can be triggered by wired or wireless interfaces, whilst the TTL function cuts off, or quenches, the flashes once correct exposure is attained. Studio flashes utilised for portraiture are triggered either by a wired standard x-jack connection on the camera body, or by a wireless radio or infra-red device connected to the hot-shoe, termed slave flash photography. Also, it is possible to control some studio flashes, similar to compact flashes, by the camera electronics using TTL metering. This requires purchasing additional camera brand specific remote controls, which allow the camera to control the flash duration of the strobes for ensuring correct exposure.

Remote Shutter Release

The camera shutter is usually released by pressing a button on the camera body. This is satisfactory for the majority of dental images, but for certain treatment modalities that require photographs from various angles of view such as aesthetic dentistry, or surgical procedures where cross-infection control is paramount, it is necessary to mount the camera onto a tripod and delegate this task to another member of the dental team. In these circumstances, it is helpful to have remote shutter triggering mechanisms that do not compromise or interfere with the clinical procedure. Several options are available, including wireless, foot control and smartphone apps, which are operated by an ancillary not directly involved with the treatment.

Lenses

The technical requirements of a lens for dental photography is that it serves a dual-purpose, first for portraiture and second for close-up or macrophotography. The ideal lens for portraiture is around 100 mm focal length, and for macrophotography is a macro facility for achieving a 1 : 1 or 1 : 2 magnification. A 1 : 1 magnification ratio means that the image recorded on the sensor is the same size as the object, whilst a 1 : 2 magnification means that the captured image is half the size of the object. Macro lenses are either available as fixed focal lengths, called prime lenses, or zooms with variable focal lengths. It is recommended to use prime lenses, rather than zooms, which are usually impractical for dental photography. Furthermore, fixed focal length macro lenses greater or less than 100 mm are unsuitable for the following reasons. To achieve a 1 : 1 magnification with a 50 mm macro lens requires moving the camera extremely close to the subject, which may be intimidating for the patient. In addition, at this close distance, the cheeks and lips block the flash lights illuminating the oral cavity. Another problem with a 50 mm lens is that portraits at close distances result in spherical distortion, making the nose or other prominent parts of facial features appear larger and less flattering. Conversely, macro lenses greater than 100 mm, say 200 mm, require greater distances for obtaining a 1 : 1 magnification. This is also a hinderance since brighter lights are necessary to correctly illuminate the subject that is now further away, plus the physical size and weight of these lens is inconvenient for hand-held cameras. Many contemporary lenses offer image sta-bilisation for preventing blurred images. However, this feature is superfluous for dental pho-tography since the high flash synchronisation shutter speeds (1/125 seconds or 1/250 seconds), and the fraction of a second flash burst 'freezes' the subject, obviating the need for image stabilisation. It is important to realise that image stabilisation is different to focusing; the for-mer compensates for involuntary micro-movements referred to as 'camera shake' (for hand-held cameras), whilst the latter is concerned with focusing a sharp image onto the sensor depending on the distance of the object from the camera.

Most dSLRs are sold with general-purpose lenses, usually variable zooms, satisfying broad photographic genres such as family shots, portraiture, landscape, sports, wildlife, etc. However, these lenses are a 'jack of all trades and master of none'. They offer acceptable resolving power, but not superlative resolution. As mentioned above, the lens is a crucial factor for determining the image quality, and its resolving power should match or be greater than the size of the pixels, which vary from 5 to 12 μm. An array of lenses is available, either the same brand as the camera, third-party, or from different brands using appropriate adapters. The same brand lenses have the advantage that they seamlessly synchronise or integrate with the camera electronics and can be updated with the latest firmware, but are usually more expensive. The market is inun-dated with third-party lenses, some inferior, and others offering even better resolution than same brand lenses. Lastly, lenses from old 35 mm film cameras can easily be fitted with rela-tively inexpensive adapters to almost any camera. These offer excellent optics since they are usually constructed of glass elements but are heavier, whereas newer versions are often made of plastic elements, with reduced acuity, but are much lighter in weight. Some high-end macro lenses have the prefix 'Apo' and 'ASPH', which eliminate apochromatic and aspherical aberra-tions, respectively. These optically corrected lenses may be the same brand as the camera or third-party lenses, with state-of-the-art optics for exceptional resolution, but come with a hefty price tag, e.g. Carl Zeiss, Schneider-Kreuznach®, Meyer-Optik Gorlitz®, Voigtlander® and Leica to name a few. In addition, a search on e-Bay™ offers many pre-owned high-end lens at a fraction of the new retail price, and with appropriate adapters, e.g. from Fotodiox® or Novoflex®, can be fitted to almost any camera body. The major disadvantage is that some electronic functions of the camera, such as AF or auto-exposure, are disabled, and therefore the lens has to be used in manual mode. Other methods for achieving macro images are using various inexpensive attach-ments on standard lenses, such as reversal rings, conversion rings, extension tubes, bellows, or Lensbaby™ macro converters. The drawbacks are a slight deterioration in image quality, and the additional weight, which may be off-putting for hand-held photography.

Irrespective of the lens, a wise precaution is to purchase a UV (ultra-violet) filter that screws onto the front of the lens for protection from dust, water or other oral effusions. In addition to offering physical protection, a UV filter eliminates unwanted 'haze', enhancing the colour rendi-tion of the image. Another useful attachment is a lens hood to eliminate flare from intense illumi-nation (e.g. direct sunlight or flashes pointing towards the camera) that causes glare on images.

A further issue to contend with is whether the focal length of the lens matches the size of the sensor. The focal length of lenses is usually quoted according to old 35 mm film cameras. If the camera has a full-frame sensor (36 mm × 24 mm), the image seen in the viewfinder will almost be identical to what is recorded on the sensor (crop factor of 1). However, if the size of the sensor is smaller, say APS-C (22.2 mm × 14.8 mm), the lens image circle is greater than the sensor size, and only the central part of the image is recorded on the sensor. For example, with an APS-C sensor the lens has a crop factor is 1.61 (see Figure 1.9). Also, for smaller sensors found in compact cameras the crop factor becomes even greater, whilst for larger sensors in medium format cameras, the crop factor reduces to less than 1. Therefore, it is desirable to have a full-frame sensor so that the focal length of the lens matches the sensor size, but the additional cost of the camera body may be prohibitive. To summarise, the choice of a lens for dental photography is empirical, dictated by personal preferences and cost, which can vary from US\$ 600 to UD\$ 1000, or more, if image quality is an absolute priority.

Lighting

There are two types of lights required for dental photography: compact and studio flashes Ahmad (2009b). Many cameras have built-in flashes that pop-up when the lighting conditions are less than optimal. This is satisfactory for general photography but ill-advised for macrophotography. First, the built-in flashes are usually not congruous with the lens axis, and at close distances cast an unwanted shadow which obscures essential parts of the image. Second, on-camera flip-up flashes are relatively weak, with low intensity, and unable to adequately illuminate the entire oral cavity.

The compact flashes are further sub-divided into ring flash (ring-light), compact off-the-camera bilateral (bi-directional or twin-light) flashes, or a single unit consisting of both ring and twin-lights (Figures 1.16 and 1.17). Compact flashes, also known as hot-shoe flashes, connect directly onto the hot-shoe of the camera body and are subsequently controlled by the camera electronics. Their intensities are measured in guide numbers at ISO 100, the higher the guide number, the brighter the light output. Typical compact flashes have a guide number ranging from 20 to 50 (100 ISO metre) or 65 to 165 (100 ISO feet). For dental use, a guide number of ISO 30 (metre) is more than adequate. All electronic flashes serve a dual purpose, first to

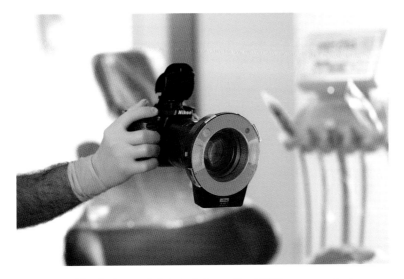

Figure 1.16 Ring flash on a digital single lens reflex (dSLR) camera system.

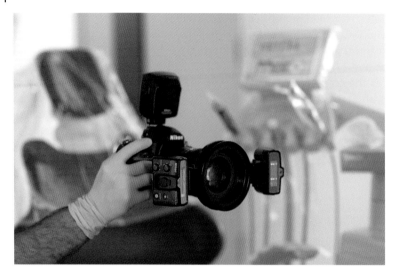

Figure 1.17 Bilateral twin flashes on a digital single lens reflex (dSLR) camera system.

provide sufficient illumination for correct exposure, and second, to 'freeze' the object being photographed due to the fraction of a second burst of light (up to 1/20 000 of a second). In addition, nearly all compact flashes (ring flash and lateral flashes) are compatible with camera brand-specific TTL metering for measuring exposure. Continuous lights sources such as daylight, tungsten lamps, fluorescent tubes and LED (light emitting diode) are capable of delivering adequate illumination but cannot 'freeze' movement. The latter is significant since the patient is unlikely to keep rigidly still during an arduous photographic session, feeling uncomfortable and claustrophobic with cheek retractors, photographic mirrors, dribbling saliva, not to mention the operator contortions with hand-held cameras. Therefore, a dental photographic session should be conducted as quickly and efficiently as possible, which is expedited by the endearing property of flashes because they allow pictures to be taken in rapid succession, simultaneously illuminating and 'freezing' the subject.

Compact ring flashes attach directly onto the front of the lens, emitting uniform (360°) shadowless illumination, which is ideal for hand-held pictures, especially in the darker posterior regions of the mouth where access for light is restricted by the surrounding cheeks and lips. The price for ring flashes ranges from US$ 100 to US$ 500, depending on the type, make and guide number. The major drawback of ring flashes is that the light is harsh, uniform and characterless. Whilst ideal for photographing posterior teeth, for anterior teeth this type of illumination produces images that are bland, boring and lacklustre. For anterior teeth, or for restorations where aesthetics are of paramount concern, ring flashes are not recommended since the uniform burst of light obliterates fine detail, translucency, surface texture, topography and subtle colour transitions and nuances within teeth or artificial restorations.

To overcome the shortcoming of ring flashes, compact bi-directional or bilateral flashes offer lighting that sculpts the object giving it a three-dimensional appearance with highlights and shadows, allowing visibility of enamel characterisations such as mamelons, cracks, staining, translucency, restorative marginal defects. Furthermore, by manipulating the light source reveals colour nuances and depth of the underlying dentine strata, which is essential for mimicking these characteristics in indirect prostheses. The intensity of individual flashes can be muted, or turned off, to enhance highlights or shadows that are ideal for capturing micro and macromorphology.

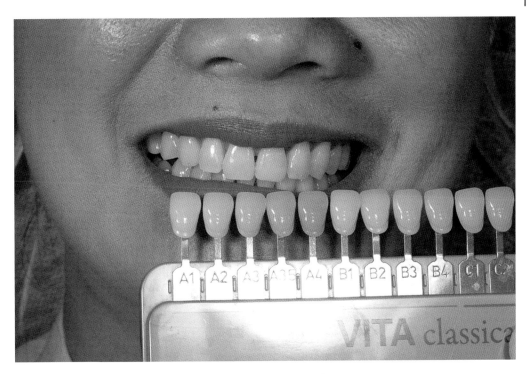

Figure 1.18 Ring flashes produce lacklustre, bland two-dimensional images.

Three are two varieties of lateral flashes. The first type attaches onto the front of the lens by an adapter and has two projecting flashes, which can be positioned right, left, top, bottom or anywhere in between. Also, since the flashes fire wirelessly, they can be detached, hand-held and positioned as desired. The negative aspect of these flashes is their proximity to the teeth, and depending on the guide number, the flash burst can be harsh, similar to ring flashes that obliterate fine detail. To circumvent this undesirable effect, the second type of lateral flashes are mounted with a bracket, or flash extension arms, beneath the camera and positioned behind the lens. These units are also triggered wirelessly but emit much softer subtle light. In addition, the light can be further attenuated by covering the flash heads with cloth or plastic diffusers to soften the output. Soft lighting adds ambience to an image, and depending on intensity and distance can reveal subtle detail by creating shadows and highlights, as well as emulating natural lighting conditions in which teeth are usually viewed. As an analogy, using ring flashes is identical to taking a picture of a subject head-on in front of car headlights, whereas lateral flashes, dampened with diffusers mimic realistic lighting of natural surroundings such as reflections and shadows from people, buildings, water, foliage, furniture, walls, etc. (Figures 1.18 and 1.19). Both types of lateral flashes, lens or bracket mounted, cost around US\$ 500.

Lastly, several unusual light sources and light modification attachments are available for dental photography. For example, ingenious contraptions such as flexible LED fibre-optic 'Medusa-like' cables for directing light into the tiniest recesses of the mouth. Also, relatively inexpensive flash accessories can be purchased to manipulate the emitted light, such as diffusers of various sizes, reflector cards of different colours (matt white, glossy white, grey, silver). Also, elaborate magnifying lenses attached to flashes can focus the light beam to highlight individual teeth or particular areas of interest.

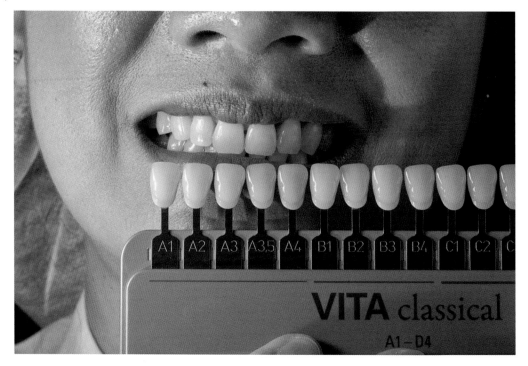

Figure 1.19 Bilateral flashes produce three-dimensional images conveying depth and vitality.

The second type of lighting is for dental portraiture, which may be hot lights, cool lights or flashes. The first two types, hot and cool lights, offer continuous illumination that is suitable for video but unsuitable for still photography. The preferred types of lights for portraits is studio flashes. Two varieties of studio flashes are available, the monolights, which connect directly to the mains, or the pack and head, which require a separate power pack and are indicated for location shooting. For dental applications, monolights are the most convenient, incorporating integral modelling lights to help position and orientate the flashes before taking a picture. A modelling light is a continuous light source that allows the photographer to visualise the lighting effect the flashes will produce, but does not affect the actual exposure (aperture and shutter speed) when the flashes are triggered. These continuous pre-flash, low-intensity lights also keep the pupils dilated, and together with 'catch lights' or Obies confer a shining aura to the subject. Catch lights are tiny reflections on the cornea that create a glint or sparkle, attracting the viewer to the eyes of an individual (Figure 1.20).

The flash intensity or output of a flash tube is measured either in watts/second (W/s), or expressed as a guide number (GN), similar to compact flashes, e.g. a 120 W/s flash has a GN of 125 (100 ISO feet) or 38 (100 ISO metre), whilst a 300 W/s has a GN of 190 (100 ISO feet) or 58 (100 ISO metre). If the flashes are intended only for head-shots of a single person, two 120 W/s flashes are sufficient. However, if pictures of small groups, bigger objects in larger spaces, or creative lighting with light-modifying attachments is required, two or more >300 W/s flashes are recommended.

Many light-modifying attachments are available for manipulating light for creative effects, e.g. reflective umbrellas, soft boxes, gels, barn-doors, honeycomb grid diffusers, reflectors, Fresnel lenses, etc. A good starting point is using two soft boxes, and once proficient, experiment with more sophisticated modifiers for conveying ambience and mood. Unlike compact

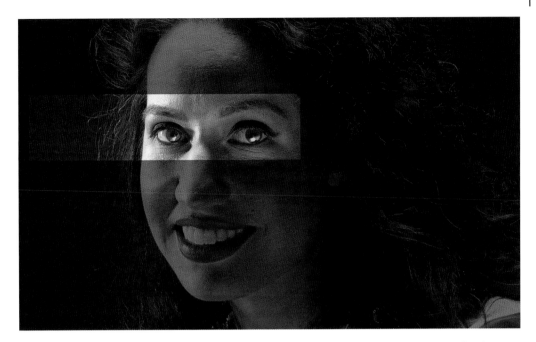

Figure 1.20 Catch lights glints representing reflections of studio flashes or reflectors that attract the observer to the eyes of the subject.

ring or lateral flashes that use TTL metering for correct exposure, studio flashes usually require manual exposure settings. The exposure can either be assessed experimentally, or precisely calculated using an incident light meter for determining the exact aperture and shutter speed. Since purchasing a light meter is an additional expense, an economical approach is taking a few test shots for determining exposure settings, distances of flashes and reflectors, which are repeatable for a given set-up. Studio flashes can either be triggered with synchronisation (or sync.) cables plugged into the standard x-jack on the camera, a radio or infra-red wireless device fitted onto the hot-shoe, or via apps from a smartphone, tablet or computer. Usually only one flash needs to be connected directly to the camera, whilst the remaining flashes are simultaneously triggered by light receiving sensors on the additional flashes. A starter studio flash kit with two monolights, two reflective umbrella or soft boxes, two air-cushioned stands or tripods and triggering mechanism costs around US$ 300–500, and is an ideal package for starting portraiture photography (Figure 1.21).

Finally, portraiture requires backdrops or backgrounds, which are limited only by the imagination. These can simply be suspended coloured cloths or elaborate stage set-ups; the choice resides with the photographer.

Supports

Most clinician and dental technicians take photographs with hand-held cameras for convenience and expediency. However, there are instances when supports are invaluable for stabilising the camera and allowing hands-free operation for precisely positioning flashes and ancillary equipment. This could be during surgical procedures, a detailed aesthetic or soft tissues analysis, and portraiture. The variety of supports available is perplexing and confusing, including

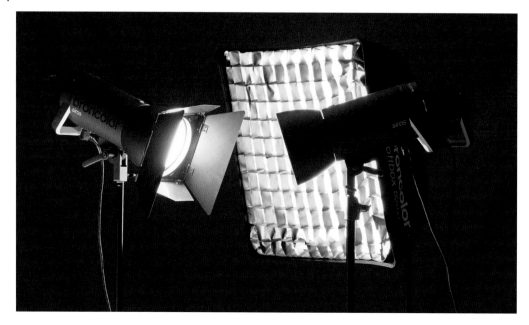

Figure 1.21 Examples of studio flashes for portraiture.

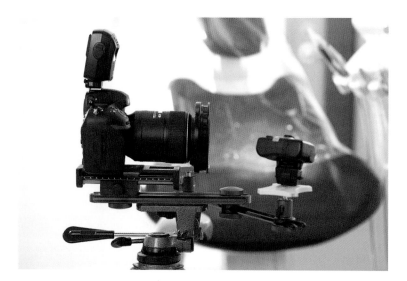

Figure 1.22 Tripod-mounted camera, compact flashes and focusing rail.

monopods, tripods, jibs, cranes, booms, cages, clamps, brackets, steady cams, rails, slides, dollies and suction pads. To simplify matters, for dental photography, a tripod with a dolly (wheels), and a four-way focusing rail (stage) for fine focusing is all that is necessary. The tripod head should have a pan (side to side) and tilt (up and down) movements, and be resilient enough to carry the payload of the camera, lens, flashes and macro focusing rail. The focusing rail is attached underneath the camera, and is indispensable for fine manual focusing at pre-determined magnifications. The cost of a tripod with a dolly, tripod head and macro focusing stage is around US$ 250 (Figure 1.22).

Table 1.2 Budget photographic equipment for dental photography[a]

Item	Cost (US$)
dSLR camera body	500
Marco lens – 100 mm (or equivalent)	600
Compact ring flash	100
Compact lateral (bi-directional) flashes (2)	500
Bracket for lateral flashes	50
Flash accessories (diffusers, reflectors)	50
Studio flash kit for portraits	300
Backdrops and reflectors for portraits	100
Tripod, tripod head, focusing stage	250
Remote shutter release	100
SD, SDHC, SDXC, CF 16 Gb storage cards (2)	30
Data storage card reader	15
Rechargeable batteries with charger for compact flashes	20
Polarising filter (circular)	50
UV bulbs	40
Total:	US$2705

[a] Prices quoted from B&H Photo, Video, Pro Audio (https://www.bhphotovideo.com/c/browse/Digital-Cameras/ci/9811/N/4288586282/1).

Other Photographic Items

Some relatively inexpensive items are also useful for completing the photographic equipment arsenal. These include rechargeable batteries, a multi-card reader for transferring images to a computer, UV bulbs for visualising fluorescence of natural teeth and artificial prostheses, or porosity defects in porcelain restorations. A polarising filter is helpful for analysing shade by eliminating specular reflections (glare) off the enamel surface. Polarising filters are available in two varieties; linear or circular, and in practice, both do the same job. The former, linear, is better suited for manual focusing but more costly, whilst the latter, circular, is cheaper and can be used in both manual and AF modes. Finally, digital photography requires a computer and processing software, and recommendations for the latter are given in Section 3, dealing with editing, exporting and managing images.

Table 1.2 itemises the essential photographic equipment necessary for dental photography. However, in the beginning, it may be prudent to start by purchasing equipment for only intra-oral photography, and eventually progressing to portraiture lighting with other ancillary equipment. On a budget, the cost of purchasing all the requisite items is US$ 2705, but if finances are unlimited, the sky is the limit.

References

Ahmad, I. (2009a). Digital dental photography. Part 4: choosing a camera. *Br. Dent. J.* 206 (11): 575–581.

Ahmad, I. (2009b). Digital dental photography. Part 5: lighting. *Br. Dental J.* 207 (1): 13–18.

Manauta, J. and Salat, A. (2012). *Layers*. Milan: Quintessenza Edizioni.

Reddy, S.P., Kashyap, B., Sudhakar, S. et al. (2014). Evaluation of dental photography amongst dental professionals. *J. Educ. Ethics Dent.* 4: 4–7.

2

Dental Armamentarium and Clinical Considerations

Besides photographic equipment, there are additional items required for taking intra-oral pictures, as well as specific clinical considerations to bear in mind. The majority of these requisite items are readily available as part of the dental armamentarium, but a few need to be acquired.

Retractors

In order to have access to the cavity, it is necessary to retract the surrounding lips and cheeks. The most frequent method for retraction is cheek retractors, which come in a variety of ingenious designs, sizes, colours and materials (Figure 2.1). The basic configurations are unilateral or bilateral, the former for quadrants or sextants and the latter for full-arch images. Also, it is helpful to keep a stock of several sizes and shapes to accommodate varying degrees of mouth opening. Cheek retractors are either made of plastic or stainless steel (SS). The plastic variety are gentler but prone to fracture, especially the bilateral variety, and some can only be cold sterilised, but single-use disposable types are also available. The SS varieties are more rigid, unlikely to fracture and are autoclavable. However, some patients object to the harsh piecing sensation of steel against their cheek and lips. The choice is a personal preference of both the clinician and the patient, but the author recommends the plastic unilateral and bilateral varieties for comfort and ease of insertion and removal. In addition, the pliable plastic cheek retractors allow easier manipulation of the cheeks from right to left sides of the mouth for lateral buccal views (Figure 2.1).

Photographic Mirrors and Contrasters

Dental photographic mirrors are used for taking pictures of the occlusal/incisal and buccal/lingual/palatal surfaces of teeth. The mirrors are available in numerous shapes and sizes catering for macroglossia and visualising almost any aspect or angle of the teeth and surrounding soft tissues (Figure 2.2). The larger mirrors are used for full-arch views, while the narrower types are more suited for quadrant and buccal or lingual surface views. Intra-oral mirrors are available in various materials including titanium, and glass with front-coated chromium, rhodium or dielectric plated for eliminating double or ghost images. The titanium varieties are more durable, costlier and usually only single sided. The glass coated varieties are slightly less expensive but have the advantage of high reflectance. For example, the reflectance of titanium is 80%, rhodium-plated mirrors 75%, chromium 65–70% and SS 50–60% (Sreevatsan et al. 2015) – Figure 2.3. Also, glass mirrors are double-sided, and if one side becomes scratched, the

Essentials of Dental Photography, First Edition. Irfan Ahmad.
© 2020 John Wiley & Sons Ltd. Published 2020 by John Wiley & Sons Ltd.

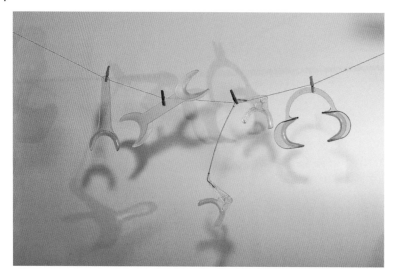

Figure 2.1 Selection of cheek retractors of various configurations and sizes.

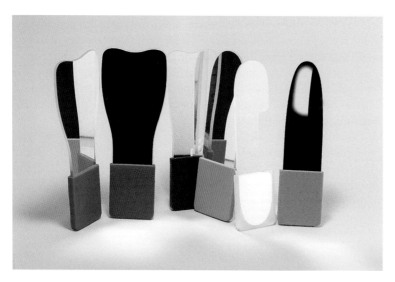

Figure 2.2 Dental photographic mirrors are available in various shapes sizes to cater for photographing various fields of view.

reverse side can be used without having to purchase a new mirror. Depending on the manufacturer, some mirrors are autoclavable, while others can only be cold sterilised. Decontamination of dental mirrors requires particular attention by using lint-free cleaning cloths and mild detergents so as not to scratch or degrade the surface coating. Another precaution is avoiding ultrasonic cleaning with abrasive or caustic disinfectant solutions, which cause irreparable damage to the front plated-surfaces.

There is a trend to photograph a section of the dental arch, especially the maxillary anterior sextant (facial and palatal aspects) with a black background for excluding distracting extraneous anatomy such as nostrils, tongue, opposing arch and soft tissues. This is achieved by using contrasters that are made from metal and coated with silicone black paint, and available in

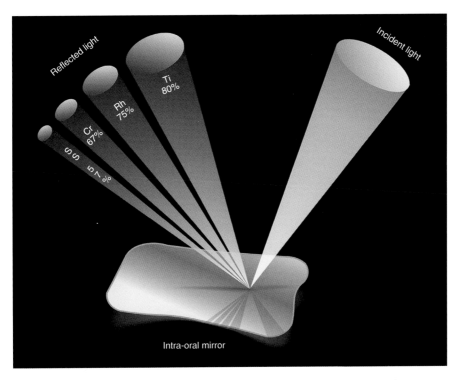

Reflected light

Incident light

Ti
80%

Rh
75%

Cr
67%

5.5%

5.1%

Intra-oral mirror

Figure 2.3 Percentage of light reflected off a mirror surface according to the type of coating.

Figure 2.4 Contrasters are made of metal with a black silicone coating.

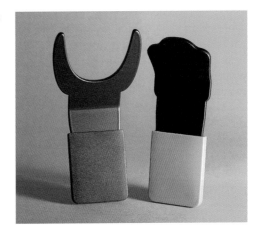

various shapes (occlusal, anterior and lateral) for various intra-oral views, and are usually autoclavable (Figures 2.4 and 2.5). They are also used for creating a black background for emphasising translucencies at the incisal edges and interproximal areas of the teeth. The contrasters are judicially placed for concealing unwanted anatomy before taking the photograph. If TTL (through-the-lens) metering is used for flash metering, the large area of a black background of the contraster confuses the camera metering system, which results in an over-exposed image. The exposure can be compensated either when taking the photograph, e.g. by moving flashes further away or reducing their intensity, or correcting the exposure in photo-editing software.

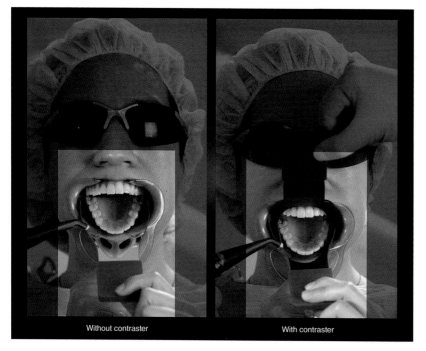

Without contraster With contraster

Figure 2.5 Contrasters are used to exclude unwanted anatomy, such as nostrils when using intra-oral mirrors.

Field of View

The field of view to photograph should be clean and clearly visible. Having displaced the lips with check retractors, it is essential to maintain a dry field during a photographic session. A dry field is required to capture details of the teeth, free gingival margin, attached gingiva and mucogingival junction, which allows accurate analysis, treatment planning and discriminating healthy and pathological changes for differential diagnosis of oral lesions.

The method used for achieving a clean and dry field depends on the clinical situation, and the type of treatment being performed. The choices are rubber dam, gingival retractor cords, cotton wool rolls, gauze, or aspiration using a slow-speed saliva ejector or high-speed suction. As well as maintaining a contamination-free environment for dental procedures, a rubber dam is also an ideal method for isolating both the anterior and posterior teeth (Figure 2.6). This is particularly relevant when documenting treatment sequences such as adhesive bonding techniques, where absolute isolation is mandatory. Although a rubber dam conceals the surrounding soft tissues, it offers an arid environment without condensation, which is particularly useful for preventing fogging of intra-oral mirrors for occlusal, buccal and lingual images.

Intermittent use of a slow speed saliva ejector and/or surgical aspiration tip is invaluable for ensuring patient comfort, and for aspirating dribbling saliva or haemorrhage while documenting surgical procedures. However, it is important to remove the ejector just before taking the picture, so it does not appear in the image. Other methods for achieving and maintaining a dry field include discreetly placing cotton wool rolls into the sulci, especially in the maxillary buccal and mandibular lingual regions at the location of parotid and submandibular salivary gland duct orifices, respectively. Gingival retraction cord, with or without a haemostatic agent, e.g. buffered aluminium chloride is an effective method for halting haemorrhaging and absorbing crevicular fluid seepage from the gingival sulcus.

Before taking the picture, all ancillary items should be made invisible, such as check retractor edges, contraster and intra-oral mirrors. The cheek retractors should be large enough to

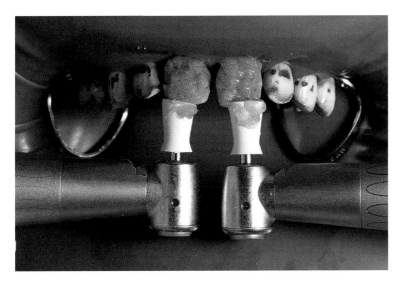

Figure 2.6 A rubber dam is ideal for isolating the teeth and for documenting clinical restorative procedures.

adequately deflect the middle part of the upper and lower lips so that they do not appear in the photograph and obscure the maxillary and mandibular frena. Any fingers holding mirrors or other dental instrumentation should be excluded from the composition. This also applies to drooping lips, glaring nostrils (in maxillary arch mirror views), flaccid tongue or double images of the actual and reflected teeth when using intra-oral mirrors. Unwanted elements can be cropped later in processing software, but it is recommended that the shot be composed correctly at the capture stage to minimise post-editing. This is particularly relevant with reflected images taken with intra-oral mirrors, as cropping can be time-consuming and onerous (The Academy of Laser Dentistry 2015).

Accumulation of surface biofilm, extrinsic stains, or food debris lodged between contract areas are annoying since they obscure the underlying enamel and dentine. Unless it is the intention to photograph these deposits, flossing and polishing with prophylaxis paste is recommended before taking photographs. Furthermore, gingival embrasures obscured by unwanted debris hinder diagnosis of interproximal carious lesions as well as accurate shade assessment for artificial restorations. The teeth should not be overly desiccated to minimise a shade shift, but gently dried to remove salivary film with compressed air from a three-in-one, or preferably a heated six-in-one, dental syringe, which also prevents condensation, or fogging, on intra-oral mirrors. In addition, air drying removes saliva droplets and trails on the teeth and gingiva (unless these are intentionally being photographed for stylistic reasons). Other methods of preventing misting of mirrors is using high-speed suction, warming mirrors beforehand or wiping the mirror surface with a surface tension reducer or anti-condensation liquid. Finally, removable dental appliances should be removed, unless their documentation serves a purpose.

For dento-facial clinical images, it is advisable to tone down or remove lurid lipstick and flamboyant make-up. However, for marketing and promotional images, make-up is justified for beautifying an individual or conveying their persona.

Cross-infection Control

Emphasising the importance of cross-infection control to dentists is preaching to the converted. There are already stringent guidelines for cross-infection control, and therefore, many would perceive it as condescending to have verbose text on this subject. However, a few key points warrant

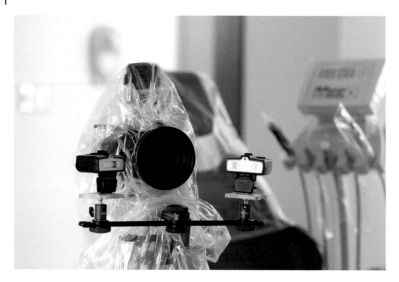

Figure 2.7 Draped photographic equipment as part of cross-infection control.

discussion (Ahmad 2009). Whenever possible, an asepsis protocol is adopted. First, the camera and lens are appropriately draped with cellophane covers, not excessively, as plastic coverings are slippery and prevent access to camera settings (Figure 2.7). Drapes are mandatory when photographing surgical procedures, but optional for routine documentation for EDP (essential dental portfolio) or EPP (essential portrait portfolio). Also, all camera, lens and flash settings are set beforehand to prevent unduly touching the equipment during a photographic session. Second, all team members participating in a photographic session should wash their hands with soap, or alcohol gel, before wearing gloves. It is generally good practice to wear gloves while taking photographs as it is often necessary to use saliva ejectors and to adjust the position of the patient's head and of ancillary equipment such as check retractors or intra-oral mirrors. In addition, the operator and ancillary staff should change gloves when pausing treatment procedures to take photographs, and subsequently wear a new pair when continuing treatment. Third, a remote camera shutter release, preferably via foot control is invaluable for hands-free operation. Photodocumentation during surgical procedures is ideally delegated to a 'dirty' dental assistant, who can operate the photographic equipment, preferably by a smartphone app. Fourth, intra-oral accessories such as retractors, mirrors, contrasters and reflectors should be appropriately sterilised, disinfected or discarded (Vasileva et al. 2017). Fifth, corrosive sterilising solutions and paper tissues are not recommended for cleaning photographic equipment, since they may cause irreparable damage. Instead, camera and flashes are wiped with moist microfibre towels (Shorey and Moore 2009). Lastly, if black and white specks or dots appear on successive images at the same position, the most likely cause is dust on the sensor. Cleaning a camera sensor is an extremely delicate task, ideally commissioned to a professional dealer. Alternately, if sensor cleaning is attempted, it is best performed using lint-free cloths and volatile liquids to avoid smears and streaks.

Health and Safety

Currently, there is a fetish for draping every piece of dental equipment with disposable cellophane sheets and covers. While laudable for cross-infection control, there are times when pragmatism should prevail. Dogmatic adherence to stringent guidelines can sometimes be counterproductive. For example, unbridled use of plastic covers hinders access to photographic equipment to change settings and are potentially hazardous, especially when wet and slippery. Also, overheated studio lights can melt, or worse ignite cellophane coverings. However, these extreme examples are not an excuse for abandoning cross-infection control, but a measure of common sense is necessary to avoid mishaps and accidents.

Other health and safety considerations include moving all mobile units, foot controls, spittoons, handpiece consoles, operatory light and chair-mounted monitor displays aside. Also, dental handpiece and suction tubes should be stored in their receptacles to avoid tripping or entangling. It is mandatory for the entire team to be aware of, and conform to, personal protection equipment (PPE), and for the patient to be offered safety sunglasses for protection and shielding from intense light burst from flashes. It is worth remembering that photographic equipment is additional to the plethora of dental armamentaria, and therefore it is prudent to place the camera in a safe and secure zone of the operatory where it can neither be knocked over, nor interfere with routine treatment, but nevertheless be readily accessible when needed. All batteries for flashes, camera and computer should always be charged in readiness. All sprawling flash or shutter triggering cables are tied or taped securely, not loosely hanging, as they are a potential hazard for trapping or entangling with dental equipment.

All unfastened clothing such as scarves or neckties is secured, and long hair tied back with disposable scrunchies. Sharp items including necklaces, rings, bracelets, extravagantly long or porcupine-like earrings are removed, so that they cannot engage with photographic cordage. In addition, facial tissues are constantly at hand to wipe excess dribbling saliva. The edges of cheek retractors and lips are liberally lubricated with petroleum jelly for facilitating insertion and removal, and avoiding chapping of the lips.

Finally, it is worth mentioning that the patient and dental team members be requested to turn off all audible mobile devices, which are obviously distracting and annoying during treatment and a photographic session.

Location

The location where dental pictures are taken is a contentious issue. For portraiture, there is little disagreement: an allocated room, or indeed a tailor-made studio away from the clinical environment. However, for intra-oral images, there is confusion, and the ideal location is debatable. Some operators prefer a non-clinical setting for placing patients at ease, and making the photographic session a relaxing experience (Davda n.d.). However, this may be counterproductive since there is no access to aspiration, compressed air, the patient cannot be reclined in the supine position for certain photographic views. Ultimately, this necessitates moving essential dental equipment to a non-clinical setting with the associated compromises in cross-infection and health and safety. There is no doubt that dental photography is a unique genre, and as discussed above, adhering to certain requirements is paramount. Therefore, it is the author's opinion that a clinical setting is best suited for intra-oral photography, fulfilling both clinical requirements and having access to essential dental armamentarium. This is particularly pertinent when photographing surgical procedures, when draping and other asepsis protocols are mandatory for avoiding contamination and ensuring treatment success. To illustrate the importance of a clinical setting for dental photography, the sequential images in Figures 2.8–2.23 demonstrate that this surgical procedure could not have been documented in a non-clinical environment.

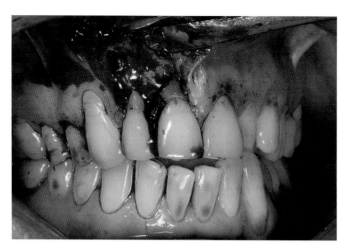

Figure 2.8 Photographing surgical procedures is particularly demanding because a strict cross-infection protocol is mandatory. This necessitates regularly changing gloves and minimising contact with photographic equipment during a surgical procedure by ensuring that camera and flash settings are optimally configured beforehand: flap elevation to reveal chronic infection associated with the right maxillary lateral and central incisors.

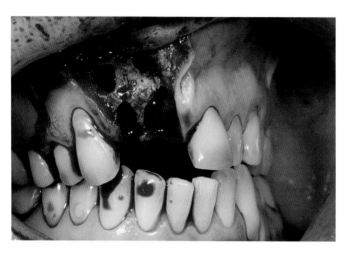

Figure 2.9 Extraction of the right maxillary incisors and curettage of the site showing substantial bone loss.

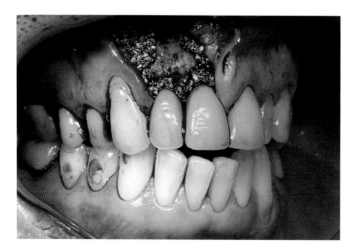

Figure 2.10 Transitional acrylic denture in-situ and grafting the site with bovine xenograft.

Figure 2.11 Suturing.

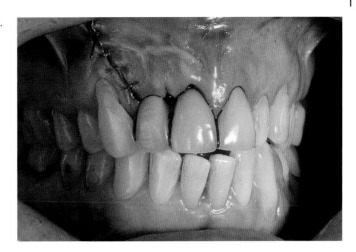

Figure 2.12 Five week healing.

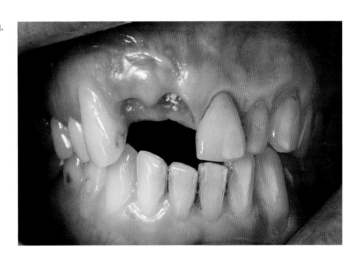

Figure 2.13 Radiopaque surgical stent for guiding flapless implant placement.

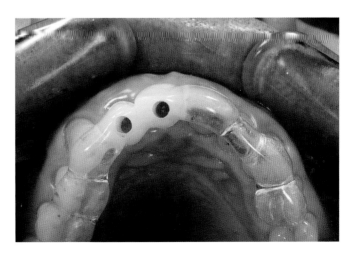

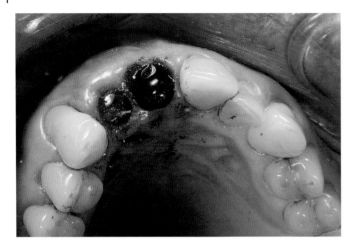

Figure 2.14 Flapless osteotomy.

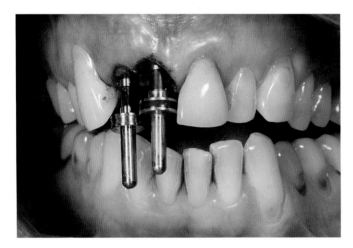

Figure 2.15 Guides for ascertaining correct implant angulation.

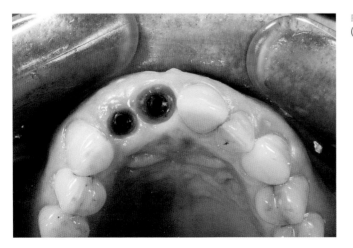

Figure 2.16 8 1/2 week healing (occlusal view).

Figure 2.17 8 1/2 week healing (facial view).

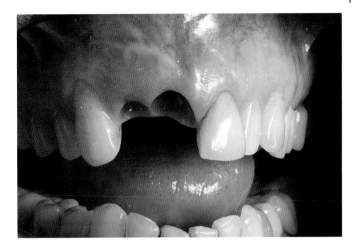

Figure 2.18 Closed tray impression abutments.

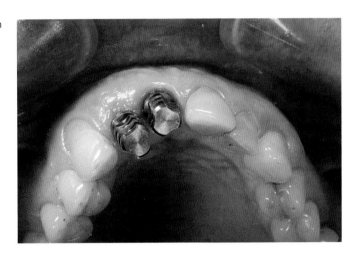

Figure 2.19 Temporary acrylic crowns.

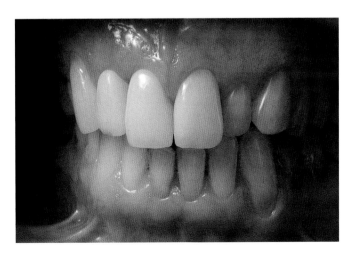

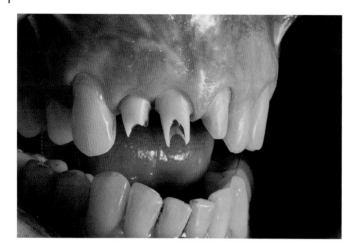

Figure 2.20 Customised CAD/CAM titanium/zirconia abutments and prepared left central incisor (right lateral view).

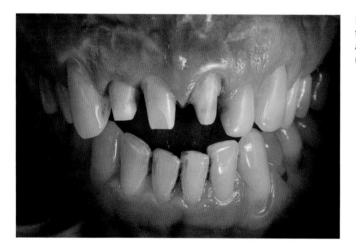

Figure 2.21 Customised CAD/CAM titanium and zirconia abutments and prepared left central incisor (frontal view).

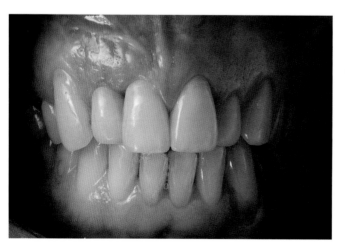

Figure 2.22 Definitive all-ceramic crowns for implants at sites #12 and #11, and replacement lithium disilicate (e-max) crown for tooth #21.

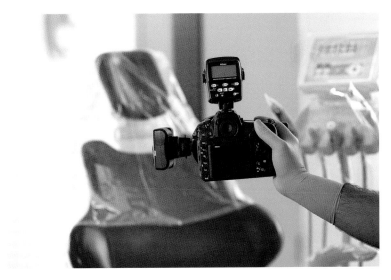

Figure 2.23 Hand-held camera with compact flashes.

Supports

Another point of disagreement is whether the camera and mounted flashes are hand-held or supported by a tripod. In this case, the answer is not so clear-cut. The advantage of hand-held cameras is manoeuvrability, and the photographer is free to position himself or herself in any position without being encumbered by a tripod. This is particularly helpful for accommodating children, or the elderly and frail, who may find a photographic session arduous and trying experience. However, if the camera is hand-held, to prevent it falling accidentally, it is advisable to use a hand and neck strap. The drawback of carrying a hefty camera and flashes is that the operator usually ends up contorting his or her body over the patient, inadvertently bumping into dental equipment, or spraining back musculature (Figure 2.23).

The tripod option offers a rigid platform, allowing the photographer to be comfortably seated, freeing the hands for precisely positioning cheek retractors, mirrors, or holding intra-oral instruments to demonstrate a particular clinical technique. In addition, if the camera is mounted onto a macro focusing stage, precise focusing is ensured. Furthermore, a series of images can be taken with similar framing for demonstrating a particular treatment protocol. The drawback of a tripod is that another piece of hardware needs to be accommodated in the clinic, which may already be restricted for space. Nevertheless, the benefits of a stable platform for consistent and standardised images outweigh the initial teething frustrations (Figure 2.24).

Ideally, it is best to use both options depending on the type of photograph being taken. In order to expedite a photograph session for compromised patients, or where access to the posterior regions of the oral cavity is limited, hand-held equipment is the best option without fettering with a tripod. Alternately, for certain dental applications where composition and framing are paramount, the solid platform of a tripod is indispensable for standardisation. Lastly, whichever option is chosen, it is helpful to draw markings on the floor for the location of the photographic equipment, the patient, photographer and assistant for repeatable positioning.

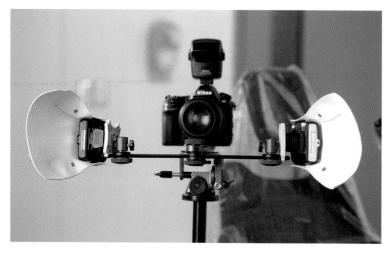

Figure 2.24 Tripod-mounted camera and compact flashes with diffusers.

Delegation

Another frequently asked question is 'Who should take the photographs?'

It is tempting to delegate photographic documentation to ancillary staff or assistants (Christensen 2005), or indeed a professional photographer (Sandler and Murray 2002). Delegating has its advantages; it frees up valuable time during a busy daily schedule to concentrate on other pertinent clinical matters. In addition, the clinician may lack competence, or be indifferent to taking pictures. However, assigning this responsibility to assistants can prove fruitless. This is not denigrating an assistance, without whom any dental procedure is arduous, and often impossible. It is simply allocating tasks that an individual is best trained for, and proficient in, for the followings reasons. First, the assignee should have adequate training in dental photography and be versed with taking both extra- and intra-oral pictures. Second, trying to explain to assistants what an image should depict, is asking for a miracle. After carrying out an examination of the patient, it is the clinician who possesses the depth of knowledge and experience for assessing the dental status, including the visual appearance of dental and oral pathology. Only he or she can decide on the type of image that is required, and more importantly, what it should convey (McKeown et al. 2005). This is similar to taking radiographs, which can only be requested by the clinical after an intra-oral examination. Asking an assistant to take on the role of the clinician is perhaps presumptuous, and also expecting too much. Therefore, before appointing a proxy, it is worthwhile asking a few questions; can the delegate differentiate between diseased and healthy tissues, assess defective restorations, perform shade analysis, and capture nuances and characterisations of teeth and restorations? Furthermore, is the ensuing frustration of unusable images, and extra time needed to repeat them, worth the hassle?

Alternately, employing a professional photographer will obviously produce technically satisfactory images, but will they be clinically satisfactory? The same comments as those for dental assistants apply to professional photographers, who are proficient in photography, but not in dentistry. In addition, the extra expense of a professional photographer will unnecessarily increase the cost of treatment for the patient. Finally, many dentists may have attended lectures or presentations by competent clinicians demonstrating superlative techniques but accompanied by poor-quality images, which fail to convey the message and wrongly reflect on the presenter's competence. This is another reason why a clinician needs to be is versed in photographic techniques for communicating his or her clinical knowledge to an audience.

Ideally, a photographic session should be performed as a team including the clinician with the help of an assistant, no different to four-handed dentistry. The clinician is responsible for operating the photographic equipment and framing the composition to include salient features, while the assistant is indispensable for ensuring patient comfort by aspirating saliva or blood, responding to concerns such as pressure from cheek retractor, preventing gagging reflex from mirrors, vigilantly adhering to cross-infection control and addressing health and safety issues. Also, an extra pair of hands is essential for positioning cheek retractors, contrasters, mirrors, flashes, reflectors, etc. In addition, the assistant is able to hold instruments adjacent to the teeth or oral mucosa that are essential as reference markers, as well as using a three-in-one syringe for maintaining a dry field of view and clearing condensation from mirrors. This applies equally to dental technicians, who should work as a team for recording a particular technique, showing intricate details they have created in artificial prostheses, or for visual communication with the clinician about clinical deficiencies such as poor impressions. Hence, in the dental laboratory, the dental technician is also the protagonist to operate the photographic equipment and frame the picture, while the assistant is responsible for ensuring that the session is conducted productively and effortlessly.

Patient Consent

There are varying opinions and ambiguity regarding guidelines about the type of consent necessary for using dental images in both the clinical and non-clinical context (Berle 2008). Some believe that no consent is necessary when the images are utilised for therapeutic purposes or for communicating with fellow professional colleagues for the benefit of the patient. This may be justified for emergency treatment, or if the patient is incapacitated by a prevailing medical condition and therefore unable to grant consent. However, when using images for non-clinical contexts, such as marketing and promotional endeavours, consent is unquestionably mandatory. Another contentious issue is responding to requests for images from criminal investigators or for forensic identification. In these circumstances, it be best to seek advice from dental professional bodies before releasing images to third parties (Kornhaber et al. 2015).

In the current climate of escalating patient litigation and increasing demand for elective dental therapies, it is wise not to tempt fate, and to obtain written consent even for the most innocuous treatment.

Therefore, before embarking on photographic documentation, patient consent is unquestionably obligatory, and without a signed consent form a photographic session should not be contemplated. In addition, the patient should be briefed about the intended use of the images, whether they are purely for clinical documentation, liaising with specialists, monitoring treatment progress, or whether the images will be used for marketing (including social media dissemination and websites), research, education, public relations, patient counselling, staff training, lecturing and publishing (Bauer n.d.). Furthermore, it is necessary to inform the patient that consent for photographic documentation is voluntary, and if declined, will in no way compromise the provision of therapy. Various consent form templates are available from defence societies, dental academies and organisations or publishers, each catering for specific uses of the images that can be tailored to suit patients' wishes.

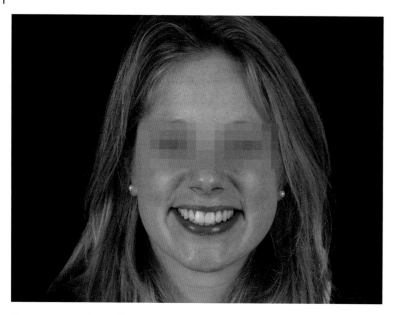

Figure 2.25 Pixelating the eyes is a simple method for concealing the identity of the patient.

For certain treatment modalities, dental photography is an essential diagnostic and communication tool. These include orthodontics, diagnosis of pathology by specialists, or shade analysis for artificial restorations, and so on. In these circumstances, if patient consent is not forthcoming, consent is still necessary, with the proviso that the images will not be used for any purpose other than the treatment in question. Also, after completing treatment, the images can either be handed over to the patient for safekeeping or permanently destroyed or deleted. Another method for ensuring anonymity is by pixelating the eyes using image manipulation software (Figure 2.25). However, if treatment involves visualising facial features for plastic surgery, reconstruction or aesthetic enhancement with local muscle relaxants and fillers, pixellation may not be a feasible option.

A cautionary footnote that cannot be overstressed, particularly involving aesthetic or elective dental procedures, is the importance of involving the patient at each and every stage of treatment. In addition, gaining written consent before starting or progressing to the next phase of therapy is imperative. This may seem fastidious, but a few signatures during a course of treatment can prevent unforeseeable future rage at a later date.

References

Ahmad, I. (2009). Digital dental photography. Part 8: intra-oral set-ups. Br. Dent. J. 207 (4): 151–157.

Bauer, R. (n.d.). *Digital Photography Made Easy*. Canada: Coordinator of Digital Media Education, Faculty of Dentistry, University of Toronto.

Berle, I. (2008). Clinical photography and patient rights: the need for orthopraxy. J. Med. Ethics 34 (2): 89–92.

Christensen, G.J. (2005). Important clinical uses for digital photography. J. Am. Dent. Assoc. 136: 77–79.

Davda, M. (n.d.). Standardization in dental photography. Dental Photography School.

Kornhaber, R., Betihavas, V., and Baber, R.J. (2015). Ethical implications of digital images for teaching and learning purposes: an integrative review. J. Multidiscip. Healthcare 8: 299–305.

McKeown, H.F., Murray, A.M., and Sandler, P.J. (2005). How to avoid common errors in clinical photography. J. Orthod. 32: 43–54.

Sandler, J. and Murray, A. (2002). Current products and practice: clinical photographs – the gold standard. J. Orthod. 29: 158–167.

Shorey, R. and Moore, K. (2009). Clinical digital photography: implementation of clinical photography for everyday practice. J. Calif. Dent. Assoc. 37 (3): 179–183.

Sreevatsan, R., Philip, K., Peter, E. et al. (2015). Digital photography in general and clinical dentistry – technical aspects and accessories. Int. Dent. J. Stud. Res. 3 (1): 17–24.

The Academy of Laser Dentistry (2015). Guidelines for Clinical Photography 3: 1–4.

Vasileva, R., Kolarov, R., and Nikolov, N. (2017). Protocol for sterile conditions using dental photography. MedInform 1: 551–558.

3

Technical Concepts and Settings

Having acquired the requisite photographic equipment and gathered the necessary dental armamentarium, the penultimate stage before taking photographs is understanding some basic photographic principles. Whenever a new piece of equipment is purchased, there is undoubtedly an eagerness to use it as soon as possible. However, instead of diving straight in and getting frustrated by disappointing outcomes, it is better to take time out for grasping some theoretical concepts and apply these to practical situations. This knowledge is invaluable for achieving predictable results at the outset, rather than wasting time rectifying mistakes. Also, for convenience, some of the information below is repeated in subsequent modules dealing with Capture, Process and Display or the CPD triad (Figure 3.1).

Every Picture Tells a Story

Photography is a synæsthetic experience (Cytowic 2003), similar to the aesthetic experience or aesthetic appreciation of beauty (Figure 3.2). Aesthetics is defined as elevating material entities, such as paint on a canvas or a sculpture carved from stone, to a psychological [usually] pleasurable experience. Therefore, similar to art, the raison d'être of a picture is 'to tell the story that needs to be told' so as to elicit a psychological response.

Hence, the aim of any picture, whether a painting or photograph, is to convey a message. All that matters is that the intentional message reaches the intended audience. If this goal is achieved, the picture has served its purpose. Essentially, all pictures are representations of objects or subjects photographed in a particular light at a given moment in time. If the light is changed, the object or subject appears different, conveying a difference message. Dental photography is no exception. Therefore, before taking a photograph, the photographer should have a lucid idea of what the image is supposed to convey, or its intended use. Without this mandate, a photograph serves little or no purpose, and the exercise deemed pointless and futile.

The intended purpose of a photograph is essential for deciding the type of imagery required; either for conveying clinical information or for inducing the desired inspiration. Hence, it is pivotal to produce images that communicate a visual dental message or tell a story, no different from watching a movie or reading a novel. Consequently, images for communicating with patients convey a different message to those for communicating with professional colleagues. The former is seductive, alluring and emotive, whilst the latter lacks figurative connotations and is instead impassive, but informative for inter-clinician tele-consultations or tele-conferencing (Manjunath et al. 2011). For these purposes, standardised imagery is essential for consistency and comparison.

Essentials of Dental Photography, First Edition. Irfan Ahmad.
© 2020 John Wiley & Sons Ltd. Published 2020 by John Wiley & Sons Ltd.

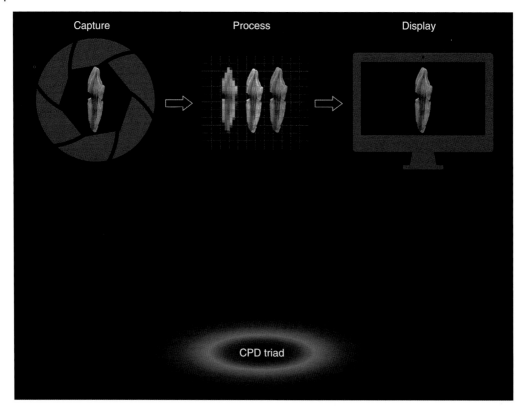

Figure 3.1 Digital photography consists of three distinct stages: capture, process and display (CPD).

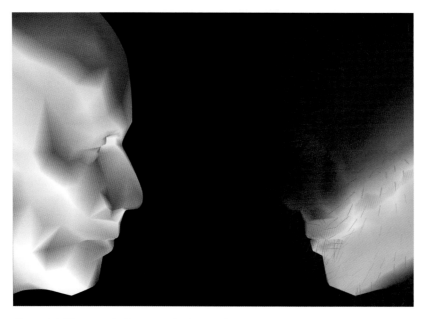

Figure 3.2 Photography is a synæsthetic experience.

Figure 3.3 Image with high marketing value, but low clinical value.

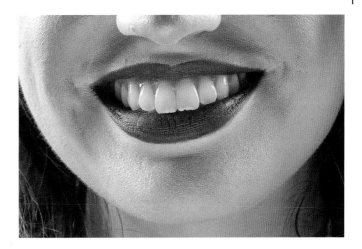

Figure 3.4 Image with high clinical value, but low marketing value.

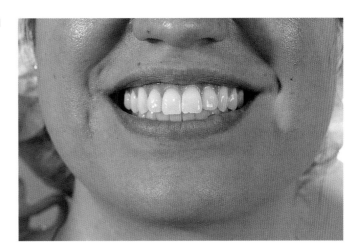

Both the dental literature and the internet are awash with dental imagery that crosses the clinical/artistic line. Furthermore, some literature on dental photography is preoccupied with clinical fidelity and dismisses artistic imagery as facile. However, as mentioned above, each type of picture serves a different purpose, and there is room for both styles (Figures 3.3 and 3.4). There is no doubt that images for marketing dental products or promoting dental services are stylistic, devoid of clinical relevance, but their intention is different from providing information for clinical diagnosis, treatment planning or treatment outcomes. Thus, the two types of images are often incongruous, but nevertheless relevant because they are appealing to different spectators. Creating stylistic, or artistic photographs depends on the creativity of the photographer rather than the type of camera or photographic equipment. The camera is merely a machine, without feelings or emotions, but it is the individual taking the photograph who adds these qualities to express his or her vision. Anyone can purchase a canvas and paints, but not everyone can produce works of art. This aspect of photography is difficult, or even impossible to teach. Artistic qualities develop with passion and time, and are beyond the scope of this publication. Therefore, the aim of this text is showing techniques specifically for dental needs, including clinical and marketing, which produce predictable and repeatable results, and most importantly, tell a dental story.

Setting the Tone

The oral cavity is a confined area of the body, and photographing it presents unique challenges. After all, we are taking pictures of relatively small objects, the largest teeth in the arch, the maxillary central incisors or molars are around 10 mm. Therefore, trying to capture details within these small objects requires a degree of perseverance, endurance and imagination. In addition, patient compliance and participation are paramount for achieving satisfactory results. Hence, creating an atmosphere of serenity and tranquillity, concealing frustrations and agitations, are prerequisites for a successful photographic session.

Lighting

Photography is light, and without light there is no photography. Photography is simply playing with light, it can emphasise or suppress details or features, create an ambience of tranquillity or excitement, evoke hopes or fears, kindle emotions or repulsion, inspire and aspire, be evocative or provocative, and elicit approval or rejection. Although this text cannot begin to do justice to what is possible with light, the discussion below outlines some basic lighting principles that are relevant for dental photography (Ahmad 2009a).

The method by which a light source illuminates an object or subject is by distribution, which is determined by its colour temperature, apparent size and direction. The colour temperature sets the tone, the direction influences the location of shadows and highlights, whilst the physical size dictates the intensity of the shadows and highlights.

The colour temperature is significant when shooting in daylight since the quality of light changes at sunrise, midday, overcast skies or sunset. However, as most flashes are configured to emit light at photographic daylight (5500 K), the ambient colour temperature is almost irreverent for dental set-ups. However, for creative imagery, the colour temperature can be altered by either placing coloured gels over the flashes, or using coloured fill-in reflectors. Reflectors are available in a variety of reflective coloured surfaces for altering the temperature of light, e.g. a gold surface reduces the colour temperature creating a warm glow, whilst a silver reflector increases the colour temperature and 'cools' the quality of light. Also, a highly reflective surface encouraging specular reflections for producing vibrant, high contrast images (Bazos and Magne 2013), compared to a matt white card that produces subtle lighting for a serene ambience.

There are two types of lighting: hard and soft. Hard lighting is harsh and usually unidirectional, creating distinct shadows and specular reflections (glare). Conversely, soft lighting is subdued with gradual transitions between darker and lighter parts of a picture. Furthermore, hard lighting emphasises edges of objects, whereas soft light attenuates, or 'irons out' details. Therefore, for portraiture, softer lighting is generally preferred as it is more flattering and glamorises the subject (Figure 3.5). Similarly, diffuse or soft lighting is ideal for capturing dentine strata characterisations and chromatic distribution within a tooth, whilst unidirectional illumination emphasises line angles and reveals enamel surface texture and lustre.

Various methods are available for achieving softer lighting. The first is moving the light source closer to the subject, the second is by using an intermediate material to diffuse the emitted light (e.g. soft box), third, bouncing the flash off reflective surfaces such as an umbrella or a reflector, and lastly, increasing the physical size of the light source. Altering the direction of a light creates a sense of depth in a composition. This type of directional lighting is used for highlighting specific features of an object, and at the same time giving a three-dimensional quality to the image.

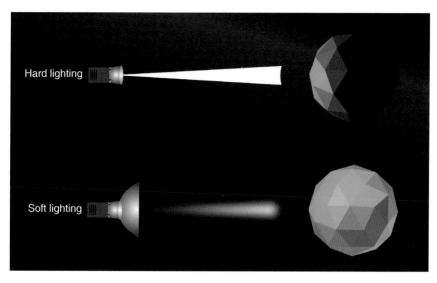

Figure 3.5 Hard lighting produces distinct shadows and highlights, emphasising edges of objects or prominent facial features, whereas soft lighting produces subtle transitions between shadows and highlights, and is more flattering by smoothing prominent facial features and wrinkles.

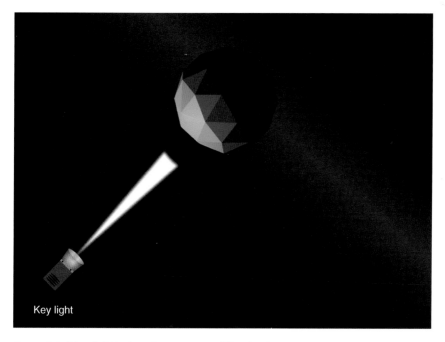

Figure 3.6 A key light is the primary source of illumination.

For any photographic set-up, the protagonist light is termed the main or key light, which is the primary source of illumination, whilst secondary light(s) are termed fill lights because they are placed on the contralateral side to literally 'fill in shadows' created by the key light. The fill light can either be ambient or natural daylight, a second flash, or a reflector that bounces light from the key light back onto the subject (Figures 3.6 and 3.7). The degree that a fill light illuminates a

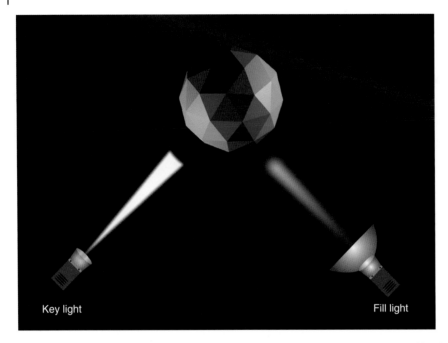

Figure 3.7 A fill light is the secondary source of illumination that fills in shadows created by the key light.

subject is expressed as a ratio of the key light. For example, if only one light is used, the ratio is 0 : 1, where 0 represents the absence of a fill light, and 1 is the key light. A 1 : 4 ratio signifies that the fill light is a quarter of the intensity of the key light. It is important to note that the smaller number always represents the fill light (Figure 3.8). Asymmetrical lighting is generally preferred, as it coveys depth with increase contrast, e.g. an acceptable ratio for portraits is 1 : 2 (Figure 3.9). An equal ratio of 1 : 1 produces a flat image (Figure 3.10), sometimes referred to as a 'high key' image, that excessively softens facial features, but is ideal for glamour shots, or pictures of children for conveying joviality and playfulness. On the other extreme, a 'low key' image emphasises shadows, giving the picture depth and character, and is ideal for portraying personality traits such as insight and wisdom. In a similar manner to the key light, the position of the fill light also produces different effects. The simplest set-up for portraiture is two studio flashes angled at 45° to the subject, and is ideal for clinical portraits. This arrangement produces consistently repeatable and standardised images, ideal for reference and comparison. Whilst these images serve the purpose of clinical reality, they are construed as bland, and unsuitable for marketing and promotional purposes. In order for a portrait to fulfil marketing criteria, more elaborate set-ups are necessary, and some ideas for these images are discussed in Module 6.

There is an ongoing debate in dentistry as to which type of lighting is best suited for intra-oral dental photographs: uniform (with ring flash) or unidirectional illumination (with bilateral flashes). The ultimate aim of flash photography is producing images where it is difficult to detect whether or not a flash was used. Due to inappropriate illumination, the major flaw with intra-oral dental photography is that it is often blatantly obvious that flashes were utilised to take the photograph. The resultant images appear flat, unnatural and totally devoid of character. In reality, teeth are illuminated by subtle ambient lighting that conveys depth, character and nuances of the dentition, rather than being 'washed out' by harsh illumination. Hence, it is necessary to decide which type of flashes are the ideal choice for a particular type of intra-oral image.

The choices available for extra-oral (dento-facial), intra-oral and bench images are either compact bilateral or ring flashes. The first option of a twin bilateral configuration with the

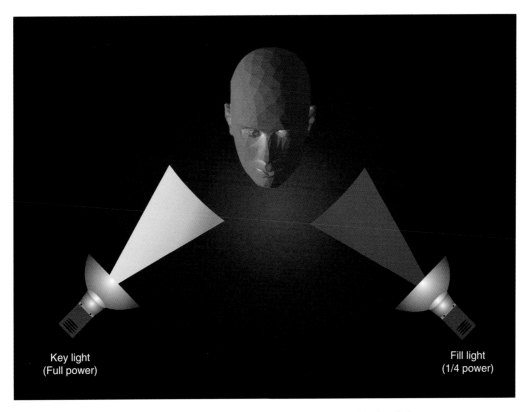

Figure 3.8 1 : 4 ratio signifies that the fill light is a quarter of the intensity of the key light.

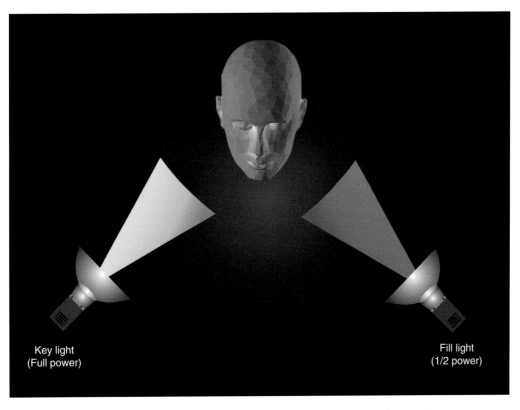

Figure 3.9 1 : 2 ratio signifies that the fill light is a half of the intensity of the key light.

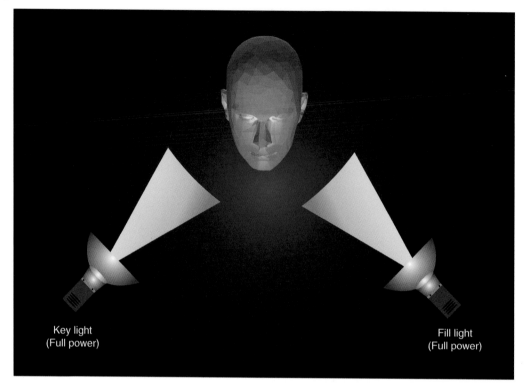

Figure 3.10 A 1 : 1 ratio signifies that the fill and key light have equal intensity.

flashes positioned 45° to the subject, using a balanced flash ratio of 1 : 1 that produces uniformly exposed images with few shadows or highlights. In effect, this set-up behaves similar to a ring flash that produces uniform and shadowless illumination. The resultant images are lifeless and appear as if they were taken with a flash. To mitigate this effect, asymmetrical unidirectional lighting using a fill flash to key flash ratio of 1 : 2 is recommended. This means that the key flash (e.g. the right flash) is set to maximum power (full duration or 1/1), whilst the fill flash output (e.g. the left flash) is muted to half its power (half duration or 1/2). Alternately, a single flash can be used with a silver reflector on the opposite side to bounce light back to fill in the shadows. This set-up produces a flash ratio of 1 : 2 that creates highlights, without completely obliterating shadows on the opposite side, resulting in an image that appears three-dimensional and realistic (Figures 3.11 and 3.12).

The second option is using ring flashes, which are available in two varieties. The first type of ring flash has a circular flash tube that delivers consistent, 360° uniform shadowless illumination. These units emit light at a predefined intensity, which is usually unchangeable. The second variety of ring flash has individual flash tubes located arounds its axis; top, bottom, right and left. In addition, the intensity of the individual flash tubes can be altered and offers flexibility for modifying the flash ratio to a desirable 1 : 2 for asymmetrical illumination.

Depth of Field

The depth of field (DoF) is the range, or linear distance, in front and behind the point of focus that appears sharp. The DoF is not abrupt, but a gradual blurring of the foreground and background around the object that is in focus. This depends on a multitude of factors including the

Figure 3.11 Symmetrical uniform lighting produces lacklustre, bland, two-dimensional imagery.

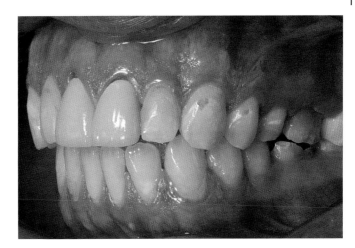

Figure 3.12 Asymmetrical unidirectional illumination produces three-dimensional imagery rich in detail and depth.

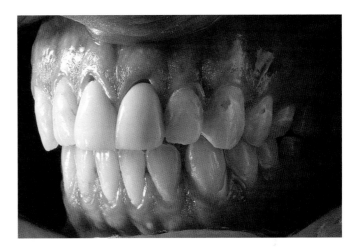

type of sensor, focal length of the lens, distance from the object, aperture, circle of confusion, diffraction, pupil magnification and hyperfocal distance. The hyperfocal distance is the area or point in a scene where focusing will result in the maximum DoF. This is particularly relevant for macrophotography to maximise sharpness by making the most of DoF. The hyperlocal distance is calculated according to the focal length of the lens, the sensor crop factor and the chosen *f*-stop. An example is photographing the maxillary anterior sextant using a 100 mm macro lens with a full-frame sensor at *f* 22. If the point of focus (PoF) is the mesial aspect of the central incisors, the posterior DoF is 'wasted' as only the centrals are sharply focused. Similarly, if the point of focus is the canines, the anterior DoF is lost. Therefore, the ideal hyperlocal distance in this composition is the mesial aspect of the lateral incisors, to maximise the DoF (Figure 3.13). Table 3.1 shows varying DoF according to different factors.

The DoF is related to the degree of magnification: the higher the magnification, the shallower the DoF. The significance of DoF for dental photography is that a macro lens is extremely close to the subject, and therefore the area of sharpness is vastly diminished, limited to only a few millimetres (shallow DoF). Since the hardware specifications (camera, lens) and visual acuity are unchangeable, the user settings that affect DoF are the aperture and distance of the object (focus distance) from the lens. However, the distance is also be unchangeable because achieving a particular magnification, e.g. 1 : 1, requires a specific distance, or minimum focusing distance

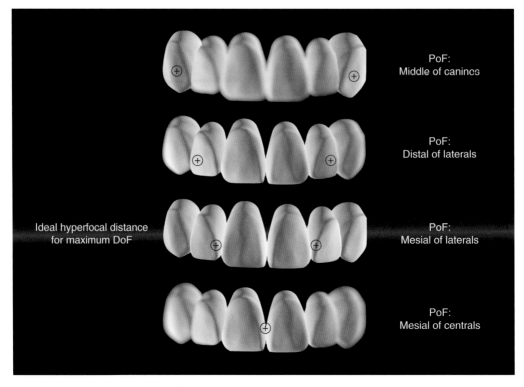

Figure 3.13 The ideal hyperlocal distance for photographing the maxillary anterior sextant is the mesial aspect of the lateral incisors, which ensures maximum depth of field (DoF) (PoF = point of focus, represented by the blue cross-line reticles).

Table 3.1 Depth of field (DoF) calculations.

Sensor	Lens focal length (mm)	Aperture (f)	Focus distance (cm)	DoF (mm)
APS	100	22	30	6
Full-frame	100	22	30	8
Point-and-shoot compact camera (1 : 2/3 in. sensor)	100	8	1	10

of a macro lens. Hence, the only parameter to manipulate is the f number, which varies inversely with the aperture opening. A large aperture opening (small f numbers) results in a shallow DoF, whilst a small aperture opening (large f numbers) results in a deep DoF (Figures 3.14–3.16). Therefore, it is essential to use small apertures (large f numbers), e.g. f 22, for ensuring that intra-oral images have as many teeth as possible, or large areas of soft tissue in focus. Table 3.2 shows increasing DoF by reducing the f numbers at a fixed focus distance of 30 cm.

Another factor to consider is that DoF varies according to the focal length of the lens. Wide angle lenses have greater DoF, but as the focal length increases, the DoF decreases. As well as altering the DoF, the focal length of the lens also changes the distribution of the DoF. For example, the DoF for a standard lens is located equally in front and behind the point of focus. Whereas, with a macro lens the DoF is distributed approximately 1/3 in front and 2/3 behind

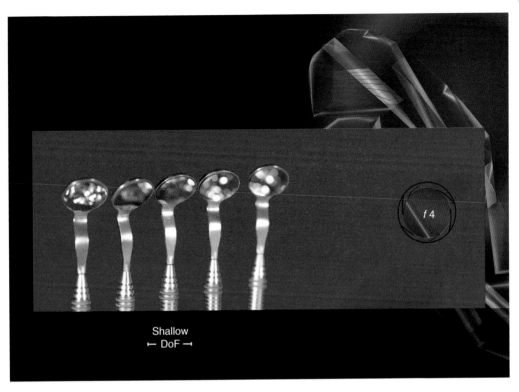

Figure 3.14 Shallow depth of field (DoF): large aperture (small *f* number), only the third mirror from the left is in sharp focus.

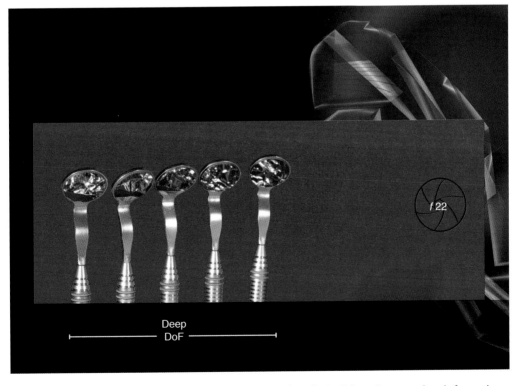

Figure 3.15 Deep depth of field (DoF): small aperture (large *f* number), all five mirrors are sharply focused.

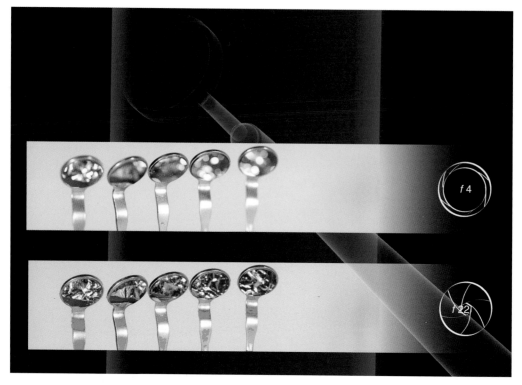

Figure 3.16 Turning on the focus mask (green areas) shows the parts of the image that are in focus.

Table 3.2 Depth of field (DoF) vs. aperture.

Sensor	Lens focal length (mm)	Aperture (*f*)	Focus distance (cm)	DoF (mm)
APS	100	2.8	30	1
APS	100	5.6	30	1
APS	100	8	30	2
APS	100	11	30	3
APS	100	16	30	4
APS	100	22	30	6

the point of focus (Ahmad 2009b) – Figure 3.17. Therefore, if the DoF is 6 mm at f 22, objects 2 mm in front, and 4 mm behind the point of focus will appear sharp. In theory, it is possible to increase the DoF by using even smaller f-stop numbers such as f 32 or f 64. However, f-stops greater than f 22 cause chromatic diffraction at the edges of objects (rainbow effect), deteriorating image resolution. Therefore, setting an aperture smaller than f 22 substantially diminishes image quality without a substantial gain in DoF. This is the reason why many high-quality macro lenses are designed with diaphragms limited to f 22. Another method for increasing DoF is by a process called focus stacking. A series of images is taken at different focus points, which are subsequently merged in dedicated focus stacking software to create a single image with a

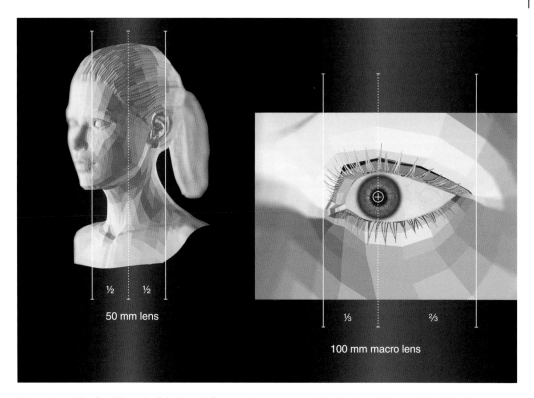

50 mm lens

100 mm macro lens

Figure 3.17 The focal length of the lens influences the range and distribution of depth of field (DoF) (PoF = point of focus, represented by the white cross-line reticles).

larger DoF. This technique is ideal for stationary still life compositions, but unsuitable for intraoral photographs.

For portraiture, the DoF is less significant, since the lens is a considerable distance from the object. For example, a camera with an APS sensor, 100 mm lens, at a focus distance of 2.5 m, will have a DoF of 15 cm at an aperture setting of *f* 5.6, almost the entire anterior–posterior distance from the tip of the nose to the ears. Hence, even with relatively large aperture openings (smaller *f* numbers), the entire face will appear in focus. Furthermore, unlike macrophotography, the DoF for portraiture is distributed evenly in front and behind the point of focus. Manipulating the DoF is useful for emphasising certain facial features, e.g. eyes or teeth, whilst throwing the remaining facial landmarks out of focus by using larger apertures, creating a pseudo-three-dimensional quality.

Exposure and Histogram

Exposure determines whether an image is too dark, too bright or just right. It is influenced by the intensity of the light source and three cameras settings; aperture, shutter speed and ISO number. The aperture is a metal diaphragm located inside the lens and controls the amount of light entering the camera, similar to the iris controlling the diameter of the pupil of the eyes. A wide aperture opening (small *f* number) allows more light to enter, whilst a small aperture (large *f* number) restricts the amount of light. The shutter is a mechanical flap, similar to the eyelids, and is either built into the lens or located in front of the sensor. Its speed is expressed in seconds or fractions of a second, and controls the duration of light falling onto the sensor. Lastly, the ISO number is the sensitivity of the sensor to incoming light. The sensor is analogous to the retina, which has rods that are extremely sensitive to light and effective for low-resolution night vision, whilst the fovea is densely packed with cones and requires brighter illumination for high-resolution daylight vision.

For dental macrophotography (both intra- and extra-oral), aperture, shutter speed and ISO are virtually unchangeable for the following reasons. In order to gain the maximum DoF, close-up images require a small aperture, usually $f22$. Since flashes are the most frequently used light sources for dental pictures, the synchronisation shutter speed, indicated by a lightning symbol on the shutter dial or the liquid crystal displays (LCD) display, is also fixed, usually at 1/125 or 1/250 seconds. Finally, a minimum ISO setting, ranging from 50 to 200, is necessary for avoiding visually noisy or grainy images. Therefore, the only part of the exposure equation that can be changed is the flash intensity and/or the distance of the flashes from the subject. Consequently, if the exposure is too dark or too bright, the only way to correct this is either increasing or decreasing flash intensity output, or moving the flashes closer or further away (Figures 3.18 and 3.19). If the image is still underexposed, then additional flashes or those with higher guide numbers are required. Adding extra flashes is not a concern with TTL metering, as the camera automatically controls the duration of flash bursts to ensure sufficient illumination. However, TTL may not always result in correctly exposed images. This is particularly significant for intra-oral photography because the highly reflective enamel surfaces against a dark background of the oral cavity often confuse the flash metering mechanism. Another problem is using black contrasters, which have the benefit of masking extraneous anatomy, but

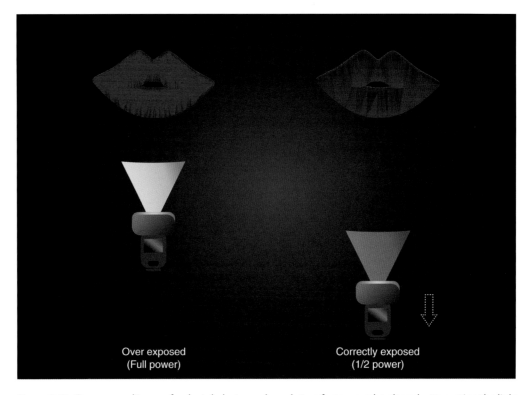

Over exposed
(Full power)

Correctly exposed
(1/2 power)

Figure 3.18 Overexposed image: for dental photography only two factors can be altered: attenuating the light intensity and/or moving the flash(es) further way from the subject.

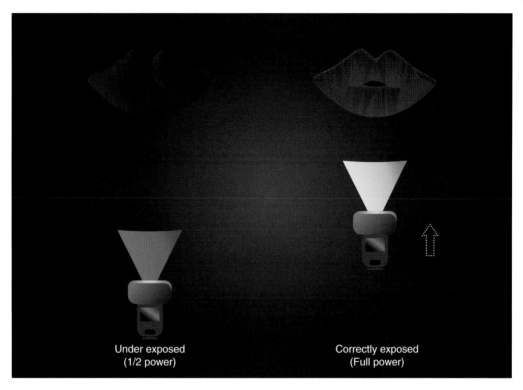

Under exposed
(1/2 power)

Correctly exposed
(Full power)

Figure 3.19 Underexposed image: for dental photography only two factors can be altered: increasing the light intensity and/or moving the flash(es) closer to the subject.

often produce overexposed images since the camera metering registers the scene as overly dark and compensates by over-illuminating the scene. This is usually inconsequential as minor over- or underexposure can be corrected in imaging software. However, significant exposure compensation in editing software will result in image quality deterioration and unwanted colour shifts. If using manual mode, the best way to control illumination is moving the flash(es) closer or further away until the correct exposure is attained. Taking a few test shots for a given set-up allows precise settings to be repeated for subsequent images.

Portraiture photography offers much more latitude for changing *f*-stops and shutter speeds, as well as altering studio flash intensity and positioning for creating the appropriate mood for capturing or creating an individual's persona.

With digital photography, the easiest method for gauging exposure is by a histogram, which is a graph consisting of peaks and troughs of light intensity within an image (Nordberg and Sluder 2013). It is often displayed on the LCD on the back of cameras, and also in image processing software. The histogram, on a continuum, shows the tonal values within an image ranging from the brightest (highlights), midtones to the darkest (shadows), on a scale of 0–255. The histogram is useful for determining several factors, but the most important are the exposure and dynamic range (DR). If the peaks are concentrated to the left side, the image is underexposed, and vice versa for overexposed images (peaks are located to the right side) – Figures 3.20– 3.23. However, for a given image, there is no ideal histogram, and its appearance depends on the subject matter or the creativity of the photographer.

The DR is a measure of the difference between the brightest and darkest part of an image, and expressed as the number of *f*-stops, represented on the *x*-axis of the histogram. Its

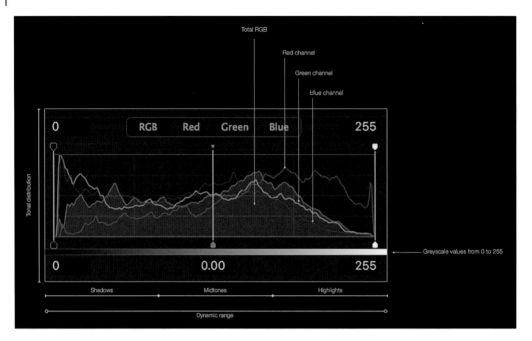

Figure 3.20 The histogram is a graphical representation of several parameters including exposure and dynamic range (DR).

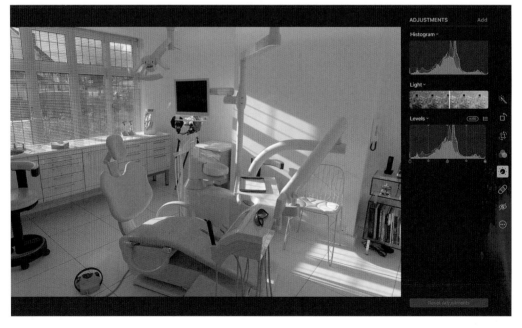

Figure 3.21 Correct exposure: the histogram of a correctly exposed image has peaks mainly confined to the midtones middle area, with a few peaks located in the shadow and highlight regions.

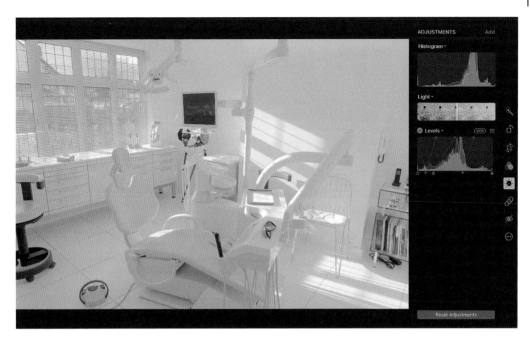

Figure 3.22 Overexposure: the peaks are located to the right side of the histogram.

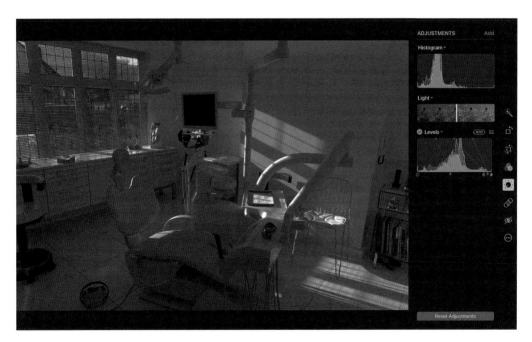

Figure 3.23 Underexposure: the peaks are located to the left side of the histogram.

significance is that detail in an image is only discerned within the DR, i.e. the larger the DR the greater the detail. The human eye has a large DR ranging from 16 to 24 *f*-stops, a high-end digital camera around 15 *f*-stops, semi-professional cameras about 5 *f*-stops, film transparency or high quality photographic print 6 *f*-stops, computer monitors 6 *f*-stops and the printing press 3–5 *f*-stops, depending on lithographic equipment and the quality of printing paper

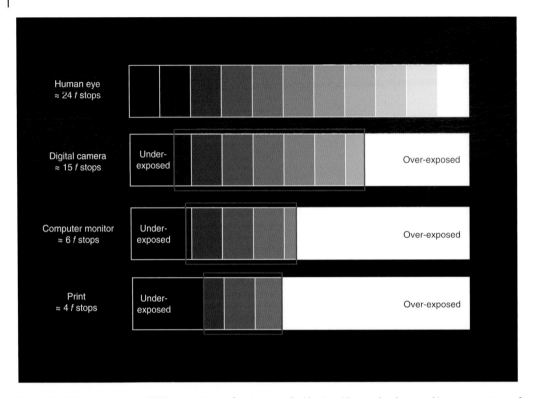

Figure 3.24 Dynamic range (DR) comparison of various media/devices (*Source:* background image, courtesy of Zayan Ahmad).

(Figure 3.24). This means that a high-end digital camera records nearly 5 *f*-stops more detail than film.

As detail is only discernible within the DR of an image, if the peaks are too much on the left side (dark) or right side (bright), detail is indiscernible, even if the image is manipulated by photo-editing software. It is very easy to move the sliders in imaging software to achieve the desired exposure, but extensive shifts in tonal range can first, deteriorate image quality, and second, result in unwanted colour casts (see Figure 1.14 in Module 1). Therefore, to avoid these eventualities, it is important to achieve the correct DR at the time of taking the photograph. The issue at the capture stage is that if the brightest part of a scene has a EV (exposure value) of 12, and the darkest part EV 1, the DR is 11. This means that the camera sensor must be capable of recording a DR of 11 to faithfully reproduce every detail in the image. However, DR range is an inherent hardware feature of the camera sensor, and if the sensor is limited to a DR of 4 *f*-stops, it is impossible to manipulate exposure to record a greater DR or enhance detail. Most camera manufacturers are coy about stating the DR because of numerous variable factors. However, independent testing reveals that most mid-range dSLRs, with APS sensors, have a DR of around 9 *f*-stops, whilst full-frame and medium format camera sensors can achieve a DR of up to 15 *f*-stops. Therefore, depending on the camera, some detail is likely to be lost due to limitations of the sensor. One approach to expand DR is by HDR (high dynamic range) photography or image hallucination technique, which 'virtually' increases the DR using post-processing software (see Module 9 for more details).

So, what is the ideal DR for an image? As mentioned above, this depends on the scene being photographed and the intended use of the image, and ultimately a compromise is necessary. If the purpose is using the image for a lecture or presentation with a projector, a high DR, nearer to the perception of the human eye, is the ideal. However, for printing purposes, a high DR is futile, since the printing process inherently degrades an image to 3–5 *f*-stops. Hence, an image with a DR of 11 will deteriorate to 4 *f*-stops when printed, losing 7 *f*-stops stops of detail. This is the reason why an image that looks vivid and vibrant on a computer monitor or auditorium screen appears dull and lacklustre when printed. Practically, it is advisable to achieve a median DR of around 6 *f*-stops, which allows acceptable screening, but also mitigates detail loss when printed or published.

White Balance

The white balance (WB) is simply 'telling the camera' about the quality, or colour temperature, of light. The term 'white balance' is used because any 'white' part in a scene should be faithfully reproduced as 'white' in the image. It is a setting that constantly changes depending on the prevailing illumination. There are three methods for setting the WB: automatic, manual or using an 18% neutral density grey card.

Using the automatic method is the simplest, and is usually displayed in the camera menu as AWB (automatic white balance). In AWB mode, the camera detects the light source and automatically sets the WB accordingly, which works well for the majority of photographic scenarios. However, extreme or subtle lighting conditions are challenging for camera detectors, and may cause unwanted colour casts of the image. This is particularly relevant for low or bright ambient light, or a mixture of different light sources in a given scene. Examples of some illumination are sunrise (2000 K), daylight (6500 K), twilight (8000 K), moonlight (4000 K), indoor lights (3000 K) and photographic flashes (5500 K) – see Figure 1.15 in Module 1. In these circumstances, the camera gauges an average of the mixed lighting conditions, which may be satisfactory, but sometimes the results are disappointing due to the dominance (or colour cast) of a single light source. AWB is not recommended for intra-oral photography since many light sources are present, including daylight from widows, ceiling lights, operating light and fibreoptic illumination of dental loupes. Any of these may confuse the WB mechanism, often resulting in capricious colour cast images, which are diagnostically useless due to the altered colour of healthy and pathological tissues.

The second method is manually setting the WB, either by selecting the quality of light, or inputing a numerical value for the colour temperature. The former involves choosing various symbols in the WB menu, representing different lighting conditions such as bright sunlight, overcast or cloudy sky, indoor halogen bulbs, fluorescent tubes, flash illumination, etc. Manually selecting a pre-set WB symbol is pure conjecture regarding the true colour temperature, perhaps acceptable for general photography, but inappropriate for clinical fidelity. The second option is inputting a numerical value in Kelvins corresponding to a particular type of illumination, for example matching the colour temperature of the flashes, which is photographic daylight at 5500 K. Numerical input of colour temperature is more predictable, but if the ambient light is overpowering or changes, this may affect colour rendering as well as confusing the TTL flash metering of some cameras.

Finally, the third method for WB setting is using an 18% neutral density grey card, which reflects all colours of the spectrum in equal proportions. This is not just any grey card, but one specifically designed for calibrating light meters or camera WB, and is available from photographic outlets. Similar grey cards are also used for shade analysis and selection of ceramic and resin-based composite restorations, and are included in ceramic and composite kits. This method of setting the WB is the most accurate, but somewhat tedious. However, for a specific

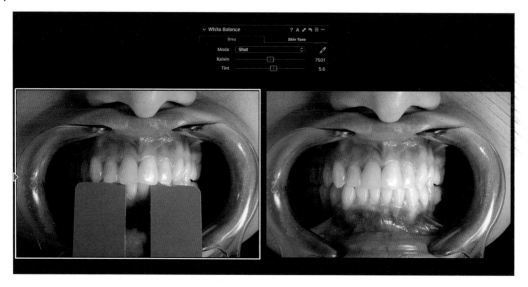

Figure 3.25 White balance (WB) setting with an 18% grey card: an initial reference picture is taken with the card in-situ. The initial colour temperature is 7501 K.

recurrent set-up, the procedure need only to be performed once. A photographic grey card is placed within the scene, making sure that it is illuminated identically to the object/subject. For intra-oral pictures, the card should be in the same plane (optical axis) as the teeth or soft tissues, avoiding shaded areas or obstructing the light source (flashes). A reference picture is then taken with the card in-situ, before proceeding with the remaining photographic session. All images of the same session are imported into a photo-editing software together with the reference picture. In the processing software, the 'neutral grey', 'neutral picker' or 'pick white balance' tool is selected (usually depicted by a pipette or eyedropper). The mouse pointer changes shape to a pipette, and the latter is placed and clicked on the grey card in the reference picture, which immediately corrects its WB. This setting is saved as a 'user preset' and subsequent applied to images with a similar photographic set-up. In this manner, multiple selected thumbnails from the session can simultaneously and instantly be corrected by recalling the saved WB settings with a single click of the mouse (Figures 3.25–3.28). Although the grey card method for WB is the most accurate and predictable, flash angulations, distance and intensity must be kept identical as for the reference picture in order to ensure consistent results. If illumination or camera setting are changed, another reference picture is required for the new set-up.

Resolution

Resolution is the quality of the captured image. The quality of an image is influenced by numerous factors, including the resolving power of the lens (Bengel 2006; Sajjadi et al. 2015), the size of the digital camera sensor (Sajjadi et al. 2016), post-capture editing and the display media. Another variable is the degree of training of the observer to discern details in an image. A trained eye can pick out details that may go unnoticed by the novice (Figures 3.29 and 3.30). For example, a dental specialist is more trained to scrutinise the dentition compared to a layperson (Ker et al. 2008). Furthermore, every observer will concentrate on different aspects of an image

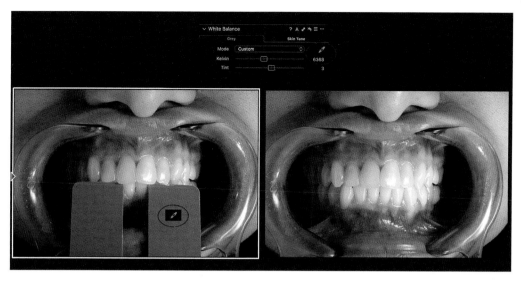

Figure 3.26 White balance (WB) setting with an 18% grey card: the neutral picker is selected in the processing software and clicked on the grey card in the reference image. The colour temperature (WB) is instantly corrected according to the reference grey card and is now 6368 K. Notice that the corrected image on the left is slightly bluish compared to the uncorrected image on right that appears more yellowish.

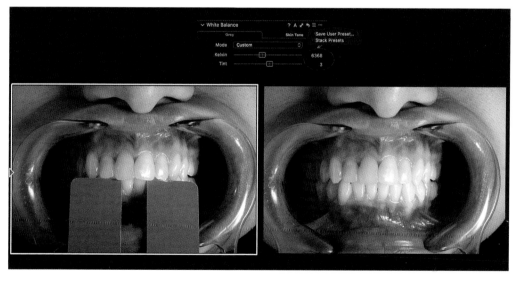

Figure 3.27 White balance (WB) setting with an 18% grey card: the WB setting is saved as a user preset (WB-30Jan18)…

depending on his education or speciality. An orthodontist concentrates on tooth alignment, a restorative dentist may be concerned with the marginal integrity of a filling, a periodontist with gingival inflammation, and so on. Therefore, the resolution of an image depends on the amount of detail required for a given speciality, and every speciality has different resolution needs. For restorative dentistry, assessing nuances in colour, dentine mamelons or incisal and interproximal translucencies is essential for mimicking these characteristics in artificial restorations, and

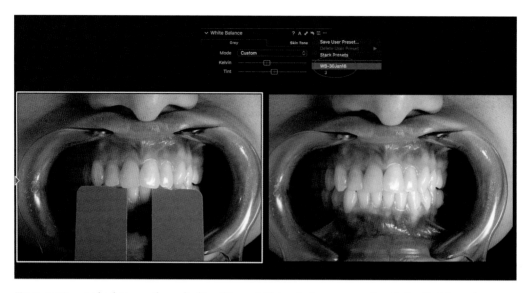

Figure 3.28 ...and subsequently applied to all image(s) taken in the same session. Notice that the colour rendering of both images is identical after correcting the white balance (WB).

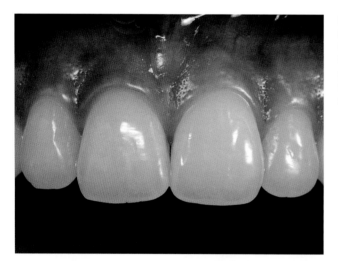

Figure 3.29 Resolution is influences by several factors including the trained eye to discern detail. The intricate capillary network within the free gingival margin surrounding the maxillary right central incisor may go unnoticed by the untrained eye.

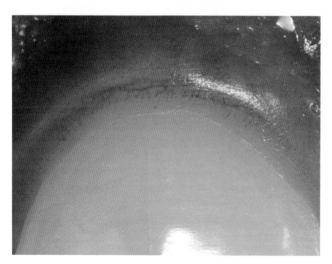

Figure 3.30 Magnified view of the cervical region of the maxillary right central incisor showing the intricate capillary network.

therefore, images with higher resolution for discerning fine detail are required. Conversely, assessing tooth alignment before and after orthodontic treatment can be achieved with relatively low resolution images. For aesthetic dentistry, the quality of an image impacts on the perception of beauty, together with treatment outcomes after aesthetic improvement. In these circumstances, a high-resolution image is beneficial for conveying beauty, irrespective of the modalities used for the aesthetic enhancement (Jacobsen et al. 2006; Tüzgiray and Kaya 2013).

Table 3.3 Synopsis of camera settings for close-up and portraiture dental photography.

Setting	Close-up or macro (intra-oral, extra-oral and bench shots)	Portraiture
Shutter speed	Compact flash synchronisation speed, either 1/125 s or 1/250 s	Any, depending on camera brand and lens, usually 1/125 s
Aperture	f 22 N.B. When using intra-oral mirrors, reduce by one f-stop to f 16 When using contrasters increase by one by one f-stop, or reduce flash intensity	For standardised clinical portraits f 11 is recommended to ensure sufficient depth of field (DoF). For non-clinical portraits, any f-stop is suitable depending on the desired effect; a good starting point is f 5.6
ISO	50–200	50–200
White balance (WB)	Manually set to 5500 K, or take reference picture with 18% neutral density grey card	Depending on type of light, for studio flashes manually set to 5500 K, or take reference shot with 18% neutral density grey card
Aspect ratio	Camera default aspect ratio	Camera default aspect ratio
Colour space	Adobe® RGB, or sRGB	Adobe RGB, or sRGB
Moiré reduction	Default setting	Default setting
Focusing	Manual focus	Manual or auto-focus
Exposure modes	Aperture priority or manual	Manual
Exposure metering	Compact flashes (TTL or manual)	Manual
Auto-exposure metering mode	Multi-field or multi-zone	Any
Exposure bracketing	None	None
Shutter drive modes	Single	Single
Image data format (file format)	Proprietary RAW, Adobe DNG (digital negative graphic)	Proprietary RAW, Adobe DNG (digital negative graphic)
Date/time format	Depending on country	Depending on country
All other settings	Default setting	Default setting
Storage/data transfer	UHS I (30 MB/s writing speed) SD card or UHS II (100 MB/s writing speed) SD card or internal RAM storage	UHS I (30 MB/s writing speed) SD card or UHS II (100 MB/s writing speed) SD card or internal RAM storage
Location (GPS – Global Positioning System)	Personal preference	Personal preference

Other Settings

Contemporary cameras offer a huge number of additional settings, many beyond the scope of this book. However, the best practice is initially keeping everything to factory default settings. After gaining confidence and experience, and guided by referencing advanced photographic literature, one can fine-tune these settings for stepping up to the next level. Table 3.3 summarises some commonly used options for dental photography and their corresponding values. These settings need only be carried out once for a specific set-up, and most cameras allow user settings to be stored as 'user presets' and recalled when required. For dental photography, two user defined settings are required, corresponding to two basic set-ups: the first for intra-oral, extra-oral and bench shots, and the second for portraiture.

References

Ahmad, I. (2009a). Digital dental photography. Part 5: lighting. *Br. Dent. J.* 207 (1): 13–18.

Ahmad, I. (2009b). Digital dental photography. Part 6: camera settings. *Br. Dent. J.* 207 (2): 63–69.

Bazos, P. and Magne, M. (2013). Demystifying the digital dental photography workflow. The big picture: facial documentation with high visual impact photography. *J. Cosmet. Dent.* 29 (1): 82–88.

Bengel, W. (2006). *Mastering Digital Dental Photography*. New Malden, UK: Quintessence.

Cytowic, R. (2003). *The Man Who Tasted Shapes*. Cambridge, MA: MIT Press.

Jacobsen, T., Schubotz, R.I., Hofel, L. et al. (2006). Brain correlates of aesthetic judgment of beauty. *Neuroimage* 29: 276–285.

Ker, A.J., Chan, R., Fields, H.W. et al. (2008). Esthetics and smile characteristics from the layperson's perspective. *J. Am. Dent. Assoc.* 139 (10): 1318–1327.

Manjunath, S.G., Ragavendra, R.T., Sowmya et al. (2011). Photography in clinical dentistry – a review. *Int. J. Dent. Clin.* 3 (2): 40–43.

Nordberg, J.J. and Sluder, G. (2013). Practical aspects of adjusting digital cameras. *Methods Cell Biol.* 114: 151–162.

Sajjadi, S.H., Khosravanifard, B., Esmaeilpour, M. et al. (2015). The effects of camera lenses and dental specialties on the perception of smile esthetics. *J. Orthod. Sci.* 4 (4): 97–101.

Sajjadi, S.H., Khosravanifard, B., Moazzami, F. et al. (2016). Effects of three types of digital camera sensors on dental specialists' perception of smile esthetics: a preliminary double-blind clinical trial. *J. Prosthodontics* 25: 675–681.

Tüzgiray, Y.B. and Kaya, B. (2013). Factors affecting smile esthetics. *Turk. J. Orthod.* 26: 58–64.

4

Composition and Standardisation

The preceding modules have concentrated on the technical aspects of photographic equipment, which are important but do not necessarily guarantee a good picture. Besides light, the second most important aspect of photography is composition. Composing a picture is no different to compositing a piece of music. After configuring the photographic equipment, similar to tuning musical instruments, the next stage is making music. Photographic composition is about framing a picture so that it has visual harmony. Put simply, it is guiding the eye to the most important part of the picture,[1] and elevating it to a psychological and synæsthetic experience.

Composition

A picture can be composed ad hoc or using a set of predefined rules. Many of the principles of composition are also used for aesthetic dentistry when designing a smile. There are several rules and principles for photographic compositions including figure-to-ground, the rule of thirds, Phi grid, Fibonacci spiral, leading lines, diagonals, the rule of direction, visual weight, symmetry, balance and image content, to name a few. Although these rules are not applicable to every photograph, and will not necessarily produce striking images, incorporating these principles while composing a picture can help to effectively tell a story. Composing can either be orchestrated before taking the picture by changing the position of the objects, subjects and the camera, or later during the processing stage in imaging software. The latter is ideal for cropping extraneous objects or positioning items so that they are spatially located in desirable positions. However, image processing cannot correct poor composition, which should be addressed while taking the picture. The following discussion suggests some food for thought for successfully composing a picture.

Dominance

The most popular method for achieving dominance is using the figure-to-ground rule. The 'figure' is the main subject, while 'ground' is the background. The idea is to enhance separation between the two by varying contrast, size, colour or selective focusing (Figure 4.1). These are effective methods for achieving dominance, similar to the maxillary central incisors that are the dominant elements of the maxillary anterior sextant due to their larger size, position in the arch and brighter colour.

The maxim, 'less is more' is worth bearing in mind when considering dominance. The content of an image plays a crucial role in visual perception, and if an image is cluttered with

---

1 https://photographylife.com/introducing-composition-in-photography

Essentials of Dental Photography, First Edition. Irfan Ahmad.
© 2020 John Wiley & Sons Ltd. Published 2020 by John Wiley & Sons Ltd.

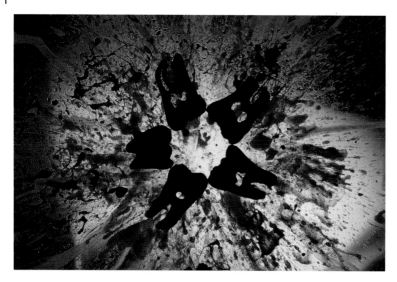

Figure 4.1 A simple but effective way to achieve figure-ground is silhouetting the subject against a bright background.

objects, the result is visual cacophony and tension since there is too much information for the eyes to analyse. Therefore, minimising the image content by selective focusing or increasing the magnification factor to frame a few objects, allows the eye to concentrate on the main point of interest (Bengel and Devigus 2006) – Figures 4.2 and 4.3. Framing or cropping is an obvious way to allow the observer concentrate on salient features without being distracted by extraneous, irrelevant objects. This is particularly relevant when documenting sequential procedures for demonstrating techniques. A series of pictures should be cropped to concentrate on the salient teeth, rather than including the whole arch (Figure 4.4). Another dental example is using a black contraster to enhance the contrast of the teeth against a dark background, and for emphasising tooth characteristics such as incisal translucency (Figure 4.5).

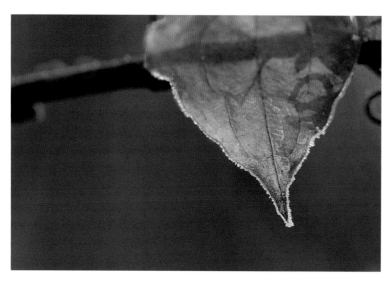

Figure 4.2 Selective focusing and selective lighting achieves a desirable figure-ground separation, e.g. focusing on the frost on a leaf, which is thrown out of focus.

Figure 4.3 Selective focusing and selective lighting achieves a desirable figure-ground separation, e.g. the sharply focused #15c surgical blade with an out-of-focus oral cavity, guiding the eye to the point of interest.

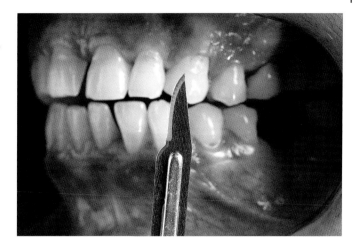

Figure 4.4 A series of images depicting a clinical technique should be framed to allow the observer to concentrate on specific teeth.

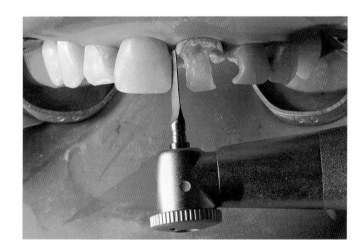

Figure 4.5 Placing a contraster behind teeth increases contrast and emphasises incisal translucency.

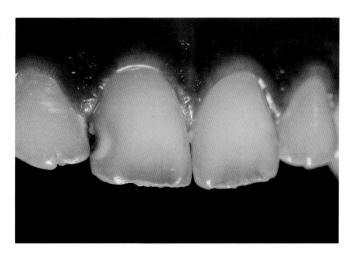

Positioning

The basic concept of composition is arranging or positioning objects within the frame so they have visual appeal. The first rule that is universally taught about composition is the rule of thirds, which helps to position elements in a frame so that they are interesting and engaging for the viewer.[2] The rule of thirds divides an image with four lines into a nine-part grid (Figure 4.6). This is the most popular grid used by camera manufacturers and is either visible through the viewfinder, or on the LCD display on the back of the camera body. If objects are placed along or at the intersection of the four lines, the image is more appealing to the observer.[3] This is because the eyes are more attracted to objects that are off-centre in a frame than those that are in the centre. Therefore, placing points of interest to one side, or at the

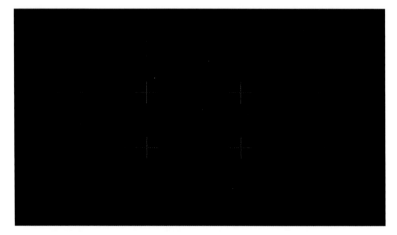

Figure 4.6 The rule of thirds grid.

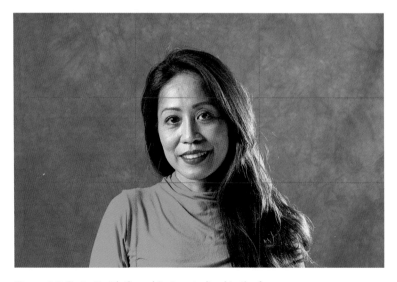

Figure 4.7 Portrait with the subject centralised in the frame.

2 Rule of Thirds – Digital Photography School, 2015
3 What is the mysterious 'Rule of Three?, https://rule-of-three.co.uk

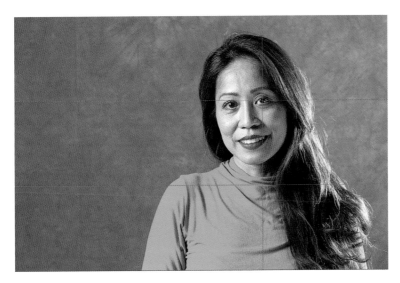

Figure 4.8 Portrait conforming to the rule of thirds, with the pupil of the subject's left eye intersecting the grid.

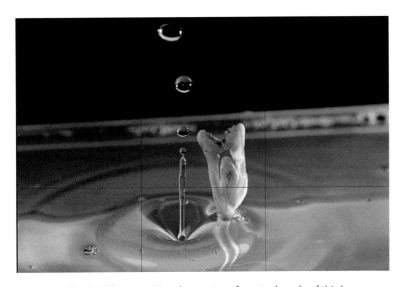

Figure 4.9 The initial composition does not conform to the rule of thirds.

intersection of the four lines, adds interest to the composition. The rule of thirds is applicable for any picture, including portraits (Figures 4.7 and 4.8), but particularly still life or bench shots, as the photographer has full control to position the objects anywhere in the composition (Figures 4.9–4.11). This rule is also relevant for intra-oral images, especially at the editing and cropping stage, when points of interest can be shifted to the intersection of the rule of third grid lines (Figures 4.12 and 4.13).

Instead of dividing the grid equally into 1 : 1 : 1 vertically and horizontally as in the rule of thirds, the Phi grid divides the frame according to the Golden Proportion (GP) into 1 : 1.618 : 1 rectangles (Figure 4.14). Similar to the rule of thirds, the Phi grid is used to compose a picture so that items of interest are located within the grid divisions or at the intersection of the lines. The choice between using the rule of thirds or the Phi grid is a personal preference, the rule of

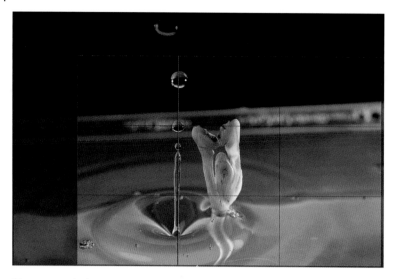

Figure 4.10 At the cropping stage, the image is cropped and moved using the rule of thirds grid to place the water droplets along and at the intersection of the grid lines.

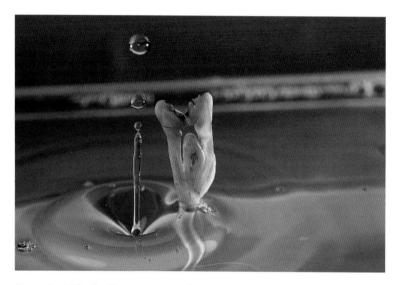

Figure 4.11 The final image composed according to the rule of thirds.

thirds is not mathematically accurate, and therefore, may be perceived as too simplistic, contrived and obvious, but in practice is easier to use. The Phi grid provides a mathematically precise and perfect composition, which may sometimes be difficult to attain. Also, the choice depends on the subject matter, what the photographer is trying to convey, and which one 'feels' right for a particular composition (Figures 4.15 and 4.16).

Another grid is the Fibonacci spiral (Figure 4.17), which is also based on the GP and is ubiquitously evident in nature such as the Milky Way, flower petals arrangements or spirals of seashells. This grid is used by artists, architects and graphic designers for arranging elements to enhance visual appeal. The principle of this grid is arranging elements along a curved path that guides the eye to the protagonist object at the 'eye' of the grid. This is an extremely effective

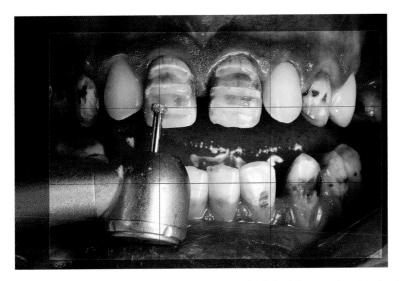

Figure 4.12 An image framed to conform to the rule of thirds by ensuring that the depth cut bur is located at the intersection of the grid lines.

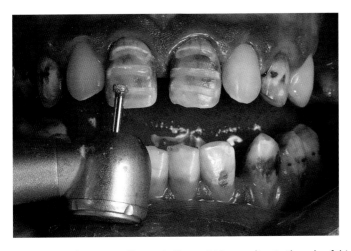

Figure 4.13 The cropped image in Figure 4.12 according to the rule of thirds.

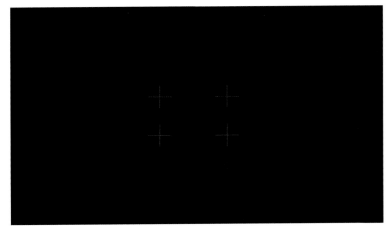

Figure 4.14 The Phi grid.

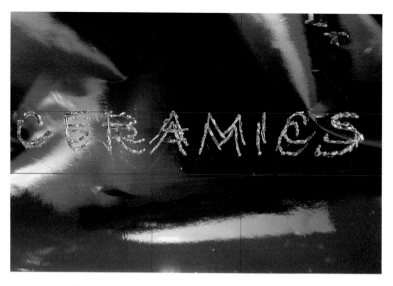

Figure 4.15 The Phi grid was used to frame this picture, ensuring that the text 'CERAMICS' was confined to the middle row of the grid.

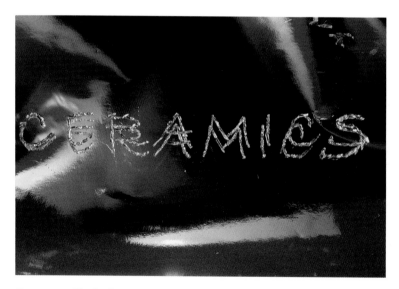

Figure 4.16 The final composition according to the Phi grid.

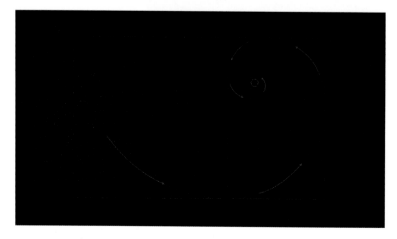

Figure 4.17 Fibonacci spiral grid.

method of framing a picture and can be carried out at either the capture, or post-processing stages. Figures 4.18–4.24 demonstrate framing a picture according to the Fibonacci spiral at both the capture and processing stages. All the above three grids are accessible in imaging software during the alignment and cropping stage, or as plug-ins and apps from vendors (Figure 4.25).

Aligning grids are a useful guide and offer a systematic approach for composing images at the capture and/or post-processing stage in editing software. However, aligning images that conform to these grids is subjective, and may not be appropriate, or desirable, for every type of image. A classic example is portraiture, when framing depends on the subject's and photographer's personal preferences, which may or may not conform to a particular grid (Figures 4.26–4.29).

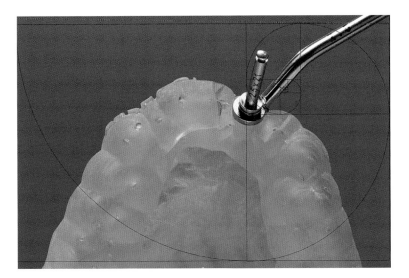

Figure 4.18 A 3-D printed surgical guide with osteotomy drill. The main point of interest is the drill, which is incorrectly framed since the 'eye' of the Fibonacci spiral does not corresponding to the position of the drill.

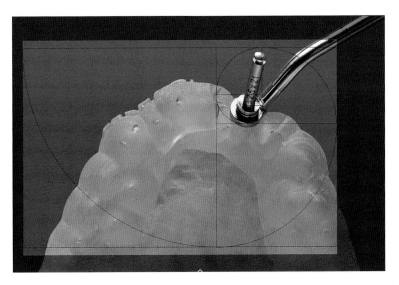

Figure 4.19 Correctly framed image with the 'eye' of the Fibonacci spiral corresponding to the position of the drill.

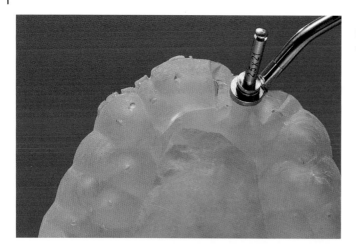

Figure 4.20 The final cropped image according to the Fibonacci spiral.

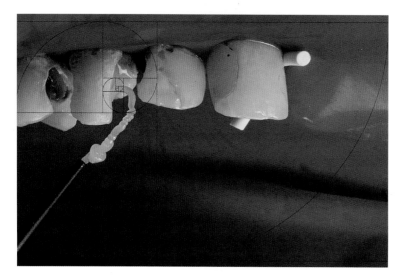

Figure 4.21 In order to frame this picture according to the Fibonacci spiral, the patient's head was moved to the left and the camera positioned to capture a lateral view ensuring that the point of interest (the tip if the flowable composite) was in the 'eye' of the Fibonacci spiral.

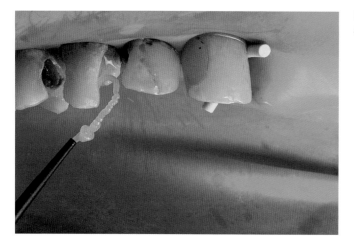

Figure 4.22 The final framed image according to the Fibonacci spiral.

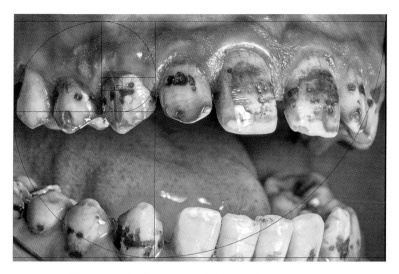

Figure 4.23 The 'eye' of the Fibonacci spiral is located at the point of interest, which is the haemorrhage emanating from the sulcus of the maxillary right canine.

Figure 4.24 The final image framed according to the Fibonacci spiral.

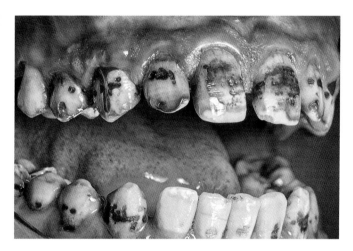

Leading the Eye

Leading the eye means guiding the eyes with imaginary or actual line(s) to the point of interest in the image. A leading line is any structure or part of an image that leads the eye to the main subject (Figures 4.30 and 4.31). This concept is predominately employed for landscape photography, but can also be creatively applied to both intra-oral and bench images (Figures 4.32 and 4.33). For example, in landscape photography, this principle is effectively applied where roads, railway lines, stairs, rivers or paths are framed in the foreground and guide the eye inwards and upwards to the main point of interest. Another method is using leading lines to convey mystery by deliberately placing the point of convergence outside the frame of the shot, which leaves the viewer wondering what lies at the end of the lines. Furthermore, leading lines add depth and perspective to a composition. For dental photography, imaginary lines such as the inter-pupillary line, Camper's plane (ala-tragus line), Frankfort plane, and dental or facial midlines give stability to an image (Figure 4.34). Another example is parallelism of the maxillary incisal

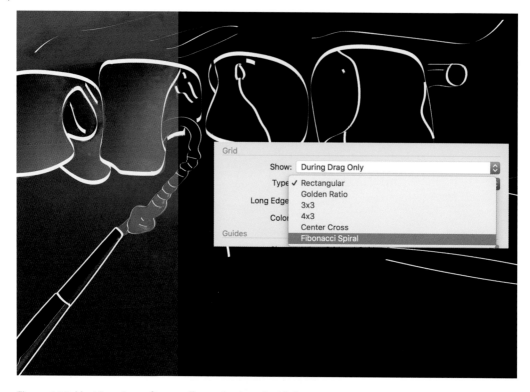

Figure 4.25 Most imaging software offer a selection of grids for composition pictures at the aligning and cropping stages.

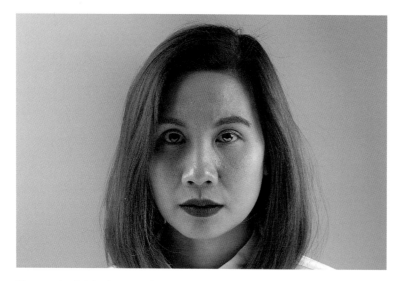

Figure 4.26 Original captured image.

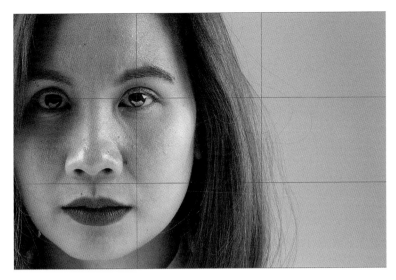

Figure 4.27 Cropping according to the rule of thirds.

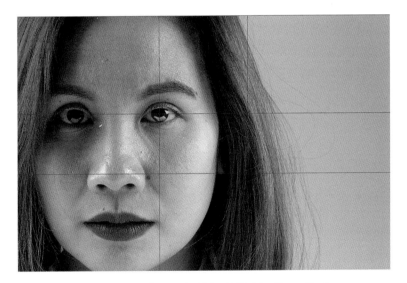

Figure 4.28 Cropping according to the Phi grid (Golden Proportion).

plane to the curvature of the mandibular lip during a relaxed smile, which adds cohesiveness to a dento-facial composition (Figures 4.35 and 4.36).

Diagonals or diagonal lines serve a similar purpose to leading lines by engaging the viewer. Whereas leading lines guide the eye to a particular destination *into* the picture, diagonal lines guide the viewer *through* the picture. As with leading lines, diagonals add a three-dimension quality to an image. An important distinction between leading (or converging) lines and diagonals is that the former creates static dramatic imagery, while the latter creates kinetic imagery by adding a sense of motion (Figures 4.37 and 4.38).

The rule of direction is yet another way of guiding the eyes. In most western cultures, reading and writing are from left to right, while the opposite is true for much of the Eastern Hemisphere

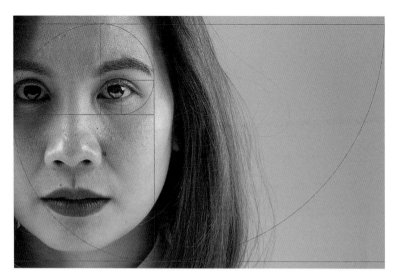

Figure 4.29 Cropping according to the Fibonacci spiral grid.

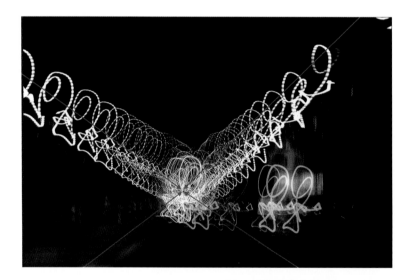

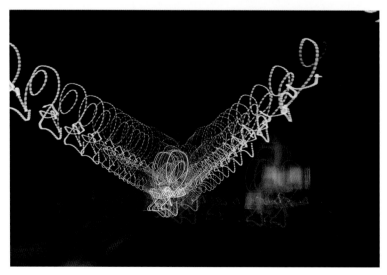

Figures 4.30 and 4.31 Leading lines draw the viewer into the picture.

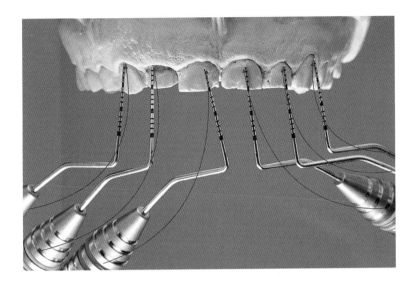

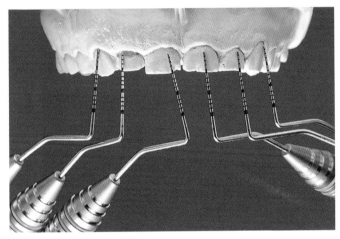

Figures 4.32 and 4.33 The periodontal probe handles guide the viewer to the tip of the probes, which are the main point of interest in relation to the short clinical crown lengths of the maxillary anterior sextant.

(Figures 4.39 and 4.40). Therefore, similar to reading a book, the climax should be at the end of the picture, and its direction should be left to right for Western societies, culminating to most important part of an image on the right side, and vice versa for right to left cultures. The rule of direction adds intrigue, allowing the observer to build up to the crescendo, rather than knowing the ending beforehand.

Balance

Visual weight ensures that the right and left, or top and bottom, parts of an image are balanced. This is achieved by placing objects to fill voids or negative spaces in a composition (Figures 4.41 and 4.42). This is achieved by either adding and incorporating objects within the frame, or by altering the colour and lighting of a scene. For example, a dark colour carries more balance that a light one, while an intense light is perceived as 'bigger' compared to a dim light.

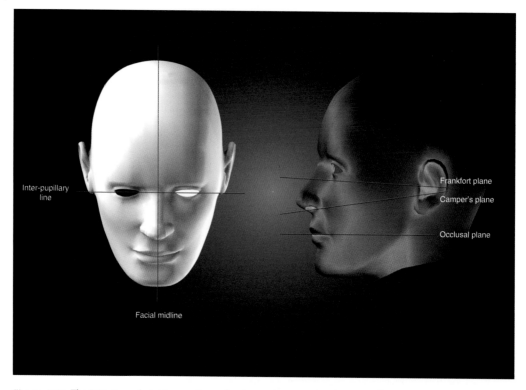

Figure 4.34 The imaginary facial lines act as cohesive and segregative forces to the facial composition.

To summarise, the basic rules for photographic compositions are guidelines, and not rigid rules cast in stone. They are useful for composing a picture, but often involve trial and error until a composition gels with the photographer's vision, which develops with time, experience and perseverance. Probably the most important factor for composing a picture is intuition, which can subconsciously direct the photographer to produce striking images. Furthermore, breaking rules can often produce innovative and visually striking results, but ignoring them may result in catastrophic failures.

Standardisation

Dental photography is basically visual dental documentation; its value lies in comparison for self and peer-critique of the same or different patients, and historical cohort studies for monitoring and research (Bengal 1985; Ettorre et al. 2006; Galdino et al. 2001).

In order to realise these objectives, some form of standardisation is prerequisite, establishing guidelines for consistency, comparison and communication (Graber 1946; Martins et al. 2013). Furthermore, standardisation starts at the capture stage when an image is composed and ends at the processing/display stage when the image is edited using computer software and reproduced with the chosen media (monitor, projector, print), respectively. There are three factors that influence standardisation; human factors, technical factors and the intended use of the image.

The human factors are the patient, assistant and the operator, usually the clinician, who is taking the photographs while the assistant ensures patient comfort and helps with positioning

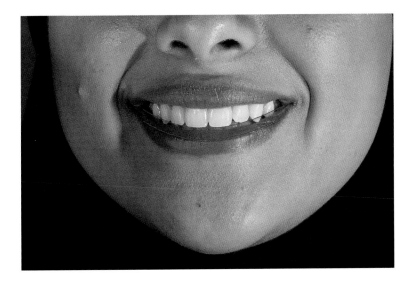

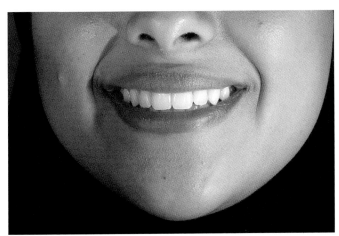

Figures 4.35 and 4.36 Cohesiveness in a composition unites elements together such as parallelism of the incisal plane to the curvature of the mandibular lip.

the dental armamentarium and photographic equipment. The operator factors include sufficient knowledge, training and experience in dental photography, and the ability to adapt to patients' idiosyncrasies to avoid jeopardising the photographic session. The patient factors include the physical and mental state of the patient, and whether they are able to fully cooperate with and endure the photographic procedures. This could mean controlling excessive salivary flow or taming involuntary gagging reflexes. In addition, paying attention to any local soft and hard tissue anatomical variations that may hinder posture in the horizontal, vertical and sagittal planes. Another issue is obtaining an unimpeded retraction of the extra-oral soft tissues for a clear field of view of the oral cavity.

The quintessential technical requirement of an image is that it is sharp, in focus, correctly composed with the proper colour balance and exposure, and records with fidelity the object(s) or subject(s) being photographed. This involves understanding basic photographic concepts outlined in previous modules, and configuring the camera and ancillary equipment settings to produce repeatable and predictable results. The technical aspects include several variables

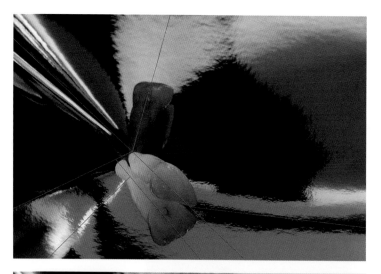

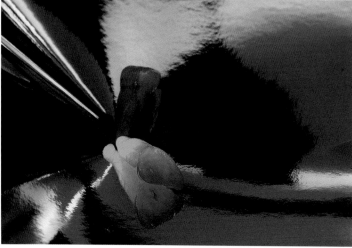

Figures 4.37 and 4.38 Diagonals add kinetic dynamism to a composition.

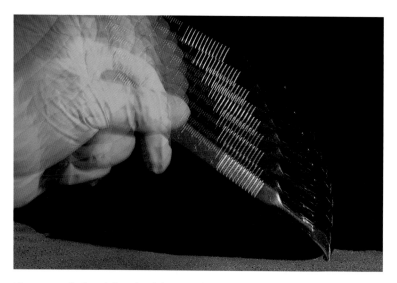

Figure 4.39 Left to right rule of direction for Western cultures: the eye is guided from left to right, culminating at the tip of the blade, which is the point of interest.

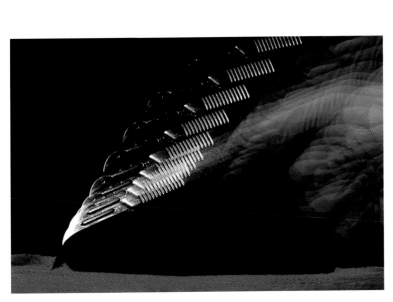

Figure 4.40 Right to left rule of direction for Eastern cultures: the eye is guided from right to left, culminating at the tip of the blade, which is the point of interest.

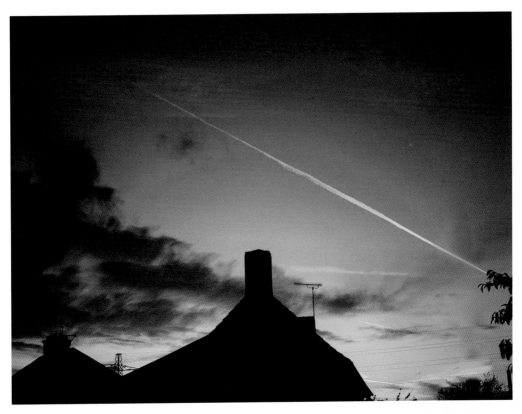

Figure 4.41 Balance is lacking in this composition due to the extensive negative space on the right side…

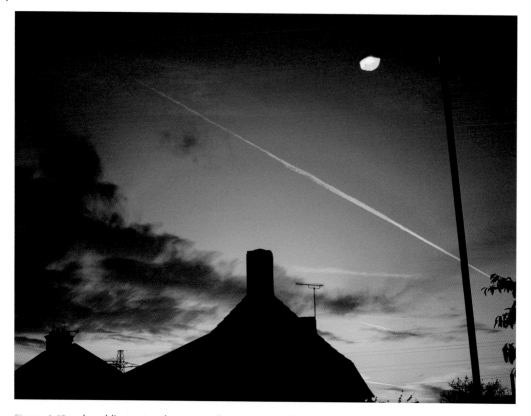

Figure 4.42 …by adding a streetlamp post, the composition becomes more balanced.

such as dental armamentarium, the camera sensor size, the focal length of the lens, equipment settings, illumination (quality and quantity), lens axis or angle of view (vertical and horizontal composition), background, and scaling or magnification.

The last factor to consider is the purpose or intended use of an image. The intended use may be clinical documentation, marketing, or educational (lecturing/publishing). Clinical documentation also depends on the particular speciality, e.g. orthodontics, periodontics, surgery, oral medicine, aesthetics, to name a few. A portfolio of stock views is adequate for basic documentation, but additional images are required depending on the speciality, or a specific treatment modality. For example, a standard set of extra- and intra-oral images are sufficient for cranio-maxillo-facial surgery (Ettorre et al. 2006), but inadequate for a ceramist who is fabricating a single unit crown to match an adjacent natural tooth. Another category is marketing and promotion, where image requirements differ from clinical reality. Marketing images serve an entirely different purpose to clinical documentation. They are intrinsically enticing, promoting a given treatment and omitting clinical procedures that may be unpalatable for laypersons, e.g. graphical depiction of surgical procedures. Lastly, recording treatment sequences and outcomes for lecturing and/or publishing are aimed at educating and inspiring a target audience. Hence, these images are different to insipid clinical documentation, and incorporate aspirational aspects for enhancing and encouraging the teaching and learning process.

In order to accomplish standardisation, two pertinent questions need to be asked. First, 'Is standardisation possible in dental photography?', and if so, 'What can, and what cannot, be standardised?'

There are certain aspects of dental photography that can be standardised. These include predefined positions of the patient, photographic equipment and operator, and configuring photographic and ancillary equipment to specific settings. However, some factors, predominantly hardware-related, cannot be standardised. These include photographic equipment that is unique to a particular manufacturer that is rarely interchangeable or inter-compatible with other brands. The market is awash with innumerable competitors with proprietary closed systems, which offers vast consumer choice, but at the expense of forgoing generic open systems. Therefore, the factors that are standardisable will produce comparable and consistent images for inter- and intra-patient documentation, but are limited to an individual dental practice or institution with specific brands of photographic equipment.

Standardisable Factors

The standardisable factors are related to photographic equipment settings, correct patient positioning (Sommer and Mendelsohn 2004), dental armamentarium and the operator taking the pictures. Ideally, a set of dental photographic protocols should be established and followed for achieving direct comparisons, even if the photographs are taken by different operators.

The technical elements for standardisation are the equipment settings for consistent exposure (Niamtu 2004), DoF, composition, framing, orientation, colour rendition, file formats, elimination of extraneous artefacts, and the requisite number of images for a given portfolio. It goes without saying that an image should be correctly exposed, neither too bright, nor too dark. This is achieved by either using flash TTL (through-the-lens) metering, or alternately, taking a few test images for identical set-ups. Another essential item is precise colour rendering, without unwanted colour casts for distinguishing healthy and diseased tissues. This is achieved by the correct white balance, periodically calibrating computer displays with calibration devices and keeping the same ICC (International Color Consortium) colour profile for all images. Although resolution cannot be standardised due to unique hardware specification, this is not an overwhelming concern since most contemporary cameras can deliver adequate resolution for the majority of dental applications. Nevertheless, a dental image should have sufficient detail for discerning salient features of hard and soft tissues. However, different specialities, or images for special applications, require specific visual information, which is elaborated in later modules. Finally, images in a standard portfolio should convey the following features with clarity and clinical fidelity (Ahmad 2009) (Figures 4.43–4.45):

- Distinction between healthy and diseased tissue, especially discriminating pathological changes
- Attached gingivae, showing degree of stippling (texture) for assessing periodontal biotypes (thick, thin) and bioforms (scalloped, flat)
- Transition between keratinised and non-keratinised oral mucosa for assessing width of keratinised tissue (attached gingivae, free gingival margin, gingival groves, clefts, scarring)
- Shade transition in teeth traversing from cervical to body to incisal edges
- Enamel characterisations, lobes, mottling, stains, chips, texture, hypoplasia, cracks, fractures and perikymata
- Incisal, interproximal translucency and mamelons
- Attrition, abrasion, erosion, abfraction lesions
- Hypocalcification, fluorosis, tetracycline staining
- Cervical dentine exposure, extrinsic, intrinsic and internalised pigmentation
- Defective restorative margins
- Secondary caries, restorative material wear, chips and discolouration

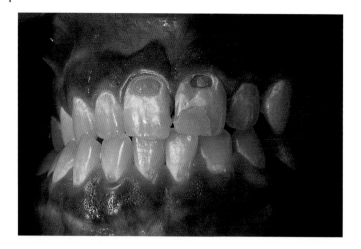

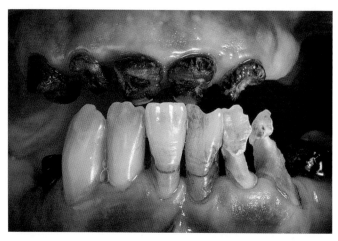

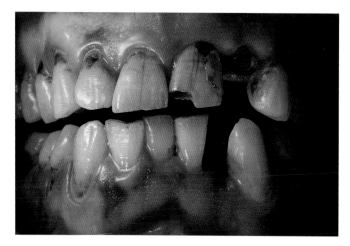

Figures 4.43–4.45 Clinical documentation should include features of diagnostic value (see above list for some salient features).

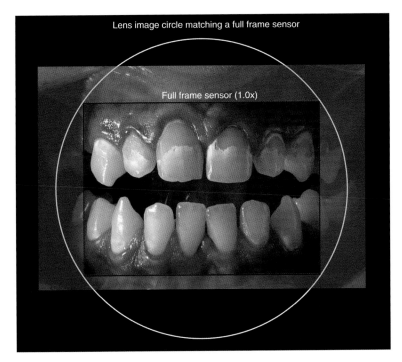

Figure 4.46 A full-frame sensor has the same magnification factor as the focal length of the lens (crop factor 1.0×).

Scaling or magnification is also a crucial aspect for ensuring consistency (Sugawara et al. 2014). The proverbially quoted magnifications for specific dental photographs – i.e. 1 : 1 and 1 : 2 for intra-oral, 1 : 5 for dento-facial compositions and 1 : 8 to 1 : 15 for full face or portraiture – is based on 35 mm film photography. All analogue 35 mm cameras used the same celluloid film consisting of identical 35 mm × 24 mm frames. Hence, for a given focal length lens, the magnification factor was always the same for all 35 mm cameras, irrespective of the brand. However, this is not the case with digital photography, since the film is replaced by sensors that have different physical dimensions (see Figure 1.9 in Module 1). Therefore, the magnification factor of a lens is only applicable for cameras that have a full-frame sensor corresponding to the size of a 35 mm film frame (Figure 4.46). If the sensor is smaller (usually) or larger than conventional 35 mm film, a crop factor is applied, which varies according to the size of the sensor. To overcome the issue of different sensor sizes and to ensure a consistent magnification, the focusing distance on the lens barrel can be pre-set for a particular view, e.g. intra-oral, dento-facial or portrait compositions.

Besides the technical issues of scaling, the physical size of facial features and intra-oral anatomy varies enormously between individuals. If the maxillary and mandibular arches are large or small, a pre-set magnification may crop vital features, or include extraneous objects such as cheek retractors, respectively. Another approach for ensuring a consistent field of view is using anatomical landmarks for composing both extra-oral and intra-oral dental images. For clinical portraiture, instead of using a predefined magnification, the background area surrounding the hairline and the auricles can be predefined with the lower margin bounded by the sterno-clavicular joint. For dento-facial views the landmarks could be the tip of the chin (menton) to the middle of the nose (rhinion) – Figure 4.47. For intra-oral images, the mucogingival junction, retracted sulci, number of posterior teeth and buccal corridor are helpful anatomical pointers

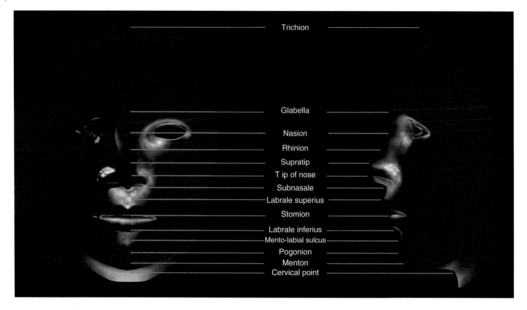

Figure 4.47 Facial anatomical landmarks are useful guides for farming a particular view.

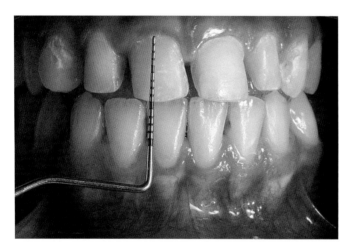

Figure 4.48 Reference makers such as periodontal probes are an ideal way to depict scale within an image.

for ensuring reproducible and consistent compositions, irrespective of the magnification scale on the lens. A useful approach for conveying scale within an image is including reference markers such as periodontal probes or rulers for indicating dimensions of teeth, restorations, soft tissue landmarks or lesions (Figure 4.48). The major items that can be standardised are summarised in Table 4.1.

Non-standardisable Factors

Although not exhaustive, the standardisable factors outlined above are sufficient to allow comparisons for the majority of inter- and intra-patient photographic documentation. However, there are several factors, mainly hardware-related, which are impossible to standardise. Factors such as resolution, colour space, bit depth, absolute colour rendition, quality and quantity of

Table 4.1 Standardisable factors for dental photography.

What?	Why?	How?
Positioning (patient, operator, assistant, equipment)	To expedite photographic session, repeatable images for diagnosis, treatment planning, sequencing outcome, and inter- and intra-patient comparisons	Patient position: seated upright, partially relined or supine (depending on the type of image required). Mount camera on tripod, makings on floor for positions of camera, lights, photographer and assistant
Image orientation	For same perspective	Landscape orientation
Spacial orientation	For same angle of view in vertical, horizontal and sagittal planes	Use orientation guides such as the horizon, Frankfort plane, Camper's line, inter-pupillary line, facial midline, camera viewing screen grids, spirit level
Composition (field of view)	Consistent views for compassion	Magnification factor, pre-set focusing distance on lens, intra-oral and extra-oral anatomical landmarks
Framing	Cropping irrelevant parts of image for concentrating on points of interest	Capture image with larger framing for subsequent cropping in imaging software
Exposure	For faithfully reproducing subjects with a given lighting set-up	For intra-oral images: manipulating intensity and distance of flashes. For extra-oral images: manipulating shutter speed, f-stop, ISO, histogram and illumination (intensity and distance)
Colour rendition	For true colour reproduction	Setting the white balance, identical ICC profiles
Shapness	For discerning details	Fast shutter seeds, flash illumination, ideal hyperfocal distance, sufficient depth of field
Extraneous objects or artefacts	For avoiding visual distractions	Judicial placement of saliva ejector, cotton wool rolls, edges of mirrors, cheek retractors and contrasters. Remove saliva, blood, biofilm, extrinsic stains, food debris. Prevent scratches, droplets, fogging (condensation) on mirrors
Number of images in portfolio	For inter-patient comparison, and comparing pre and post-operative treatment outcomes	Predefining the number of images according to the dental discipline or specific application
Post-capture processing	Consistent criteria for comparisons	Use same photo-editing software for exposure correction, orientation, cropping extraneous artefacts or parts of image
Metadata	For recall and archival	Date, patient details, camera and software settings
Image data format (file format)	Different formats for different needs	Small JPEG files for internet communication, large TIFF files for publishing and archiving

illumination are all device-specific, with little standardisation between different brands. It is worth noting that although the relative colour rendition for a given computer display can be standardised using colour calibration devices and ICC profiles, absolute colour rendition between different monitors presents a challenge. Nowadays, images are disseminated and exchanged rapidly through the internet and viewed on innumerable mobile devices such as smartphones, tablets or smart televisions. The colour space for all these displays is unique, and therefore an image will have a different colour rendition, which is virtually impossible to standardise. A simple method for circumventing different colour rendition on display devices is to include a reference picture taken with a neutral density grey card when transmitting a particular portfolio. The reference image can be used by the recipient to calibrate all images within a portfolio to ensure correct colour rendition.

In addition, post-capture image processing by in-camera processors and various imaging software all yield disparate results depending on their unique algorithms (Bister et al. 2006). Lastly, human fallibility also plays a part in standardising, e.g. patient and operators factors. Young children, the elderly and patients with limited mouth opening or debilitating illness may be unable to endure, or fully participate in, a photographic session. This includes maintaining a particular position or tolerating cheek retractors and other intra-oral dental armamentarium for correct image framing and composition. Also, the operator taking the pictures should be versed in dental photography, and most importantly, have the aptitude for tolerating and accepting negative prevailing eventualities.

The last aspect to standardise is honesty (Schaff et al. 2006). Current photo-editing software allows even a novice with little or no computer knowledge to transform the 'girl next door' into a 'Mona Lisa'. Whilst this frivolity is harmless narcissism, manipulating clinical documentation is potentially bordering on criminality. This could involve concealing pre-preoperative pathology or enhancing post-operative treatment results by camouflaging defects (Chowdhry 2016). In addition, altering images for publishing or lecturing for personal advancement is obviously deceitful. To reiterate, photographs are essentially visual dental documentation, no different to dental records or radiographs. Therefore, strict adherence to medical ethics is paramount, and as professionals, we ultimately rely on fellow colleagues to follow a code of conduct befitting our vocation. Put succinctly, honesty is professional de rigueur.

References

Ahmad, I. (2009). Digital dental photography. Part 1: an overview. *Br. Dent. J.* 206 (8): 403–407.

Bengal, W. (1985). Standardization in dental photography. *Int. Dent. J.* 35 (3): 210–217.

Bengel, W. and Devigus, A. (2006). Preparing images for publication: part 2. *Eur. J. Esthet. Dent.* 1: 112–127.

Bister, D., Mordarai, F., and Aveling, R.M. (2006). Comparison of 10 digital SLR cameras for orthodontic photography. *J. Orthod.* 33: 223–230.

Chowdhry, A. (2016). Seeing is no longer believing. *Indian J. Dent. Educ.* 9 (2).

Ettorre, G., Weber, M., Schaaf, H. et al. (2006). Standards for digital photography in cranio-maxillo-facial surgery – part I: basic views and guidelines. *J. Craniomaxillofac. Surg.* 34: 65–73.

Galdino, G.M., Vogel, J.E., and Vander Kolk, C.A. (2001). Standardizing digital photography: it's not all in the eye of the beholder. *Plast. Reconstr. Surg.* 108: 1334–1344.

Graber, T.M. (1946). Patient photography in orthodontics. MSD thesis. Northwest University Dental School.

Martins, R.F.M., Costa, L.A., Bringel, A.C.C. et al. (2013). Protocol for digital photography in orthodontics. *Rev. Clín. Orthod. Dental Press* 12 (4): 102–111.

Niamtu, J. (2004). Image is everything: pearls and pitfalls of digital photography and PowerPoint presentations for the cosmetic surgeon. *Dermatol. Surg.* 30: 81–91.

Schaff, H., Streckbein, P., Ettorre, G. et al. (2006). Standards for digital photography in cranio-maxillo-facial surgery – part II: additional picture sets and avoiding common mistakes. *J. Cranio-Maxillofac. Surg.* 34: 366–377.

Sommer, D.D. and Mendelsohn, M. (2004). Pitfalls of nonstandardized photography in facial plastic surgery patients. *Plast. Reconstr. Surg.* 114: 10–14.

Sugawara, Y., Saito, K., Futaki, M. et al. (2014). Evaluation of the optimal exposure settings for occlusal photography with digital cameras. *Pediatr. Dent. J.* 24: 89–96.

Section 2

Photographic Set-ups

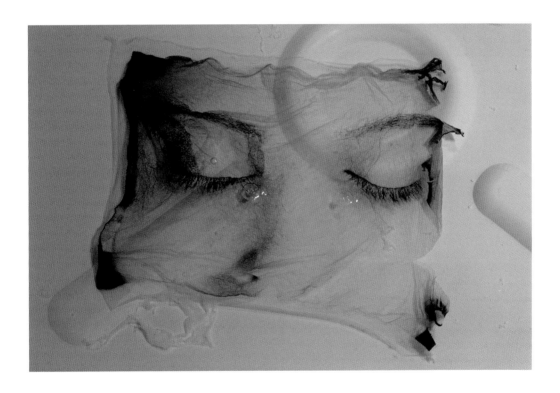

5

Extra-Oral and Intra-Oral Images

This module covers the most frequently documented images in dentistry; extra-oral and intra-oral compositions (Ahmad 2009). The former is also referred to as the dento-facial composition since it includes the lips, extra-oral soft tissues and their relationship to the intra-oral dentogingival elements.

Positioning

As discussed in Module 2, unlike conventional photography, dental photography has additional factors to consider, such as cross-infection control, health and safety and confidentiality. Therefore, optimal settings of the camera, flashes and ancillary equipment, outlined in Module 3, are repeated in this module for convenience. Before starting, it is worth browsing through Module 3 for a detailed analysis of cameras settings, and Module 4 about composing and standardising images. Besides these fundamental requirements, positioning the patient, photographer, assistant, photographic equipment, flashes and dental adjuncts are crucial for extra- and intra-oral pictures.

The position of the patient is pivotal, and synergistically determines the position of the photographer, assistant and equipment (Devigus 2012). The type of image dictates the position of the patient, who can be seated upright, partially reclined or supine. For the majority of standardised extra-oral and intra-oral images, the ideal position of the patient is seated upright. This position is repeatable, whereas the degree of recline varies, and compromises standardisation. However, for promotional and marketing images, positioning is somewhat lackadaisical, since a rigid posture is perceived as uptight and possibly confrontational.

For the majority of extra- and intra-oral clinical images, the patient's head and the camera axis is perpendicular to the facial midline and parallel to the horizon (Figures 5.1–5.3). The lens axis is centred exactly at the mesial contact point areas of the maxillary centrals. Using orientation facial landmarks, such as the inter-pupillary or inter-commisure lines for orientation, prevents eschewed or incorrect alignment of the incisal plane and/or dental midlines. In the sagittal plan, the head should neither be pointing up, nor down, i.e., parallel to the ala-tragus (Camper's line) or Frankfort plane and perpendicular to the lens axis (Figure 5.2). Maintaining a perpendicular lens axis ensures correct perspective; if the lens axis is superior or inferior, the teeth appear elongated or shortened, especially the maxillary and mandibular anteriors. In addition, if a ring flash is mounted on the front of lens, a superior or inferior lens axis will unduly illuminate the 'red' oral mucosa, and the light reflected back onto the palatal aspects of the teeth will make them appear more reddish, conveying an incorrect colour rendition that may affect precise tooth shade evaluations. Also, it is important to avoid using

Essentials of Dental Photography, First Edition. Irfan Ahmad.
© 2020 John Wiley & Sons Ltd. Published 2020 by John Wiley & Sons Ltd.

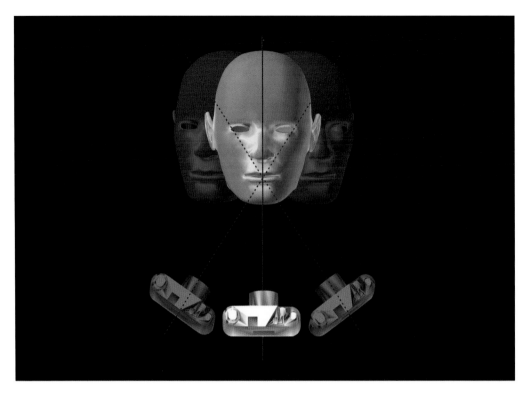

Figure 5.1 Incorrect angulation of the camera or the patient's head in the vertical plane causes distortion of perspective or unwanted shadows.

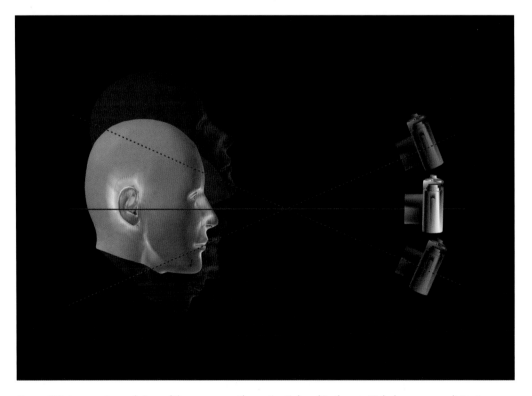

Figure 5.2 Incorrect angulation of the camera or the patient's head in the sagittal plane causes distortion of perspective, unwanted shadows and/or conveys a reddish colour rendition of the teeth that are unintentionally illuminated by the reflected 'red shadows' of the oral cavity.

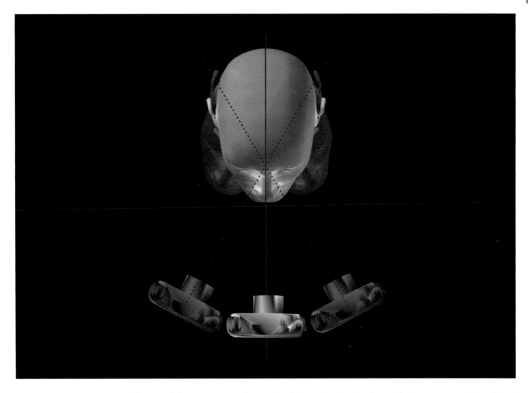

Figure 5.3 Incorrect angulation of the camera or the patient's head in the horizontal plane causes distortion of perspective or unwanted shadows.

the occlusal or incisal planes for orientation as the latter may be misaligned, and instead use the horizon for alignment for recording the true inclination, which is essential for diagnosing cants of the maxilla or altered eruption patterns.

After orientating the patient, the photographer positions himself/herself accordingly with the photographic equipment, depending on the angle of view to be recorded. The assistant stands either to the right or left of the patient, ensuring easy access to an aspirator, three-in-one dental syringe and other dental armamentarium. Alternately, the assistant may stand behind the patient for holding two unilateral cheek retractors for displacing the lips and cheeks. However, the latter ties up the assistants' hands, and therefore may require another assistant for aspiration, etc. Since there are several different types of images with different angles of views, the section below graphically depicts the set-ups required for each type of photograph. In addition, each set-up is accompanied by the necessary photographic equipment settings and technical notes for expediting the photographic session.

The Essential Dental Portfolio

Depending on the discipline in question, different dental organisations and clinicians advocate varying number of images for a dental portfolio (Bengel 2006; Ettorre et al. 2006; Evans et al. 2008; Haddock et al. 2018; Pani 2017; Steel et al. 2009–2013). In addition, extra images are required according to individual patient needs, clinical findings and the proposed treatment. This module concentrates on an essential dental portfolio (EDP) that caters for most dental applications, irrespective of the discipline. Since the intended use of an EDP is clinical photodocumentation, standardisation is mandatory, and the guidelines below are intended to ensure that intra- and inter-patient comparisons are possible. Furthermore, an EDP should form part of the patient's dental records, no different to charting or radiographic documentation. This portfolio serves as a record, even if no treatment is contemplated, and is an invaluable reference if the patient suffers acute trauma, especially involving the anterior teeth, as a guide for restitution of the traumatised dentition. Furthermore, an EDP is vital for forensic identification, should the patient befall a fatal tragedy.

The EDP consists of nine basic dental views (Figure 5.4); three extra-oral (dento-facial) and six intra-oral compositions, as follows:

- EDP Image #1: extra-oral, frontal habitual or 'rest' lip position
- EDP Image #2: extra-oral, frontal relaxed smile
- EDP Image #3: extra-oral, frontal laughter
- EDP Image #4: intra-oral, frontal view in maximum intercuspation (MI)
- EDP Image #5: intra-oral, frontal view with separated teeth
- EDP Image #6: intra-oral, right lateral view in MI
- EDP Image #7: intra-oral, left lateral view in MI
- EDP Image #8: intra-oral, occlusal full-arch maxillary view
- EDP Image #9: intra-oral, occlusal full-arch mandibular view

The full face, or clinical portraiture, is excluded from the EDP since some patients may withhold consent for photographing their face due to personal, social, cultural or religious reasons. However, if this is not a concern, seven full face images of the essential portrait portfolio (EPP) can be added to the EDP, bringing the total number to 16 images, see Module 6: Portraiture.

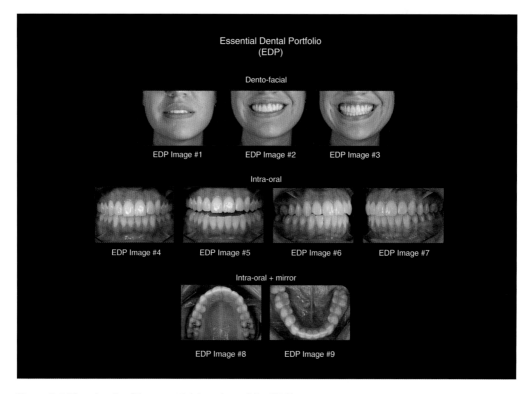

Figure 5.4 Thumbnails of the essential dental portfolio (EDP).

Extra-Oral (Dento-Facial) Compositions

- EDP Image #1: Extra-oral, frontal habitual or 'rest' lip position

An extra-oral or dento-facial composition centres on a commissure-to-commissure view of the lips in static and kinetic states. The static position is often referred to as the 'rest position'. However, this is erroneous, since the oro-facial muscles are contracting to maintain this position and are not truly at rest. The true rest position is whilst sleeping, when all the oro-facial muscles are completely relaxed, and the mandible drops down, causing the mouth to open. A better terminology to describe the so-called 'rest position' is the habitual lip position, e.g. whilst ambling or concentrating on a task. This view is usually the starting point for most dental portfolios, and its set-up is similar to that for subsequent intra-oral views. Dento-facial images, together with portraits, are the most appealing and relevant to patients' aesthetic sense. Furthermore, most laymen assess the outcome of aesthetic dental treatment by these compositions, rather than clinical intra-oral images. The best method for attaining the habitual lip position is asking the patient to iterate the letter 'm' or 'Emma' and then relaxing to achieve an inter-labial gap or habitual lip separation. The composition is framed to include the tip or rhinion of the nose above, and the menton below (Figure 5.5). This allows assessment of the dental midline in relation the facial midline (philtrum), and the axial inclination of the maxillary anterior teeth during a relaxed smile. The mesial axial inclinations of the teeth in maxillary anterior sextant should ideally converge at the menton (Figure 5.6).

The patient is seated upright in the dental chair and asked to turn around 90° towards the camera. The positioning of the photographer and assistant are shown in Figure 5.7 (sagittal

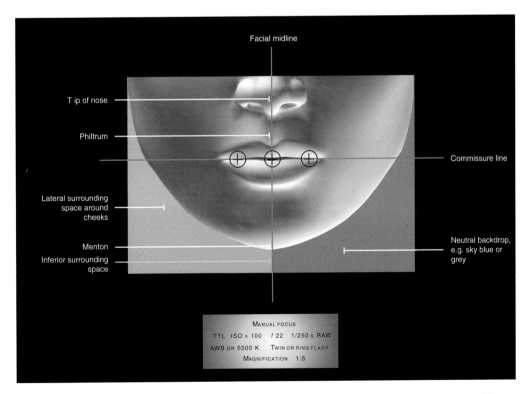

Figure 5.5 Photographic settings and field of view for dento-facial compositions, essential dental portfolio (EDP) images #1, #2 and #3. (PoF [point of focus] = blue cross-line reticle. NB. For a relaxed smile the PoF is the central incisors and for laughter the PoF is the canine tips.)

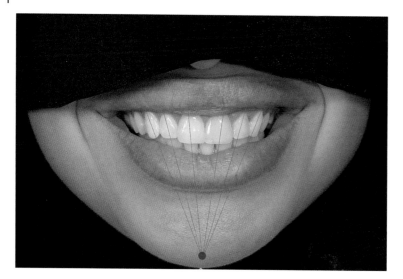

Figure 5.6 Imaginary lines representing the mesial axial inclination of the maxillary anterior teeth converging at the menton.

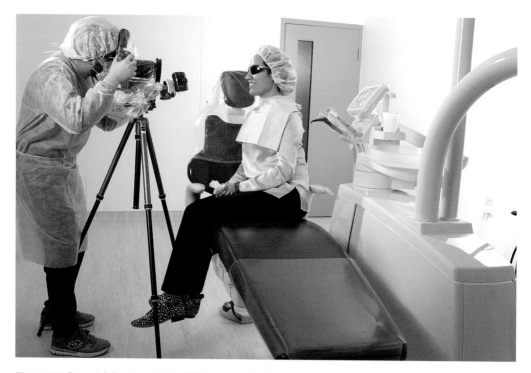

Figure 5.7 Essential dental portfolio (EDP) Images #1, #2 and #3 set-up: The patient is seated upright facing the camera, the camera is tripod-mounted with bilateral flashes. The assistant is out of the frame, but standing to the side ready to assist and ensure patient comfort (sagittal view).

view), Figure 5.8 (bird's-eye view) and Figure 5.9 (photographer's point of view (PoV)). It is advisable to take the extra-oral pictures first before moving onto the intra-oral images to avoid transient creasing or redness of the lips caused by the cheek retractors, which may be apparent in the photographs. Also, the flashes, either twin bilateral, or ring flashes, should have the facility of altering the light intensity output to enable the flash ratio to be adjusted to 1 : 2 (fill flash: key

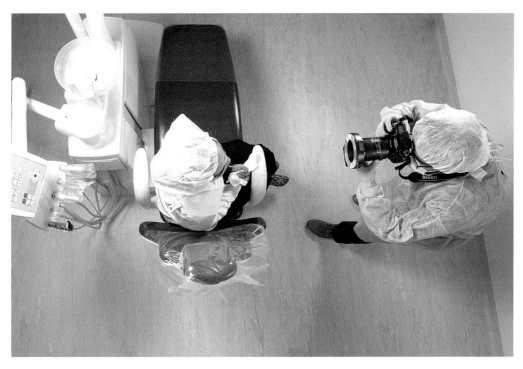

Figure 5.8 Essential dental portfolio (EDP) Images #1, #2 and #3 set-up: The patient is seated upright facing the camera, the camera is hand-held with a ring flash (bird's-eye view).

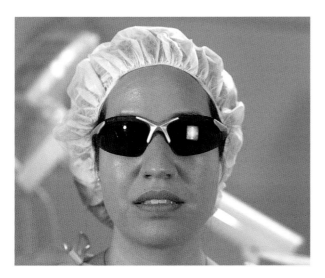

Figure 5.9 Essential dental portfolio (EDP) Images #1, #2 and #3 set-up: Photographer's point of view (PoV).

flash) for producing three-dimensional images with highlights and subtle shadows. The technical settings and guidelines for extra-oral images #1, #2 and #3 are summarised in Table 5.1, and EDP Image #1 is shown in Figure 5.10.

- EDP Images #2 and #3: Extra-oral, frontal relaxed smile and laughter

The next two extra-oral images are a relaxed and exaggerated smile (laughter). The degree of contraction of the lips influences elevation of the commissure line, smile line parallelism, oral

Table 5.1 Settings and guidelines for extra-oral essential dental portfolio (EDP) images #1, #2 and #3.

Item	Setting/description	Notes
Focus	Manual	
Exposure metering	TTL or manual	Manual: take a few test shots to ascertain correct exposure, or use histogram
ISO	50–200	
Aperture	$f22$	
Shutter speed	1/125 s or 1/250 s	Flash synchronisation speed depends on a specific camera brand
Image data format (file format)	RAW or DNG	
White balance	AWB (automatic white balance) 5500 K or manual	Manual: numerical value input, or take a reference image with an 18% neutral density grey card
Flash	Twin bilateral with diffusers angled 45°, or ring flashes	Adjust fill light: key light ratio to 1 : 2. If images are too bright or too dark, adjust intensity of flashes, or move flashes closer or further away until correct exposure is achieved (only applicable for bilateral flashes as ring flashes are usually fixed on the front of the lens)
Magnification factor	1 : 5	Only relevant for full-frame sensors, or set predefined focusing distance on lens, or use anatomical landmarks (see Field of view below)
Point of focus (PoF) represents the ideal hyperfocal distance for maximum DoF (depth of field)	Habitual lip position: central incisors Relaxed smile and laughter: canine tips (The PoF will depend on the shape of the face, if parts of the image are out of focus, change the PoF either anterior or posterior to the suggested areas.)	Hand-held cameras: for predefined magnification or focusing distance, move camera backwards and forwards until focus is obtained, or use anatomical landmarks for composing (see Field of view below) Tripod-mounted camera: for predefined magnification or focusing distance use macro stage for focusing, or use anatomical landmarks for composing (see Field of view below)
Field of view (composing)	Anatomical landmarks	Right/left: lateral aspects of cheeks (with surrounding lateral space) Superior/inferior: tip of nose to menton (if possible, with surrounding inferior space) Anterior/posterior: tip of nose to lateral aspects of cheeks
Background	Variable	Standardised clinical images: Neutral, e.g. sky blue or grey Promotional images: Vivid colours – carte blanche

mucosa visibility (bilateral negative spaces), tooth display and amount of gingival exposure, which is particularly relevant for disciplines such as orthodontics, cranio-maxillo-facial surgery, periodontics and dental aesthetics. However, the smile is highly contentious, since many patients train themselves to smile in a particular way to enhance their personality. This may involve concealing dental anomalies such as excessive gingival display (gummy smile), diastemata, imbrications, discolourations, decay, fractured teeth or poor-quality dentistry

Figure 5.10 Essential dental portfolio (EDP) Image #1.

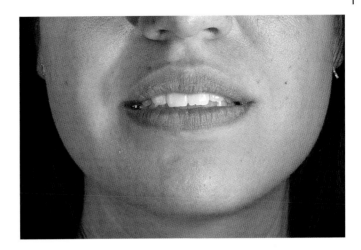

Figure 5.11 Forced, contrived smile with little diagnostic value.

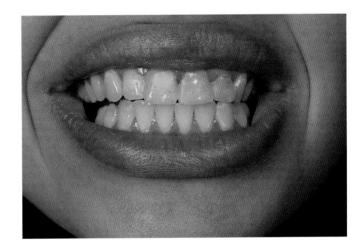

(unsightly fillings, crowns, veneers, etc.). Therefore, capturing a relaxed smile is challenging, and may require several attempts until the patient feels comfortable and builds up a professional confident relationship with the dental team. Nevertheless, it is important to capture smiles that have diagnostic value, including a relaxed smile as well as laughter, so that all relevant factors are visible for assessment and treatment planning (Figures 5.11 and 5.12). These include incisal embrasures whilst the teeth are separated, as well as the incisal plane inclination relative to the curvature of the mandibular lip (essential for elucidating maxillary or incisal plane cants), and dental midline shifts in relation to the facial midline. This is another reason for including that the tip of the nose and chin in the dento-facial composition for assessing the relationship of the facial midline to the dental midlines (maxillary and mandibular). The set-up and settings are identical to photographing the habitual lip position shown in Table 5.1, and EDP Images #2 and #3 are shown in Figures 5.13 and 5.14.

Intra-Oral Compositions

- EDP Image #4: Intra-oral, front view in MI
- EDP Image #5: Intra-oral, front view with separated teeth

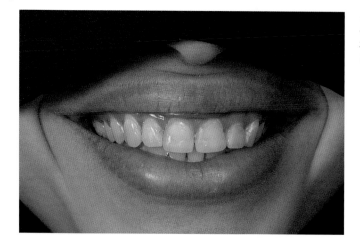

Figure 5.12 Relaxed smile showing contralateral asymmetrical gingival zeniths of the maxillary lateral incisors and canines.

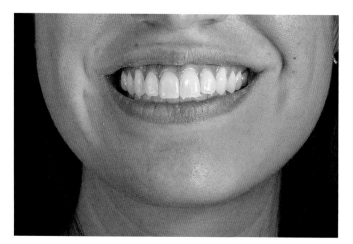

Figure 5.13 Essential dental portfolio (EDP) Image #2.

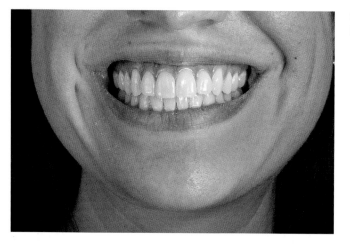

Figure 5.14 Essential dental portfolio (EDP) Image #3.

The first two intra-oral images are frontal views showing the teeth in MI (Kandasamy et al. 2018; Keys and Agar 2002), and separated approximately 5 mm to show the incisal edges, occlusal plane inclination, curves of Spee and Wilson, sphere of Monson and incisal embrasures angles, which are particularly relevant if tooth wear or tooth surface loss (TSL) is suspected due to attrition or other aetiology. Both these views require cheek retractors to displace the lips and cheeks for a clear view of the oral cavity, and the assistant ready with aspiration and a three-in-one dental syringe. The set-up and settings are similar to those for extra-oral images, with a few exceptions such as magnification factor, field of view and background, summarised in Table 5.2 and Figures 5.15 and 5.16. The set-up from various perspectives are shown in Figures 5.17–5.19, and the EDP Images #4 and 5 in Figures 5.20 and 5.21.

Table 5.2 Settings and guidelines for intra-oral essential dental portfolio (EDP) images #4 and #5.

Item	Setting/description	Notes
Focus	Manual	
Exposure metering	TTL or manual	Manual: take a few test shots to ascertain correct exposure or use histogram
ISO	50–200	
Aperture	f 22	
Shutter speed	1/125 s or 1/250 s	Flash synchronisation speed depends on a specific camera brand
Image data format (file format)	RAW or DNG	
White balance	AWB (automatic white balance) 5500 K or manual	Manual: numerical value input, or take a reference image with an 18% neutral density grey card
Flash	Twin bilateral with diffusers angled 45°, or ring flashes	Adjust fill light: key light ratio to 1 : 2. If images are too bright or too dark, adjust intensity of flashes, or move flashes closer or further away until correct exposure is achieved (only applicable for bilateral flashes as ring flashes are usually fixed on the front of the lens)
Magnification factor	1 : 2	Only relevant for full-frame sensors, or set predefined focusing distance on lens, or use anatomical landmarks (see Field of view below)
Point of focus (PoF)	Maxillary canine tips (The PoF will depend on the shape of the arches, if all teeth are not in focus, change the PoF either anterior or posterior to the canines.)	Hand-held cameras: for predefined magnification or focusing distance, move camera backwards and forwards until focus is obtained, or use anatomical landmarks for composing (see Field of view below) Tripod-mounted camera: for predefined magnification or focusing distance use macro stage for focusing, or use anatomical landmarks for composing (see Field of view below)
Field of view (composition)	Anatomical landmarks	Right/left: buccal corridors (negative bilateral spaces) Superior/inferior: apical to maxillary and mandibular mucogingival junctions and showing labial frenum attachments Anterior/posterior: as many teeth as possible from central incisors to second or third molars
Background	n/a	

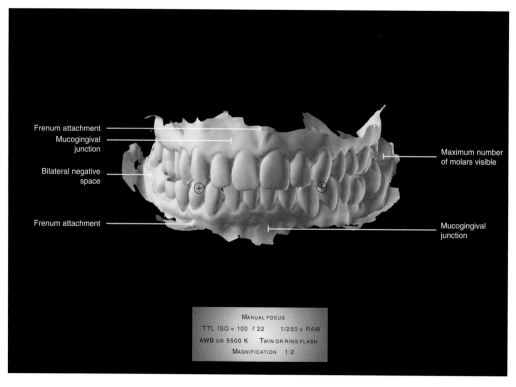

Figure 5.15 Settings and field of view for intra-oral compositions, essential dental portfolio (EDP) images #4 (point of focus [PoF] = blue cross-line reticle).

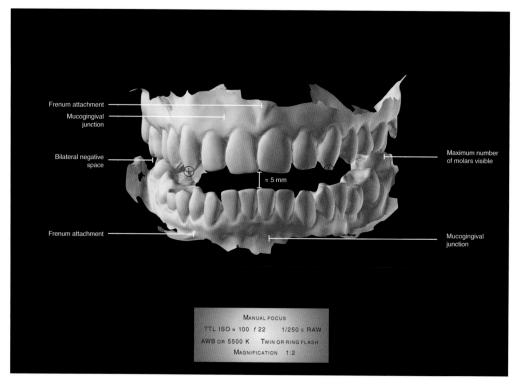

Figure 5.16 Settings and field of view for intra-oral compositions, essential dental portfolio (EDP) images #5 (point of focus [PoF] = blue cross-line reticle).

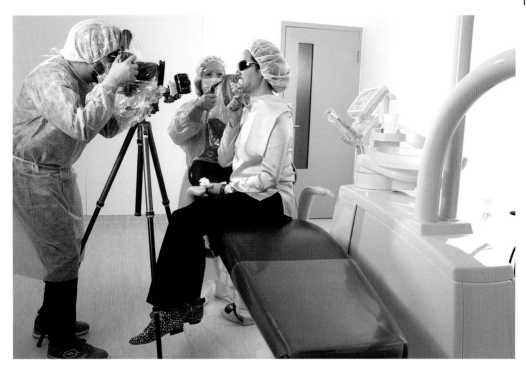

Figure 5.17 Essential dental portfolio (EDP) Images #4 and #5 set-up: The patient is seated upright facing the camera and holding the bilateral plastic cheek retractors, the camera is tripod-mounted with bilateral flashes. The assistant holds the saliva ejector and three-in-one dental syringe (sagittal view).

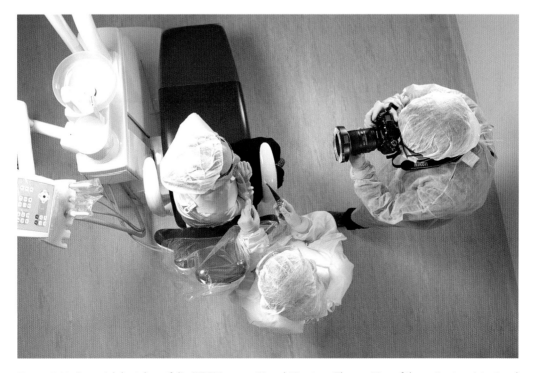

Figure 5.18 Essential dental portfolio (EDP) Images #4 and #5 set-up: The position of the patient, assistant and photographer with hand-held camera and ring flash (bird's-eye view).

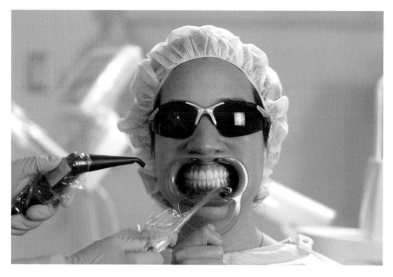

Figure 5.19 Essential dental portfolio (EDP) Images #4 and #5 set-up: Photographer's point of view (PoV).

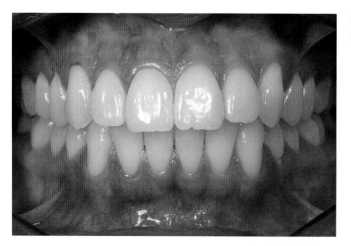

Figure 5.20 Essential dental portfolio (EDP) Image #4.

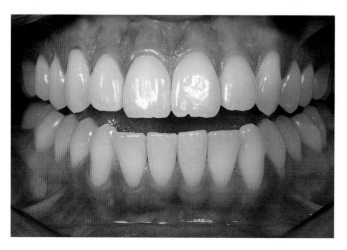

Figure 5.21 Essential dental portfolio (EDP) Image #5.

- EDP Image #6: Intra-oral, right lateral view in MI
- EDP Image #7: Intra-oral, left lateral view in MI

The next two intra-oral images are a repetition of EDP image #4, the only difference is that they are photographed from the right and left sides to show the lateral (or buccal) aspects of the teeth. Hence, the field of view is different, and ideal for showing Angle's molar, canine and incisal relationships, curve of Spee, over-erupted teeth and available interocclusal space for replacing missing teeth. There are two method for capturing lateral views: direct and indirect. The direct method is simply asking the patient to turn their head to the opposite side to the side being photographed, and rotating the cheek retractor on the side being photographed to reveal the buccal aspects of as many posterior teeth as possible. The lens axis is positioned 45° to the dental midline (Figures 5.22 and 5.23). The indirect method is using a narrow or lateral intra-oral mirror to reflect the buccal surfaces of the teeth. This involves placing a unilateral buccal cheek retractor on the contralateral side to be photographed, and then sliding a mirror into the buccal corridor on the side to be photographed to displace the cheek for capturing the reflection of the lateral surfaces of the teeth. The lens axis is positioned and aimed at the centre of the intra-oral mirror (Figures 5.24–5.26). Table 5.3 and Figure 5.27 detail the salient differences to previous EDP images, and EDP Images #6 and #7 are shown in Figures 5.28 and 5.29. Also, the reflected images need to be laterally inverted (flipped) in imaging software for ensuring the correct perspective.

- EDP Image #8: Intra-oral, occlusal full-arch maxillary view
- EDP Image #9: Intra-oral, occlusal full-arch mandibular view

The last two EDP images are full-arch occlusal views of the maxillary and mandibular arches, These are the most challenging pictures for the clinician, and the most claustrophobic and

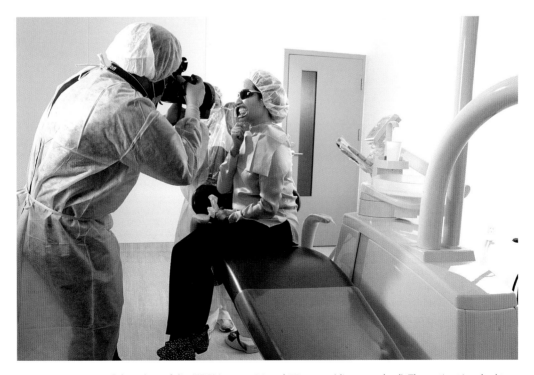

Figure 5.22 Essential dental portfolio (EDP) Images #6 and #7 set-up (direct method): The patient is asked to rotate the cheek retractors laterally to the side being photographed. The photographer moves 45° to the side, whilst the assistant holds the saliva ejector and 3-in1 dental syringe (sagittal view).

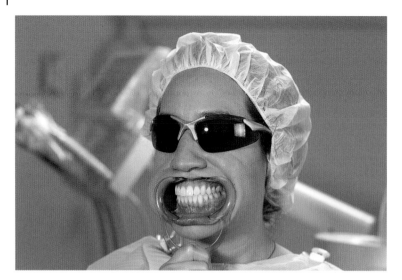

Figure 5.23 Essential dental portfolio (EDP) Images #6 and #7 set-up (direct method): Photographer's point of view (PoV).

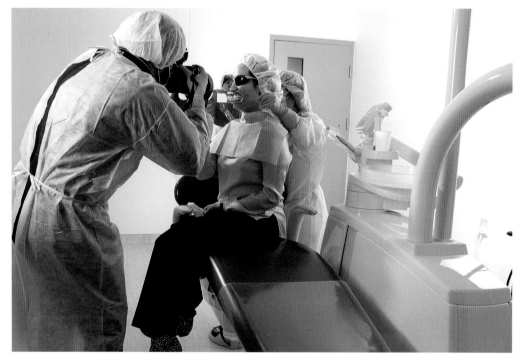

Figure 5.24 Essential dental portfolio (EDP) Images #6 and #7 set-up (indirect method): A narrow intra-oral lateral mirror is placed on the side to be photographed and held by the patient. The assistant holds a unilateral cheek retractor on the opposite side, and prevents condensation on the mirror by blowing air from a three-in-one dental syringe. The photographer moves 45° to the side, aiming the lens axis to the centre of the lateral mirror (sagittal view).

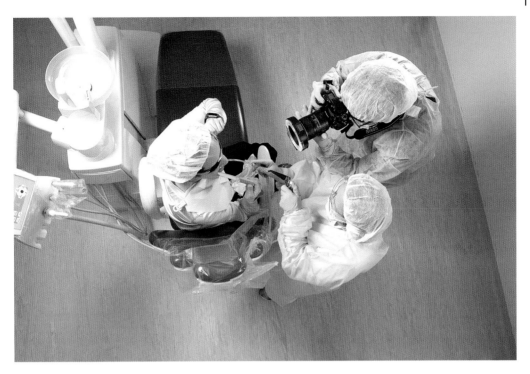

Figure 5.25 Essential dental portfolio (EDP) Images #6 and #7 set-up (indirect method): Alternately, the patient can hold both the mirror and cheek retractor, whilst the assistant holds a saliva ejector and three-in-one dental syringe (bird's-eye view).

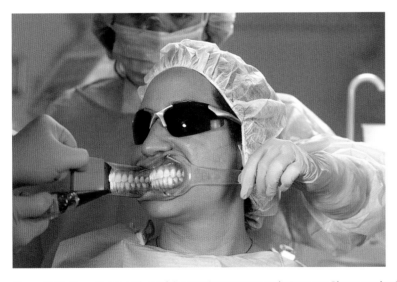

Figure 5.26 Essential dental portfolio (EDP) Images #6 and #7 set-up: Photographer's point of view (PoV).

cumbersome for the patient. For both arches, the mirror is positioned so that the incisal edges or cusp tips are clearly visible. Also, the sulci are sufficiently deflected so that the lips are off the buccal surfaces of the teeth, with a clear view of the buccal gingiva. Furthermore, whenever possible, the cheek retractors and intra-oral mirrors should not be visible in the picture.

Table 5.3 Salient differences for lateral view essential dental portfolio (EDP) Images #6 and #7.

Item	Setting/description	Notes
Aperture	ƒ 22 (direct method) ƒ 16 (indirect method)	Reduce aperture by 1 ƒ-stop to compensate for using intra-oral mirror with the indirect method
Point of focus (PoF)	Maxillary first premolar cusp tip (The PoF will depend on the shape of the arches, if all teeth are not in focus, change the PoF either anterior or posterior to the first premolars)	Hand-held cameras: for predefined magnification or focusing distance, move camera backwards and forwards until focus is obtained, or use anatomical landmarks for composing (see Field of view below) Tripod-mounted camera: for predefined magnification or focusing distance use macro stage for focusing, or use anatomical landmarks for composing (see Field of view below)
Field of view (composition)	Anatomical landmarks	Right/left: Extending from second or third molars to the canine on the opposite side Superior/inferior: apical to maxillary and mandibular mucogingival junctions and showing labial frena attachments Anterior/posterior: Contralateral buccal mucosa background to buccal surfaces of the molars on the side being photographed

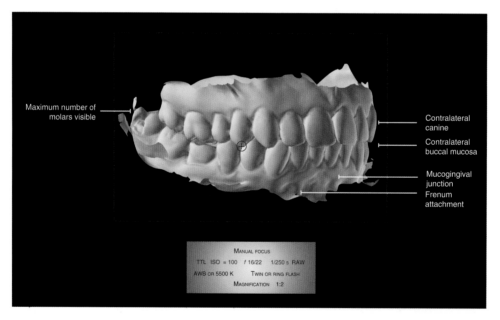

Figure 5.27 Settings and field of view for intra-oral compositions, essential dental portfolio (EDP) image #6 (point of focus [PoF] = blue cross-line reticle).

For maxillary occlusal views, the nostrils should be obscured by using a contraster (see Figure 2.5 in Module 2). Also, the reflected EDP Images #8 and #9 need to be laterally inverted (flipped) and rotated in imaging software for ensuring the correct perspective.

For the maxillary arch, EDP Image #8, the patient is asked to open as wide as possible and point their chin downwards. The reverse surface of the mirror touches the mandibular anterior teeth and the lens axis positioned 45° to the centre of the mirror in order to capture an image that

Figure 5.28 Essential dental portfolio (EDP) Image #6.

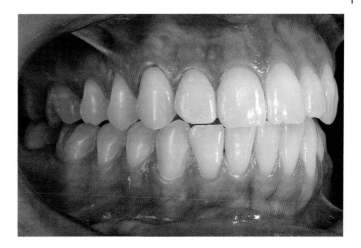

Figure 5.29 Essential dental portfolio (EDP) Image #7.

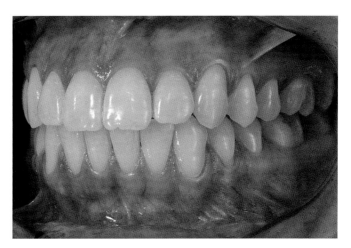

appears to be taken perpendicular to the occlusal plane of the maxillary arch. If mouth opening is limited, the resulting shallow or reduced intra-oral mirror angle will alter perspective and prevent visualisation of buccal and lingual surfaces of the teeth. (Figures 5.30–5.32). Table 5.4 details the salient differences between EDP Images #8 and #9 and other EDP images, The settings and field of view for EDP Image are shown in Figure 5.33, EDP Image #8 is shown in Figure 5.34.

For the mandibular arch, EDP Image #9, the patient is asked to point the chin upward, allowing the reverse surface of the mirror to touch the maxillary anterior teeth, with the lens axis 45° to the centre of the mirror. The tongue is gently elevated and pushed back with the mirror to exclude it as much as possible from the frame so that the lingual surfaces of the teeth are visible (Figures 5.35 and 5.36). The settings and field of view for EDP #9 are shown in Figure 5.37, and EDP Image #9 is shown in Figure 5.38.

Optional Compositions

Depending on the speciality, in addition to the EDP, several optional extra- and intra-oral images may be required. These can either be deferred to a later date, or preferably taken at the same session to make use of the photographic set-up of the EDP. The optional dento-facial images are similar to the first three EDP images, but the lips and teeth are viewed from

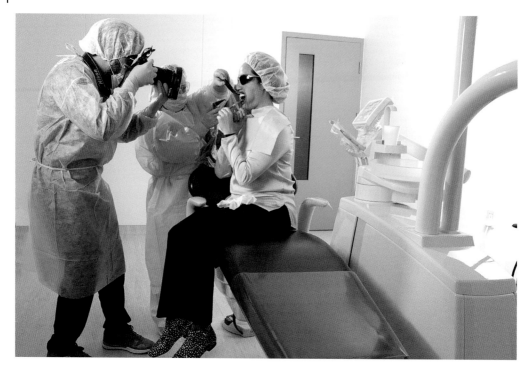

Figure 5.30 Essential dental portfolio (EDP) Images #8 set-up: The patient's head is titled downward. The patient holds the intra-oral occlusal mirror, whilst the assistant holds the contraster and three-in-one dental syringe to blow air onto the mirror. The photographer aims the lens axis 45° to the mirror (sagittal view).

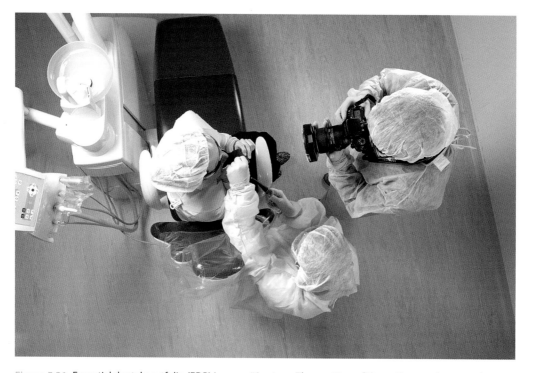

Figure 5.31 Essential dental portfolio (EDP) Images #8 set-up: The position of the patient, assistant and photographer with hand-held camera and ring flash (bird's-eye view).

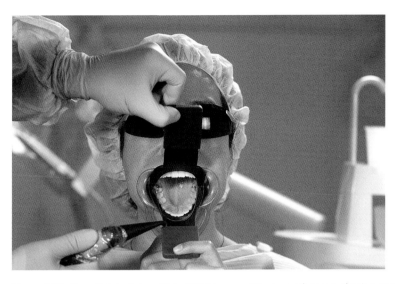

Figure 5.32 Essential dental portfolio (EDP) Images #8 set-up: Photographer's point of view (PoV).

Table 5.4 Salient differences for occlusal view essential dental portfolio (EDP) Images #8 and #9.

Item	Setting/description	Notes
Aperture	f 16	Reduce aperture by 1 f-stop to compensate for using intra-oral mirror
Magnification factor	1 : 2 or 1 : 3 (depending on size of the arches)	Only relevant for full-frame sensors, or set predefined focusing distance on lens, or use anatomical landmarks (see field of view below)
Point of focus (PoF)	Maxillary and mandibular occlusal surfaces of second premolars (The PoF will depend on the shape of the arches, if all teeth are not in focus, change the PoF either anterior or posterior to the second premolars.)	Hand-held cameras: for predefined magnification or focusing distance, move camera backwards and forwards until focus is obtained, or use anatomical landmarks for composing (see Field of view below) Tripod-mounted camera: for predefined magnification or focusing distance use macro stage for focusing, or use anatomical landmarks for composing (see Field of view below)
Field of view (composition)	Anatomical landmarks	Right/left: buccal sulci Superior/inferior: bordered by labial sulcus to soft palate or deflected inferior surface of tongue Anterior/posterior: incisal edges or cusp tips to buccal attached gingiva

different angles. These compositions are useful for assessing lip competence, maxillary incisal edge position and inclination in relation to the mandibular lip, aesthetic analysis such as smile line, excessive gingival display (gummy smile), curves of Spee and Wilson, sphere of Monson and over-erupted teeth. The optional extra-oral images are as follows:

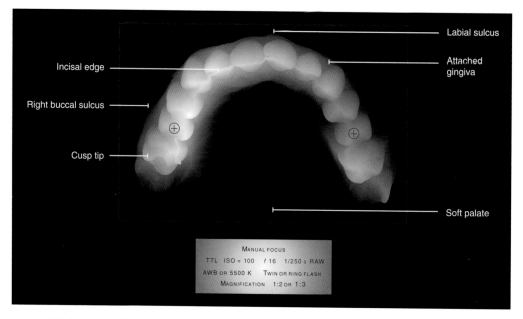

Figure 5.33 Settings and field of view for essential dental portfolio (EDP) image #8 (point of focus [PoF] = blue cross-line reticle).

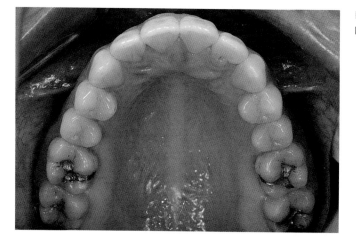

Figure 5.34 Essential dental portfolio (EDP) image #8.

1) Extra-oral: right profile view – habitual or 'rest' lip position
2) Extra-oral: right profile view – relaxed smile
3) Extra-oral: right profile view – laughter
4) Extra-oral: left profile view – habitual or 'rest' lip position
5) Extra-oral: left profile view – relaxed smile
6) Extra-oral: left profile view – laughter
7) Extra-oral: right oblique view – habitual or 'rest' lip position
8) Extra-oral: right oblique view – relaxed smile
9) Extra-oral: right oblique view – laughter
10) Extra-oral: left oblique view – habitual or 'rest' lip position
11) Extra-oral: left oblique view – relaxed smile
12) Extra-oral: left oblique view – laughter

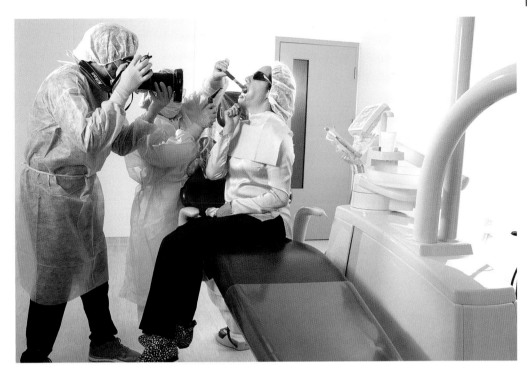

Figure 5.35 Essential dental portfolio (EDP) Images #9 set-up: The patient's head is tilted upwards. The assistant holds the intra-oral occlusal mirror and three-in-one dental syringe to blow air onto the mirror. The photographer aims the lens axis 45° to the mirror (sagittal view).

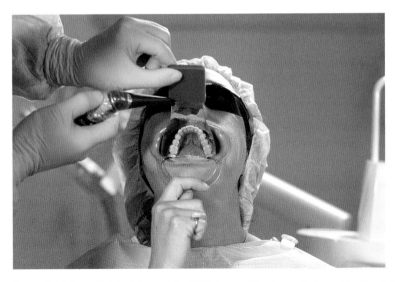

Figure 5.36 Essential dental portfolio (EDP) Images #9 set-up: Photographer's point of view (PoV).

The set-up and setting are identical to those shown in Table 5.1, but the patient is asked to turn their head right or left for the profile or oblique views (Figure 5.39). The oblique images are also termed the 3/4 or 45° view. For each view, both static and kinetic states are photographed. The oblique view is particularly useful for assessing phonetics, since people usually speak from an angle rather than head-on. Examples of a few of these compositions are shown in Figures 5.40–5.45.

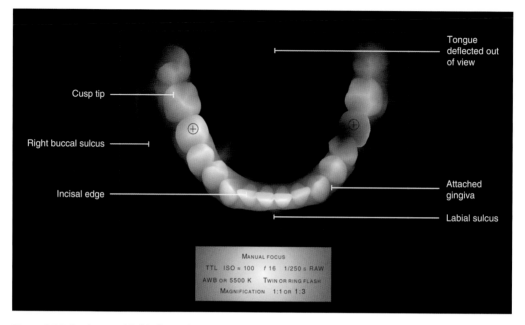

Figure 5.37 Settings and field of view for essential dental portfolio (EDP) image #9 (point of focus [PoF] = blue cross-line reticle).

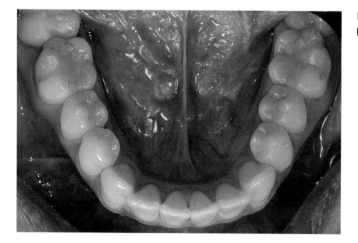

Figure 5.38 Essential dental portfolio (EDP) image #9.

The next optional images are intra-oral compositions, including lateral views with the teeth separated and detailed anterior sextant and quadrant views for visualising various tooth surfaces. These perspectives allow assessment of marginal integrity of restorations, gingival recession and calculus deposits. The first two optional intra-oral images are lateral views, which are identical to EDP images #6 and #7, but with the teeth separated:

13) Intra-oral, right lateral view with separated teeth
14) Intra-oral, left lateral view with separated teeth

The set-up and setting for optional intra-oral images #13 and #14 are the same as those shown in Table 5.3, and can either be taken with the direct method or indirect method using a lateral (buccal) mirror.

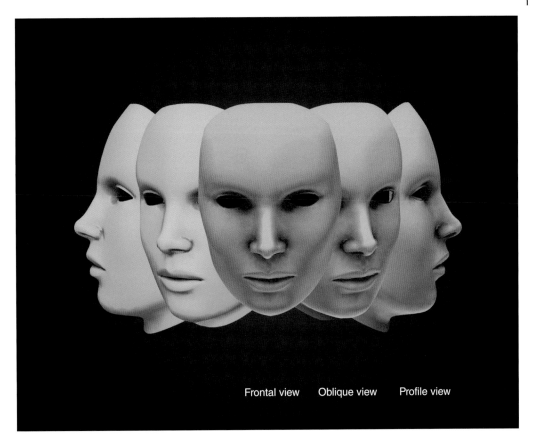

Frontal view   Oblique view   Profile view

Figure 5.39 Positioning the patient's head for oblique and profile views.

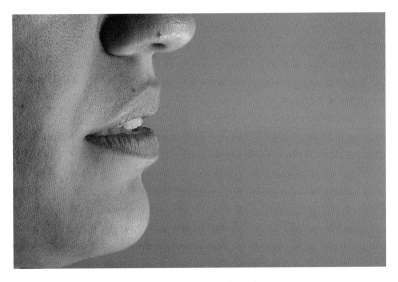

Figure 5.40 Optional image #1 (right profile habitual).

The sextant and quadrant views can be obtained by enlarging EDP images #5, #8 and #9, respectively. However, this depends on the quality of the initial images, which is predominantly influenced by the photographic hardware. If the initial images can withstand enlargement and cropping of a segment without losing resolution, additional sextant and quadrant images are

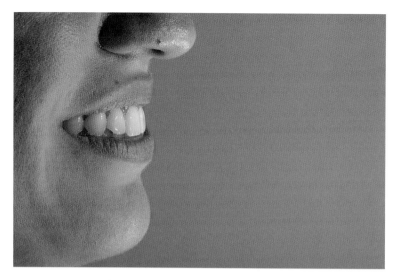

Figure 5.41 Optional image #2 (right profile relaxed smile).

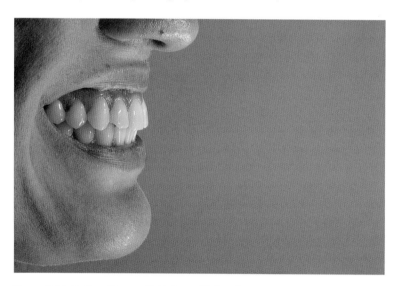

Figure 5.42 Optional image #3 (right profile laughter).

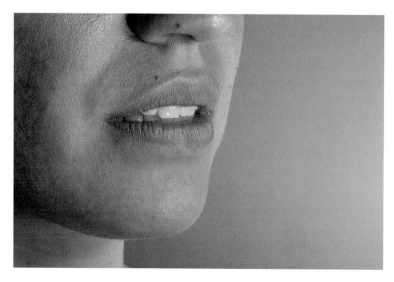

Figure 5.43 Optional image #7 (right oblique habitual).

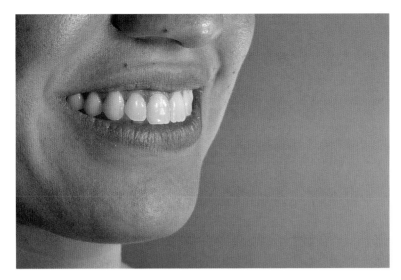

Figure 5.44 Optional image #8 (right oblique relaxed smile).

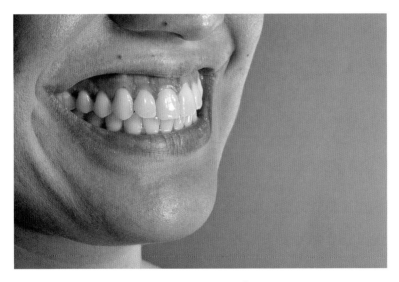

Figure 5.45 Optional image #9 (right oblique laughter).

superfluous (unless buccal and/or lingual surfaces of the teeth are required). However, if the resolution of the lens is insufficient and/or the camera sensor is small with a reduced pixel count, enlargement may substantially deteriorate the image quality, making them useless for diagnosis. Therefore, capturing only a sextant or quadrant exploits the maximum potential of the photographic hardware, irrespective of its specifications.

The optional anterior maxillary and mandibular sextant images concentrate on the buccal and palatal (lingual) surfaces of the anterior teeth:

15) Intra-oral: anterior sextant – maxillary buccal aspect with separated teeth
16) Intra-oral: anterior sextant – mandibular buccal aspect with separated teeth
17) Intra-oral: anterior sextant – maxillary palatal aspect of teeth
18) Intra-oral: anterior sextant – mandibular lingual aspect of teeth

These views are invaluable for visualising various lesions including palatal surface erosion of the maxillary teeth due to gastric regurgitation, calculus deposits on the lingual surfaces of mandibular teeth (Figure 5.46), gingival recession, palatal fistula and abscesses, tori, as well as defective restorations that otherwise may be overlooked (Figure 5.47). The increased magnification is also ideal for documenting treatment sequences in a particular region of the mouth, or on a specific tooth. The first two images (buccal surfaces) have the same set-up as EDP image #5 (Table 5.2), but the magnification factor is increased to 1 : 1 to concentrate on the anterior sextant of both arches. The next two images (lingual/palatal surfaces) utilise intra-oral mirrors, similar to EDP images #8 and #9, but the angle of the mirror is manipulated to reveal the palatal or lingual surfaces with a magnification factor of 1 : 1. Whilst EDP images #8 and #9 capture the entire arch and are centred on the incisal edges or cusp tips, the optional images 17 and 18 are restricted to only the anterior six teeth and capture detailed views of the palatal/lingual aspects.

The last of the intra-oral optional images are three perspectives of the right and left quadrants of each arch, making a total of 12 images. Each of the four quadrants are photographed from three perspectives: occlusal, buccal and palatal/lingual. The entire set of 12 images are not necessary for every patient, and may be limited to certain quadrants depending an individual needs. Similar to the anterior sextant views, the quadrant views concentrate on capturing

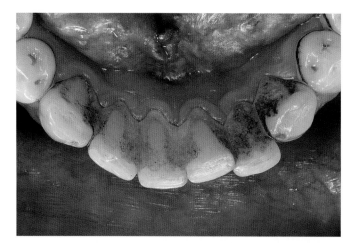

Figure 5.46 Mandibular lingual sextant view showing calculus deposits.

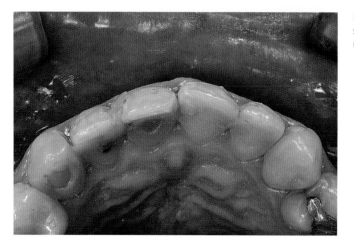

Figure 5.47 Maxillary palatal sextant view showing defective restorations.

detailed views of different perspectives for assessing healthy and diseased hard and soft tissues, and for documenting treatment sequences isolated to a specific region of the mouth.

19) Intra-oral: quadrants – maxillary right occlusal/incisal aspect of teeth
20) Intra-oral: quadrants – maxillary right buccal aspect of teeth
21) Intra-oral: quadrants – maxillary right palatal aspect of teeth
22) Intra-oral: quadrants – maxillary left occlusal/incisal aspect of teeth
23) Intra-oral: quadrants – maxillary left buccal aspect of teeth
24) Intra-oral: quadrants – maxillary left palatal aspect of teeth
25) Intra-oral: quadrants – mandibular right occlusal/incisal aspect of teeth
26) Intra-oral: quadrants – mandibular right buccal aspect of teeth
27) Intra-oral: quadrants – mandibular right lingual aspect of teeth
28) Intra-oral: quadrants – mandibular left occlusal/incisal aspect of teeth
29) Intra-oral: quadrants – mandibular left buccal aspect of teeth
30) Intra-oral: quadrants – mandibular left lingual aspect of teeth

The quadrant shots are best accomplished with the patient in the supine position. The photographer is positioned either on the same or contralateral side to be photographed depending on which side of the mouth is being photographed. The assistant holds the lateral (buccal) mirror angling it until the desired surface is in view. Since illuminating the posterior regions of the mouth is challenging, a ring flash is the ideal light source, ensuring uniform illumination (Figures 5.48 and 5.49) Also, the magnification factor varies from 1 : 1 to 1 : 2 depending on the number of teeth in the frame and the configuration of the arches.

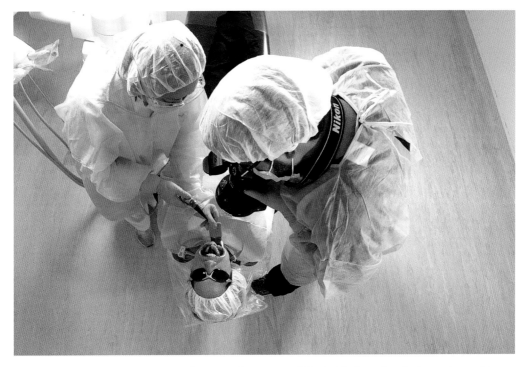

Figure 5.48 Maxillary quadrant view: This view is best accomplished with the patient in the supine position, the photographer on one side and assistant on the opposite side, holding a lateral intra-oral mirror and a three-in-one dental syringe (bird's-eye view).

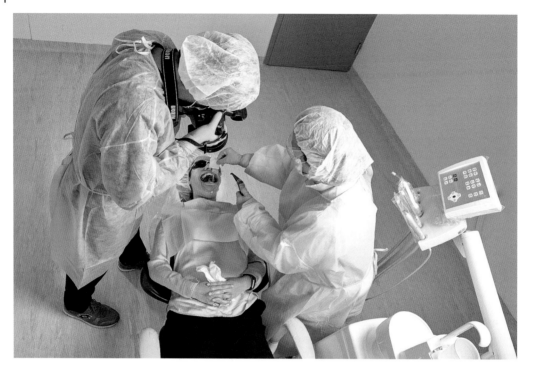

Figure 5.49 Mandibular quadrant view: This view is best accomplished with the patient in the supine position, the photographer at the front and assistant on the opposite side, holding a lateral intra-oral mirror and a three-in-one dental syringe (bird's-eye view).

An entire quadrant, a group of teeth, or a single tooth can be framed or subsequently cropped in imaging software. As stated above, the quality of the cropped images depends on the specifications of the photographic hardware. The difference in settings between for EDP images #8 and #9 (full-arch) and quadrant images are summarised in Table 5.5 and Figure 5.50, whilst Figure 5.51 shows examples of some quadrant images.

Although not exhaustive, the EDP and optional compositions outlined in this Module serve as a comprehensive and invaluable photographic record for photodocumentation, publishing, marketing and teaching (Figures 5.52–5.61). The following modules discuss portraits, bench images and special applications, which expands dental photographic documentation for further needs and uses.

As a closing comment, it is worth remembering that to obtain textbook standard images requires an ideal patient, ideal nurse, ideal photographer, ideal equipment, ideal temperament and ideal environment. However, in reality, these utopian conditions are elusive. Therefore, a compromise is inevitable. This may include accepting less than ideal fields of view, visible edges of cheek retractor or mirrors, poor angulations, copious saliva or fogging of mirrors, to name a few fallibilities. Whilst poor photographic technique is unforgivable, even an intrepid operator may be confronted with unsurmountable hurdles such as uncooperative patients, limited mouth opening, technical issues with equipment and so on. Although certain mistakes such as poor exposure or visible extraneous objects can be corrected at the editing stage, other errors including poor framing, eschewed perspectives, gross blemishes due to saliva or blood droplets, or excessive condensation on intra-oral mirrors are impossible to rectify. Hence, a degree of pragmatism is necessary, and although the aim is to produce flawless images, sometimes seeking this Xanadu may prove enigmatic.

Table 5.5 Salient settings for optional quadrant images #19–30.

Item	Setting/description	Notes
Aperture	f16	Reduce aperture by 1 f-stop to compensate for using intra-oral mirror
Flash	Ring flash	Set flash to maximum intensity burst, alter intensity, if necessary, to obtain correct exposure
Magnification factor	1 : 1 to 1 : 2 (depending on width and length of the arches and number of teeth being photographed)	Only relevant for full-frame sensors, or set predefined focusing distance on lens, or use anatomical landmarks (see field of view below)
Point of focus (PoF)	Variable: start with the maxillary and mandibular second premolars, and alter as necessary (The PoF will depend on the shape of the arches, if all teeth are not in focus, change the PoF either anterior or posterior to the second premolars, or focus on the specific tooth of interest.)	Hand-held cameras: for predefined magnification or focusing distance, move camera backwards and forwards until focus is obtained, or use anatomical landmarks for composing (see Field of view below) Tripod-mounted camera: for predefined magnification or focusing distance use macro stage for focusing, or use anatomical landmarks for composing (see Field of view below)
Field of view (composition)	Anatomical landmarks	Right/left: buccal sulci and palatal or lingual mucosa Superior/inferior: depending on perspective, i.e. occlusal, buccal or palatal/lingual surfaces bounded by attached gingiva and mucosa Anterior/posterior: Depending on the number of teeth being photographed. For an entire quadrant, the central incisor to the second or third molars

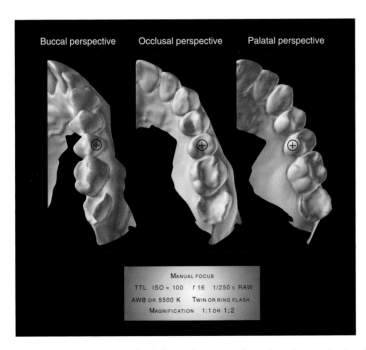

Figure 5.50 Settings and field of view for optional quadrant images (point of focus [PoF] = blue cross-line reticle). Each quadrant is photographed from three perspectives: buccal, occlusal and palatal/lingual.

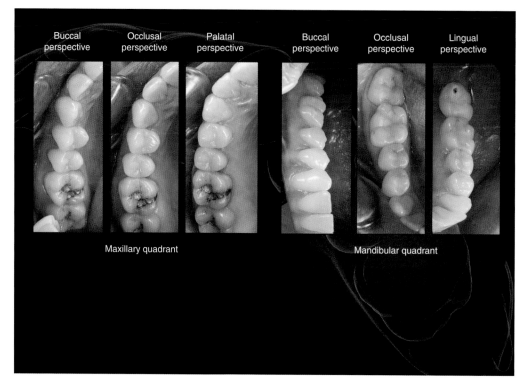

Maxillary quadrant   Mandibular quadrant

Figure 5.51 Examples of some maxillary and mandibular quadrant images.

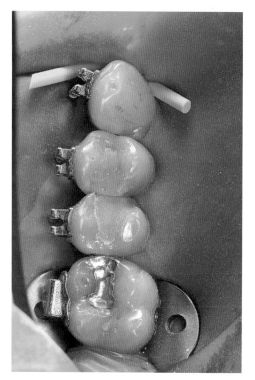

Figure 5.52 Quadrant images are ideal for showing a technique by concentrating on a few teeth.
The defective composite fillings in the maxillary right premolars require replacement.

Figure 5.53 After removing the fillings, gross decay is evident.

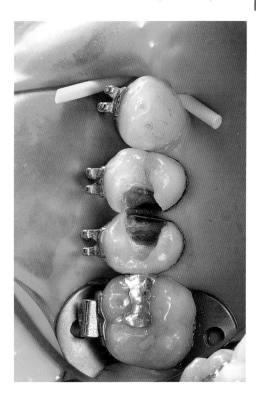

Figure 5.54 The decay is judicially removed, avoiding pulpal exposure.

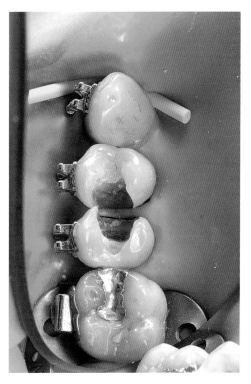

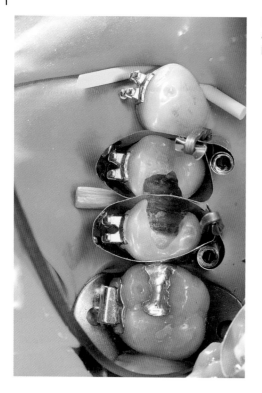

Figure 5.55 Steel matrices with an interdental wedge are placed to create transient separation of the premolars for building tight contact areas.

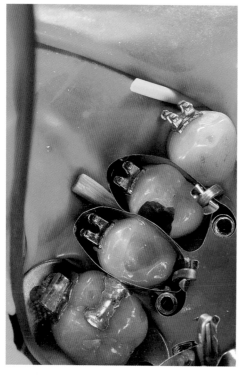

Figure 5.56 The mesial interproximal wall of the second premolar is built-up with resin-based composite (RBC) after the requisite etching and bonding stages. The initial RBC increments convert the prevailing Class II cavity to a Class I cavity.

Figure 5.57 Further increments are added to restore occlusal morphology of the second premolar.

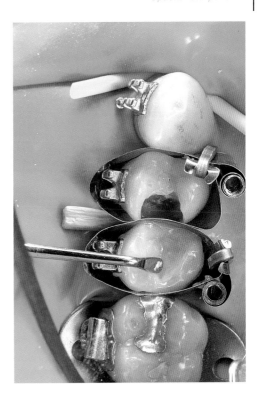

Figure 5.58 The process is repeated for the first premolar, starting with application of a dentine bonding agent…

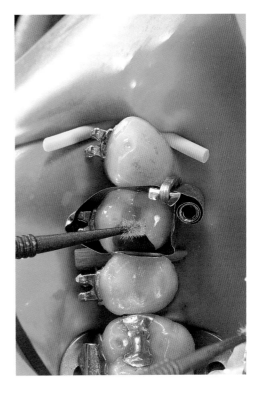

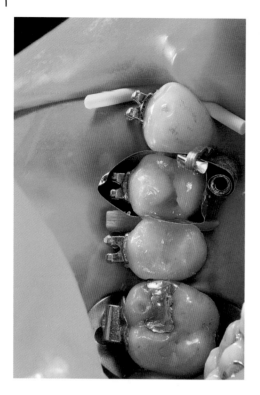

Figure 5.59 …followed by resin-based composite (RBC) incremental layering.

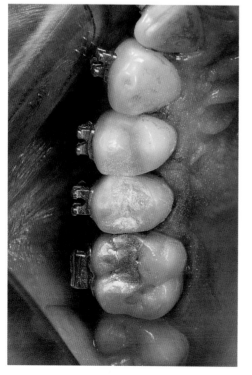

Figure 5.60 The penultimate stage is removing the rubber dam, checking occlusion and refining morphology.

Figure 5.61 A week later, the final stage involves checking the shade, refining occlusion and morphology before finishing and polishing the fillings.

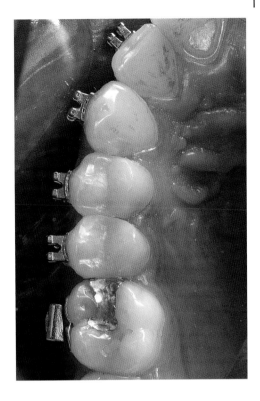

References

Ahmad, I. (2009). Digital dental photography. Part 8: intra-oral set-ups. *Br. Dent. J.* 207 (4): 151–157.

Bengel, W. (2006). *Mastering Digital Dental Photography*. London: Quintessence.

Devigus, A. (2012). A picture is worth. *J. Cosmet. Dent.* 28 (1): 82–88.

Ettorre, G., Weber, M., Schaaf, H. et al. (2006). Standards for digital photography in cranio-maxillo-facial surgery – part I: basic views and guidelines. *J. Craniomaxillofac. Surg.* 34: 65–73.

Evans, S., England, P., Jones, M. et al. (2008). Orthodontic Photography IMI National Guidelines, 1–27.

Haddock, F.J., Hammond, B.D., and Romero, M.F. (2018). Guide to dental photography. *Decisions in Dentistry* 4 (12): 1–4.

Kandasamy, S., Greene, C.S., and Obrez, A. (2018). An evidence-based evaluation of the concept of centric relation in the 21st century. *Quintessence Int.* 49: 755–760.

Keys, L.G. and Agar, J.A. (2002). Documentation of maxillomandibular relationships during dental photography. *J. Prosthet. Dent.* 87 (4): 466.

Pani, S. (2017). A review on clinical digital photography. *Int. J. Appl. Res.* 3: 10–17.

Patient photographic records (2012). Patient photographic records. http://aligntechinstitute.com/GetHelp/Documents/pdf/PhotographicQSG.pdf (accessed 25 September 2012).

Steel, C., Behle, C., Bellerino, M. et al. (2009–2013). *Photographic Documentation and Evaluation in Cosmetic Dentistry: A Guide to Accreditation Photography*. Madison, WI: American Academy of Cosmetic Dentistry.

6

Portraiture

The salient question regarding portraiture is, 'Should it depict harsh reality, or enhance attractiveness?'

The answer is both.

There are two types of portraits, clinical and non-clinical. The former yields unadulterated information that is essential for analysis and diagnosis, whilst the latter is seductive and alluring, tainted by the subject's wishes and the photographer's vision. Since clinical portraiture is harsh reality, standardisation is essential for comparison, interdisciplinary communication, as well as gauging treatment progress and monitoring treatment outcomes. Alternately, non-clinical portraiture enhances attractiveness and is primarily narcissistic. Both types of images serve different purposes, clinical portraits deliver reality, whilst non-clinical portraits steers into glamour, fantasy, artistic and surreal territory. Therefore, for clinical portraiture, adhering to strict guidelines is mandatory, while for the non-clinical variety, the rule book is discarded. The photographer has carte blanche, and depending on his or her artistic slant, is free to experiment and 'paint' a unique picture of the patient's persona (Ahmad 2009a; Jung 1933) – Figure 6.1.

Lighting for Portraiture

The crucial factor for portraits, irrespective of whether they are clinical or non-clinical, is understanding and manipulating light. Throughout this book, the subject of lighting is mentioned as the quintessential element for photography, and nowhere is this more relevant than with portrait photography, which can literally depict a person in a 'different light'. Therefore, the discussing below focuses on fundamental principles of lighting a subject, and shows how this crucial entity can be tailored for conveying different messages (Ahmad 2009b).

The three basic lights to consider for portraiture are:

- Key light
- Fill light
- Background light (if necessary)

All the above may be utilised simultaneously, individually, or in any combination for creating innumerable types of images with a particular ambience, or emphasising specific facial features. The protagonist light is termed the main or key light, which is the primary source of illumination. This can be natural sunlight, or artificially generated continuous or flash lights placed anywhere in the composition depending on the intended type of portrait. A 'fill light' is perhaps a misnomer since these secondary 'light(s)' are not always another light source, but can be reflectors bouncing light from the key light back onto the subject. They are mainly used as counter

Essentials of Dental Photography, First Edition. Irfan Ahmad.
© 2020 John Wiley & Sons Ltd. Published 2020 by John Wiley & Sons Ltd.

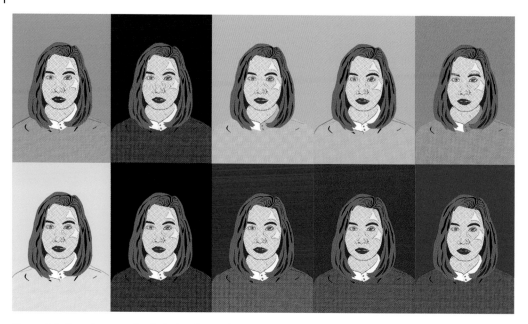

Figure 6.1 Portraiture can be clinical and non-clinical. The non-clinical variety offers the photographer and patient to express themselves without limits.

illumination to literally 'fill in' shadows cast by the key light. Finally, a third light, if necessary, is used to illuminate the background. The background light not only illuminates the backdrop or scenery, but visually separates the subject from the background for conveying a three-dimensional quality to the photograph (Figure 6.2).

Manipulating Light

The method by which a light source illuminates an object or subject is by distribution, which is influenced by its colour temperature, direction, intensity and apparent size (Portraiture light 2005–2017). The colour temperature sets the mood, the direction determines the location of highlights and shadows, whilst the intensity and physical size determines the intensity of the highlights and shadows.

Colour Temperature

The colour temperature is more relevant when shooting in daylight, for example at sunrise, mid-day, overcast skies or at sunset, as the colour temperature of the light varies depending on the time of day. However, when shooting indoors with studio flashes, the colour temperature is less important. This is because most electronic flashes (or strobes) are configured to emit photographic daylight around 5500 K, and when using a fast synchronising shutter speed, the ambient light plays little or no part in illuminating the subject. However, for creative imagery, the colour temperature can be altered either by placing coloured gels over the flashes, or using fill-in reflectors of different colours. Reflectors are available in a various reflective coloured surfaces, for example gold, which reduces the colour temperature and conveys a warm skin tone. Alternately, a silver reflector increases the colour temperature and 'cools' the quality of light Figure 6.3. Besides altering the colour temperature, the surface finish (or texture) of the reflector also affects the

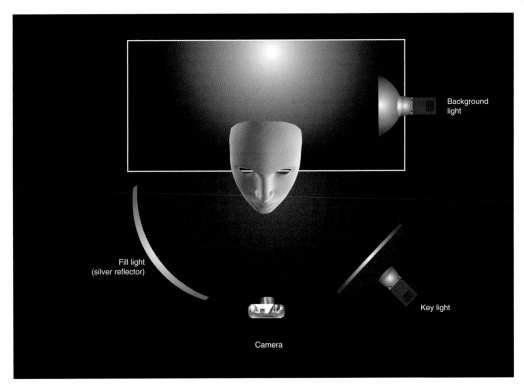

Figure 6.2 A typical portrait lighting set-up consisting of a key light, fill light and background light.

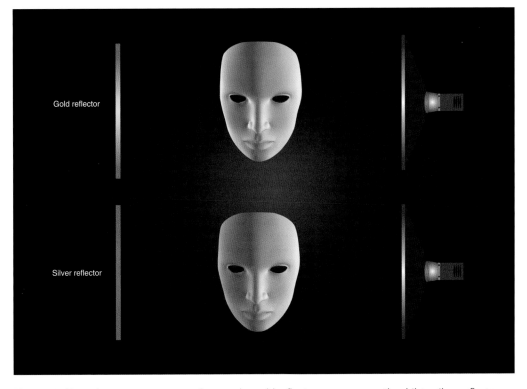

Figure 6.3 The colour temperature sets the mood, a gold reflector conveys warmth, whilst a silver reflector conveys a cool ambience.

mood of the scene. A highly polished surface not only increases colour temperature but also encourage specular reflections that result in vibrant high contrast images (Bazos and Magne 2013). Alternately, using a matt white reflector also increase colour temperature, but yields subtle lighting that depicts a serene ambience.

Direction: Key Light

The location of the illumination, or its relative position to the subject's face allows sculpting of facial features, either emphasising, or camouflaging anatomical structures. Furthermore, directional lighting creates shadows that conveys depth, both in a physical and metaphorical sense. Although the position where a light is placed is endless, there are several 'tried and tested' positions for portraiture.[1]

These positions are useful for understanding basic lighting principles, and once the fundamentals are grasped, the photographer can be adventurous and expand his/her creativity for achieving more artistic or personalised effects.

The simplest way to learn about manipulating light is starting with a single light source, which is the key light, or main source of illumination. Once the key light positions are mastered, additional light sources can be added to complement and create the desired effect. The first position of the key light is above the head, which casts shadows below the eyes ('bags under the eyes'), with an indistinct jaw line, making the person appear tired or sleepy (Figure 6.4). When the light is placed below, it emphasises unflattering features such as a prominent chin, glaring nostrils, or upper eyebrow ridges. Hence, an inferiorly located light

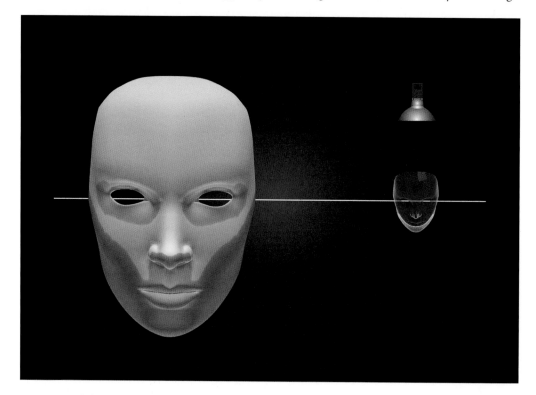

Figure 6.4 A light placed above the head conveys a sleepy appearance.

---

1 Cinematic lighting techniques: Part 1. https://www.youtube.com/watch?v=eZ5hpcn6tIM

source conjures a sinister appearance, and should be avoided, unless the intention is portraying a satanic persona (Figure 6.5).

A light positioned head-on renders a flat image, similar to using a ring flash for taking intra-oral images. This is the least dramatic set-up with a single light source, but ideal for beautify shots as blemishes, warts and wrinkles magically disappear by the uniform, lacklustre illumination that is devoid of shadows (Figure 6.6). However, the images appear two-dimensional, conveying frivolity and superficiality.

If the light source is moved upwards from the head-on position until a 'butterfly' shadow appears below the nose, the effect is termed papillon lighting. This lighting pattern is preferred for feminine portraits since it accentuates the cheek bones with subtle shadows below the zygomatic process (Figures 6.7 and 6.8). However, if the light is incorrectly positioned from above, the effect is unwanted long shadows cast by the eyebrows and nose, obscuring the eyes and lips, respectively.

Another position is altering the light angle from above until the nose casts a loop shadow on the opposite side (Figure 6.9). Loop lighting is ideal for round faces because it makes the face look slimmer and longer. Continuing to move the light further will connect the nose shadow with the cheek shadow and result in Rembrandt lighting, used by the Dutch artist in several of his portrait paintings. This is the most widely used lighting for portraiture, and is sometimes referred to as 'front upper side' lighting, as the light is positioned slightly above the face to one side (right or left) and 45° from the camera. The position achieves drop shadows on the contralateral side by forming a triangle of light. The shape of the 'triangle' depends on the position of the light and individual facial contours. Rembrandt lighting produces a dramatic effect with substantial depth for a three-dimensional quality to a portrait (Figures 6.10–6.12). Also, the set-up smoothly sculpts facial features and produces

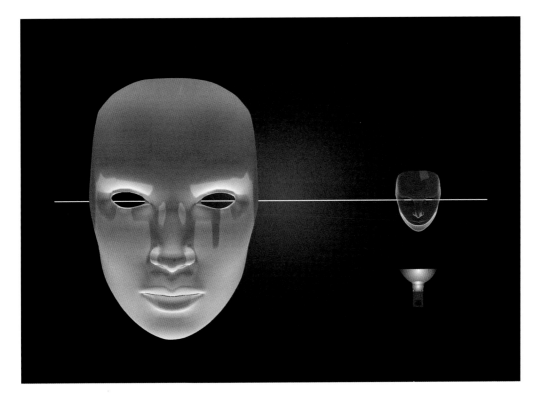

Figure 6.5 An inferiorly located light conjures up a sinister appearance.

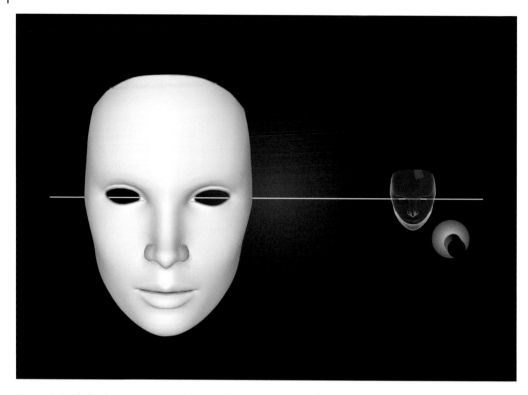

Figure 6.6 A light shone head-on produces a flat, two-dimensional image.

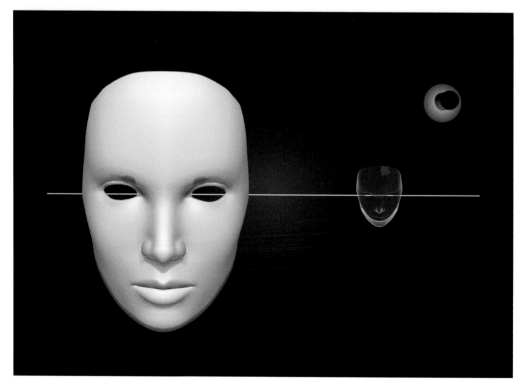

Figure 6.7 Papillon lighting is defined by the appearance of a butterfly shadow below the nose, and is ideal for feminine shots.

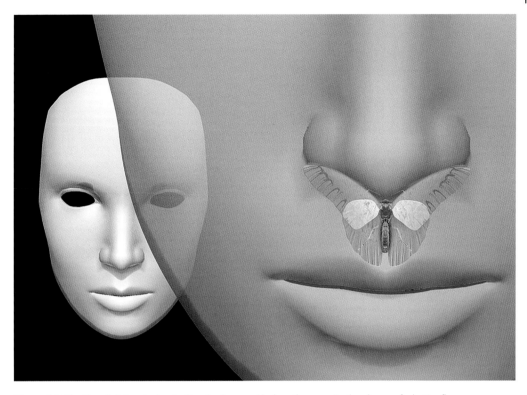

Figure 6.8 Papillon lighting is due to the shadow cast below the nose in the shape of a butterfly.

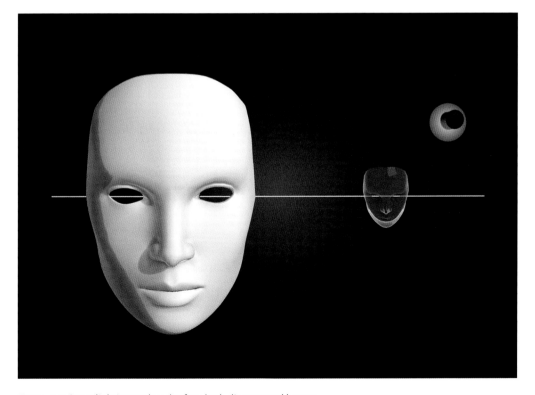

Figure 6.9 Loop lighting makes the face look slimmer and longer.

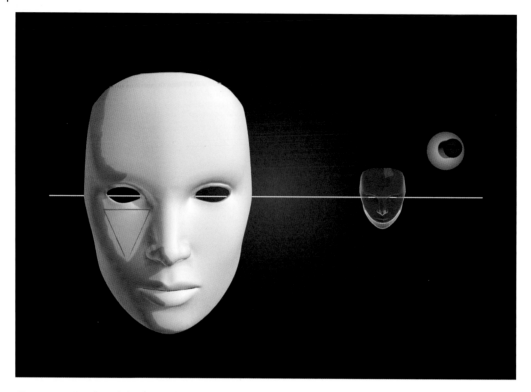

Figure 6.10 Rembrandt lighting is the most popular lighting for portrait photography.

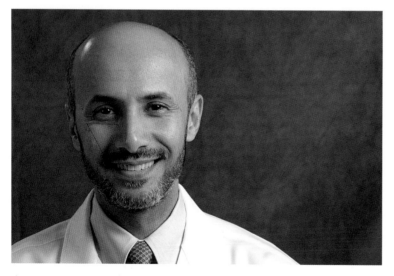

Figure 6.11 Rembrandt lighting is distinguished by the classic triangle of light below the eye on the contralateral side of the key light.

soft skin tones. However, this lighting position is subjective, and not suited for every face, but nevertheless, is a good starting point for achieving portraits with visual impact. Another endearing feature of Rembrandt lighting is that it creates beautiful catch lights, which further enhances the image and attracts the viewer to the subject. Catch lights are reflections

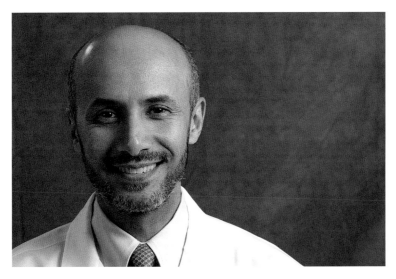

Figure 6.12 Rembrandt lighting produces a sculpted three-dimensional portrait.

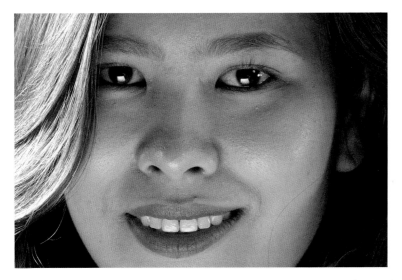

Figure 6.13 Square catch lights, which represent reflections of a square reflector placed just below the chin.

of flashes or reflectors on the cornea of the eyes, symbolising vitality and liveliness; in a manner of sense 'seeing the light in someones eyes' (Figure 6.13). The shape of the catch lights is identical to the shape of the light source, for example, round lamp, ring flashes, square soft boxes, octagon soft boxes, round reflectors, or reflective umbrellas. Finally, the position of the camera determines whether the broad light (light source side), or the opposite darker side of the face, termed short light (or dark side), is photographed. Broad lighting is obviously brighter, whilst short lighting (the dark side), as its name implies, creates more depth (Figure 6.14).

The next position is called split lighting, where the light is placed on one side of the face to completely throw the opposite side in total darkness. Compared to papillon lighting that is ideally suited for feminine shots, split lighting is 'tougher' and emphasises features as rugged, and is therefore, more appropriate for conveying masculinity (Figure 6.15). Lastly rim light is a light

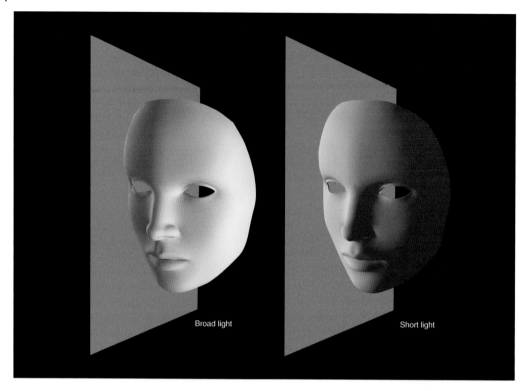

Figure 6.14 Broad lighting vs. Short lighting.

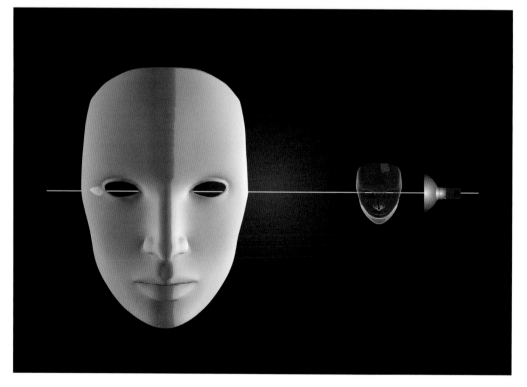

Figure 6.15 Split lighting emphasises facial features and is suited for masculine portraits.

source that is located behind the subject for a contre-jour effect, either sunlight or artificial light that illuminates the outline or boundary of objects. In portraiture, a rim, edge or hair light is used for creating a glow around the subject's head by a rim of light around the hair or scalp (for bald individuals). The light source is pointing towards the camera, placed hidden behind or to the side of the subject's head. The emanating glow creates an angelic halo around the head, giving the person an evangelical or virginal quality (Figure 6.16).

A summary of the various types of portrait lighting using a single light source is shown in Figure 6.17.

Intensity and Size

While the direction of lighting determines the position of the highlights and shadows, the power and size of the illumination determine the intensity of the highlights and shadows. It is important to realise that the intensity or power of electronic flashes is determined by the duration of output; the longer the duration, the greater the power.

The intensity of the light in relation to its distance is determined by the inversely square law:

$$\text{Intensity of light} = 1 / \text{distance}^2$$

This means that doubling the distance of the light source reduces its intensity by 75%. In practical terms the light drop-off from 1 to 2 m is significant at 75%, but as the distance increases the drop off becomes less significant, e.g. from 6 to 7 m the reduction in intensity is only 1%. Therefore, for portraiture, to create intense sharp [closed] shadows, the light source needs to

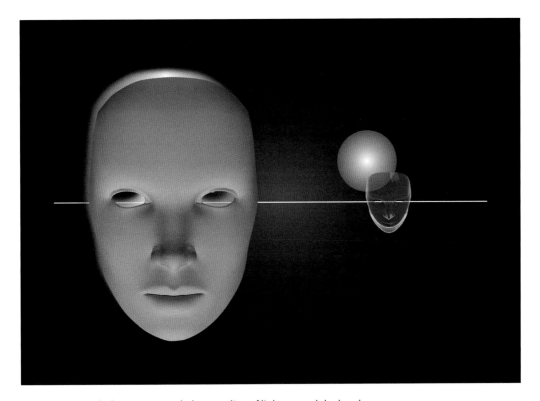

Figure 6.16 Rim lighting creates a halo or outline of light around the head.

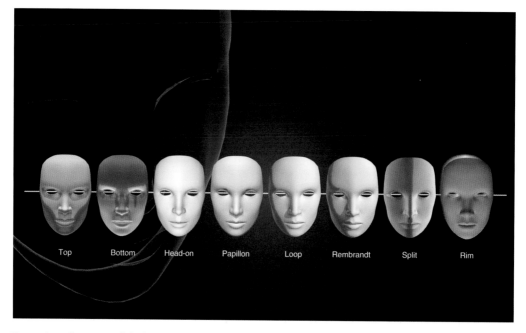

Figure 6.17 Summary of the basic types of lighting for portraiture using a single light source.

be smaller or further away from the subject, and for softer edges [open] shadows the light source needs to be closer or larger. The distance of the light from the subject also affects the background illumination. If the subject remains stationary whilst the light is moved away, the background becomes darker (Figure 6.18).

Light is classified as hard or soft. Hard lighting is harsh, smaller size and usually unidirectional for creating distinct shadows with specular reflections. It is characterised by sharp shadow outlines accompanied by areas of burnt out (or clipped) highlights. Conversely, soft lighting is larger and diffuse, creating indistinct (blurred) shadows with subtle and gradual transitions between darker and lighter parts with softer highlights. Hard lighting emphasises details such as skin blemished, pores and wrinkles, whereas soft light attenuates, or 'irons out' details, and is generally more flattering. Therefore, for portraiture, softer lighting is generally preferred to glamorise the subject (Figure 6.19). There are several methods for achieving softer lighting. The first is moving the light source closer to the subject (potentially making it brighter and larger), the second by using an intermediate material to diffuse the emitted light (e.g. soft box), third to bounce the flash off reflective surfaces such as an umbrella or a reflector, and lastly, increasing the physical size of the light source. Moving the light closer to the subject also has the effect of creating a greater subject-to-background separation, which is advantageous for emphasising a figure-ground relationship and conveying a three-dimensional quality.

There are innumerable light shaping attachments for modifying light. The most popular is attaching various reflectors or diffusers onto the flash heads for altering the emitted output. For example, if hard light is required, a silver bowl reflector with or without a honeycomb grid will suffice. However, to limit hard light to a spot, lens and fresnel dishes are attached to focus a beam of light to a specific size. To soften light, umbrellas and soft boxes are the preferred choice. Umbrellas are either reflective, or translucent catering for varying degrees of light softness. Soft boxes diffuse light as well as increasing the apparent size of the light source. The

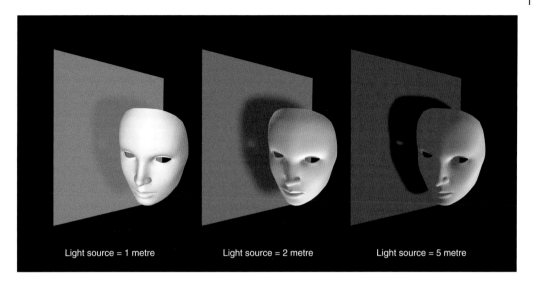

Light source = 1 metre   Light source = 2 metre   Light source = 5 metre

Figure 6.18 Inverse square law: if the subject remains stationary and the light source moves further away, the following occur:
1) background becomes darker
2) shadow of the face on the background becomes intense and sharper
3) facial shadows close up [become softer] and reveal fewer facial features on the contralateral side of the illumination

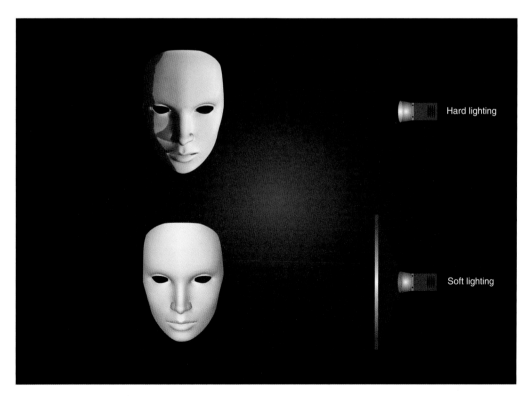

Figure 6.19 A hard light, produced by a naked light source, emphasises facial features (notice the shadows on the right side of the face contralateral to the light source), whilst soft light attenuated by diffusers, such as soft boxes, tends to smooth out detail.

shapes and sizes of soft boxes on the market is staggering, made of different materials that allows innumerable modifying effects. Added to this are beauty lights, sting lights, snoots, coloured gels, to name a few. However, unless one is contemplating photography as a profession, for dental use, a bowl reflector with two or three honeycomb grids and a couple of soft boxes (or umbrellas) is all that is necessary, which are often included in a two or three studio flash kit from several manufacturers.

Fill Light

The secondary lights are termed fill lights because they are placed on the contralateral side to 'fill in shadows' from the key light. The fill light can be ambient lighting or natural daylight, a second flash, or a reflector that bounces light from the key light back onto the subject (Figure 6.20). The degree that a fill light illuminates a subject is expresses as a ratio of the key light. For example, if only one light is used, the ratio is 0 : 1, where 0 represents absence of a fill light, and 1 is the main or key light. A 1 : 4 ratio signifies that the fill light is a quarter of the intensity of the key light. It is important to note that the smaller number always signifies the fill light. An acceptable ratio for portraits is 1 : 2, whereas an equal ratio of 1 : 1 totally eliminates shadows and is referred to as a 'high key' image. A high key image excessively softens facial features, but is ideal for glamour shots or pictures of children for expressing joviality and playfulness (Figures 6.21 and 6.22). On the other extreme, a 'low key' image emphasises shadows, giving the picture depth and character, and is ideal for portraying personality traits such as insight and wisdom (Figures 6.23 and 6.24). The computer company Apple* predominantly uses high key images to promote its

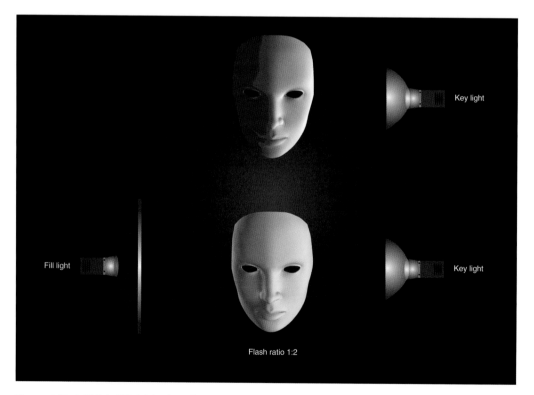

Figure 6.20 A fill light 'fills in' shadows from the key light (notice the pronounced shadows on the right side of the face without a fill light). A flash ratio of 1 : 2 (fill light: key light) is a good starting point for portraiture.

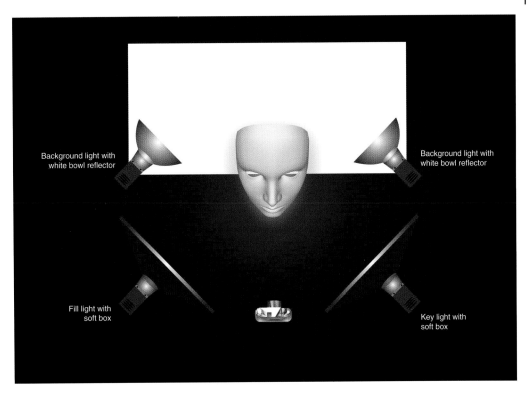

Figure 6.21 High key portrait lighting set-up with white backdrop.

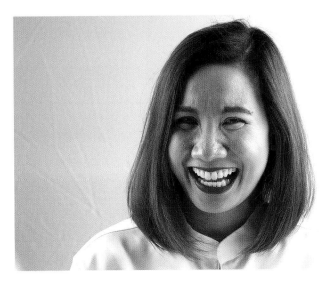

Figure 6.22 A high key portrait.

glittering and shiny products. Conversely, Baroque period painters such as Caravaggio use low key lighting that is unidirectional for conveying drama, depth and realism.

In a similar way to positioning the key light, the location of the fill light also creates different effects. The simplest set-up is two studio flashes angled 45° towards the subject, which is a fool

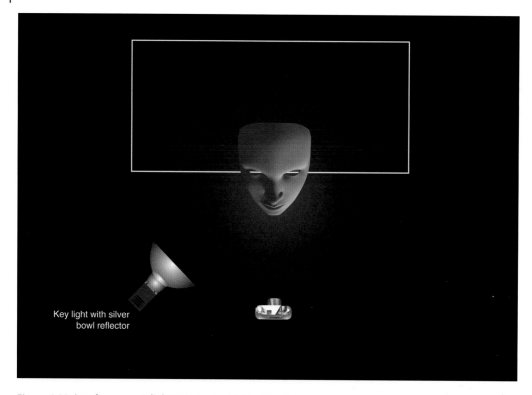

Key light with silver
bowl reflector

Figure 6.23 Low key portrait lighting set-up with black backdrop.

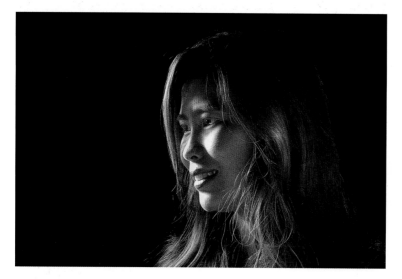

Figure 6.24 A low key portrait.

proof arrangement and ideal for clinical portraiture. This set-up produces consistently repeatable and standardised portraits for reference and comparison. Whilst these images serve the purpose of clinical fidelity, they are construed as bland, and usually unsuitable for marketing and promotional purposes. However, a little flair, combined with a vivid imagination, can position both key and fill lights to create emotive and seductive compositions, which are inspirational for both marketing and lecturing.

Background Light

As well as illuminating the subject, lights are also necessary for illuminating the background for subject-background or figure-ground separation for simulating a three-dimensional effect. All backgrounds, with the exception of black, require some form of illumination, which may be extraneous light fall-out from the key or fill lights, or extra strobes directed to a suspended cloth or other backdrop. Backlit illumination also avoids projection shadows cast by the key light onto coloured backdrops, and for ensuring a smooth, evenly lit and non-distracting background (Figure 6.25).

Finally, it is worth turning on modelling lights, if available on the studio flashes. Most contemporary studio lights, or strobes, are equipped with continuous halogen modelling lights. These low-level lights serve two purposes. First, the continuous light avoids the distracting 'red eye' phenomena, and second, it allows pre-visualisation of the effect of flash positioning and intensity on facial features before taking the picture (Glazer 2009).

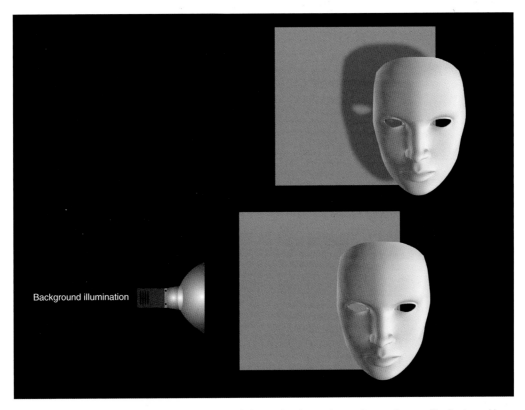

Figure 6.25 A projection shadow cast by the key light can be distracting and annoying, and is eliminated by illuminating a coloured background with an additional flash.

Clinical Portraiture Set-Up

Before embarking on portrait photography, as discussed in Module 2, a signed consent from the patient is prerequisite. More than any form of dental photography, consent is essential for portraiture. If consent is forthcoming, the ensuing pictures should be treated with the utmost confidentiality, and archived safely and securely. However, if consent is withheld, the portrait session should be abandoned.

The ideal location for taking portraits is a dedicated room, or an allocated space within a dental clinic, preferably remote from the clinical environment. This allows a relaxed and unfettered atmosphere to put the patient at ease. Music soothes the soul, and an appropriate melody does wonders for setting the mood. This is particularly important for taking non-clinical portraits when the patient needs to feel comfortable to express his or her true inner self.

For clinical portraits, the patient is seated upright in a revolving chair, hair tied back to expose the auricles, ostentatious jewellery removed and cosmetic make-up muted or washed off to capture natural skin tones and texture. There are several reference lines that are useful for orientating the head in the vertical and horizontal planes, including the inter-pupillary and facial midlines, ala-tragus line (Camper's plane), or Frankfort plane (Figure 6.26). However, it is important not to rely on the incisal or occlusal plane as a reference, as this may be eschewed and result in pseudo-alignment. The photographer is situated behind camera, which can be tripod-mounted [ideal for standardisation] or hand-held about 1–2 m away from the patient. The camera is adjusted so that the lens axis is at the same level as the middle of the face (see Figures 5.1–5.3 in Module 5). The dental assistant is at hand helping set up the photographic equipment, acting as a chaperone, and keeping a vigilant eye on the patient for ensuring their comfort.

The photographic inventory for clinical portraits consists of three studio flashes with light-modifying soft boxes or umbrellas, trigger mechanism for simultaneously firing the flashes, and a cloth or paper backdrop. The preferred backgrounds are neutral sky blue or grey, which

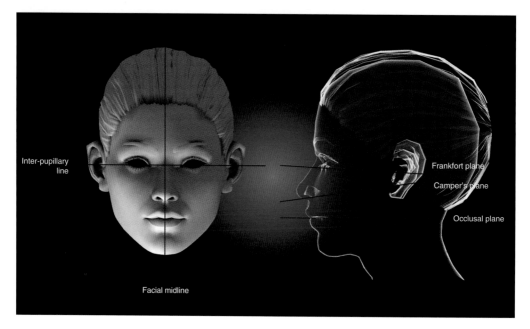

Figure 6.26 The imaginary facial lines are useful guides for orientating the head in the horizontal and vertical planes.

complement patients' complexion. White or black backgrounds should be avoided since the former creates annoying shadows, while the latter is not conductive for patients with darker skin tones (Ettorre et al. 2006). The patient is positioned sufficiently in front of the background to avoid distracting projection shadows, and to throw the background out of focus for greater visual separation between the subject and background.

As disused in Module 1: Photographic Equipment, portraiture requires slave flash photography. The electronic flashes output photographic daylight at a colour temperature of around 5500 K. They are either triggered wirelessly by radio controllers and apps, or cables connected from the flashes to the sync cord pin on the camera. The exposure is usually calculated manually, using an incident light meter, or taking test shots at a given aperture and shutter speed, and adjusting the distance or power of the flashes until the correct exposure is attained. Some studio flashes offer TTL (through-the-lens) metering using an adapter mounted onto the hot-shoe of the camera that controls the flash bursts for ensuring correct exposure. This is similar to camera mounted compact flashes controlled by TTL metering.

The location of the studio lights is determined by available space and funds. There are two options, the first is mounting the flash heads onto tripods placed on the floor, and the second, more elaborate and expensive, is suspending the flashes from ceiling mounted tracks. The retractable ceiling mounts are advantageous as they eliminate cables trailing on the floor, but need a room with sufficient ceiling height. Tripod-mounted units have the advantage of greater mobility, especially if mounted on a dolly, but require substantial floor space. In both circumstances, a minimum of three flashes are required, two angled 45° towards the patient with a fill light: key light ratio of 1 : 2, and the third directed to the backdrop (Figure 6.27). The key and

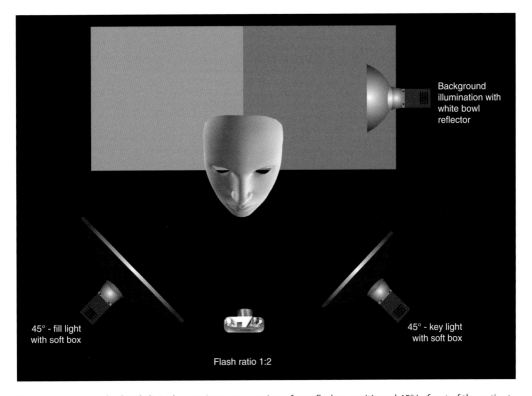

Figure 6.27 A standardised clinical portrait set-up consists of two flashes positioned 45° in front of the patient with a flash ratio of 1 : 2, and a third flash to illuminate the background, which is usually neutral sky blue or grey.

fill light output is muted to soft light by attaching soft boxes or umbrellas onto the flash heads, whilst the third flash has a white bowl reflector for uniformly illuminating the background. This set-up is very 'clinical', devoid of distinct shadows or highlights, producing a relatively flat image. However, the remit of clinical portraiture is to convey reality, without glamourising or denigrating the subject, and therefore, this lighting set-up is fit for the intended purpose. The predefined positions of the patient's revolving chair, camera, flashes and backdrops should be marked on the floor (or ceiling) with markers or adhesive masking tape so that their location is repeatable. The studio set-up for clinical portraiture is shown in Figures 6.28.

The Essential Portrait Portfolio

While the essential dental portfolio (EDP) concentrated primarily on the teeth, the essential portrait portfolio (EPP) consists of basic full face images and the relationship of the teeth to the

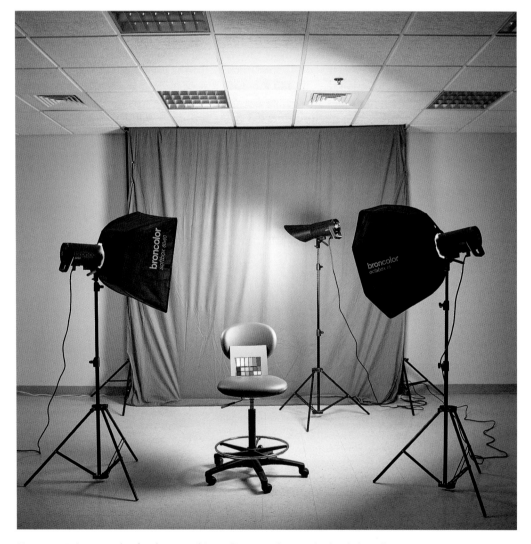

Figure 6.28 An example of a photographic studio set-up for standardised clinical portraiture.

face. The EPP is quintessential for a variety of dental disciplines including orthodontics, prosthodontics, periodontics, restorative dentistry, implantology, peadodontics, smile analysis, smile design, facial enhancement, and cranio-maxillio-facial procedures. The clinical portraits were previously excluded from the EDP since some patients are reticent to give consent to photograph their face due to personal, social, cultural or religious reasons. However, if this is not a concern, and appropriate consent is obtained, the EPP can be added to the EDP, see Module 5: Extra-oral and Intra-oral Images.

The EPP consists of seven views (Figure 6.29), as follows:

EPP Image #1: Fontal view with inter-labial separation
EPP Image #2: Fontal view – relaxed smile
EPP Image #3: Fontal view – biting wooden spatula

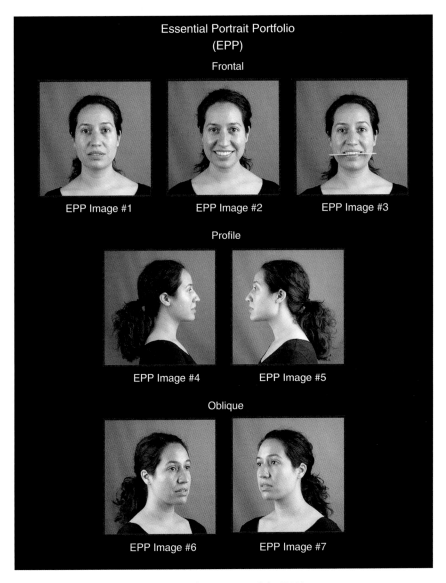

Figure 6.29 Thumbnails of the essential portrait portfolio (EPP).

EPP Image #4: Profile right side – inter-labial separation
EPP Image #5: Profile left side – inter-labial separation
EPP Image #6: Oblique right side – inter-labial separation
EPP Image #7: Oblique left side – inter-labial separation

The photographic equipment settings for standardised clinical portraits are as follows. The magnification factor ranges from 1 : 8 to 1 : 15, depending on the size of the patient's physical build and whether the camera has a full-frame sensor. An alternate approach is setting a predefined focusing distance on the lens barrel, or framing the picture according to the field of view. A f11 aperture is recommended for adequate depth of field with a 1/125 or 1/250 seconds shutter speed to eliminate the influence of ambient light. The salient camera/flash settings and guidelines for these views are outlined in Table 6.1.

Table 6.1 Settings and guidelines for standardised clinical portraits.

Item	Setting/description	Notes
Focus	Manual or auto-focus	
Exposure metering	Manual or through-the-lens (TTL)	Manual: use light meter, histogram or take test shots to ascertain correct exposure
ISO	50–200	
Aperture	f11	
Shutter speed	1/125 s or 1/250 s	Flash synchronisation speed depends on a specific camera brand
Image data format (file format)	RAW or DNG	
White balance	Automatic or manual	Manual options: numerical value input (5500 K), or take a reference image with an 18% neutral density grey card
Flash	Two studio flashes with soft boxes or umbrellas, angled 45° towards patient, third flash to illuminate background	Set the two flashes aimed at patient to a fill light: key light ratio of 1 : 2, alter intensity or distance of flashes to achieve correct exposure
Magnification factor	1 : 8 to 1 : 15	Only relevant for full-frame sensors, or set predefined focusing distance on lens, or see below for Field of view
Point of focus (PoF)	The PoF will depend on the angle of view, e.g. rhinion or bridge of the nose for frontal views	Hand-held cameras: for predefined magnification or focusing distance, move camera backwards and forwards until focus is obtained, or use anatomical landmarks for composing (see Field of view below)
		Tripod-mounted camera: for predefined magnification factor or focusing distance use macro stage for focusing, or use anatomical landmarks for composing (see Field of view below)
		If using auto-focus, ensure that the lens axis is centred on the tip of the nose for frontal views
Field of view (composition)	For frontal full face images	Right/left: bounded by background space Superior: bounded by background space Inferior: sterno-clavicular joint Anterior/posterior: tip of nose to auricles
Background	Variable	Clinical images: Neutral, e.g. sky blue or grey

The frontal views, EPP Images #1, 2 and 3, are taken with the patient looking straight towards the cameras, while for profile and oblique views the patient is asked to turn on the revolving chair until the desired angle of view is obtained. Similar to the dento-facial compositions discussed in the previous module, inter-labial separation is achieved by asking the patient to iterate the letter 'm' or 'Emma'. For EPP image #2, a relaxed smile is captured [usually accompanied by narrowing of the inter-eyelid spaces]. The EPP image #3 is biting into a wooden spatula with the head positioned to the horizontal. The angulation of the spatula is ideal for assessing incisal/occlusal plane alignment to the inter-pupillary line.

The field of view, or composition, depends on the aspect ratio setting on the camera, or the aspect ratio used in imaging software to crop the image. For portraiture, the chosen aspect ratio determines the amount of background space at the upper, right and left borders of a composition (the lower border is bounded by the sterno-clavicular joint). There are two options, the first is to be consistent with the EDP and use a landscape aspect ratio, which ensures standardisation for both the dental and EPPs. However, landscape orientation for portraits results in larger empty spaces right and left sides of the face compared to the upper border. The second option is to frame/crop the images with reduced amounts of background on the right and left sides, using the so-called 'portrait' aspect ratio, but the framing is obviously disparate with the EDP (Figure 6.30).

The point of focus (PoF) also differs according to the angle of view. For frontal views, the PoF is usually the rhinion or bridge of the nose (Figures 6.31–6.34). For profile views, EPP Images #4 and #5, the contralateral side should be totally invisible and the PoF is on the ala-tragus

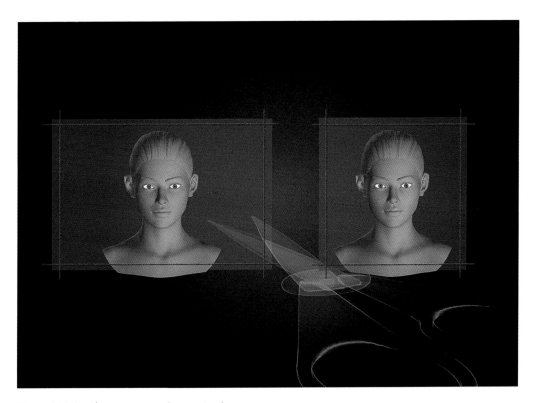

Figure 6.30 Landscape vs portrait aspect ratios.

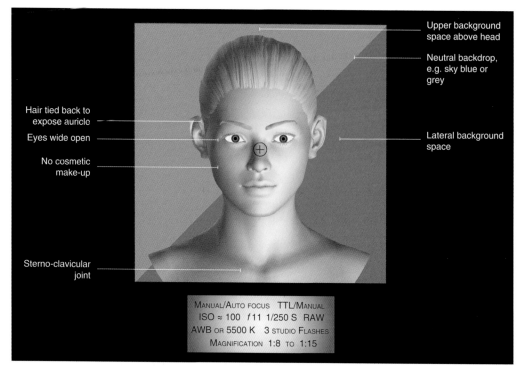

Upper background
space above head

Neutral backdrop,
e.g. sky blue or
grey

Hair tied back to
expose auricle

Eyes wide open

No cosmetic
make-up

Lateral background
space

Sterno-clavicular
joint

MANUAL/AUTO FOCUS   TTL/MANUAL
ISO ≈ 100   *f* 11 1/250 S RAW
AWB OR 5500 K   3 STUDIO FLASHES
MAGNIFICATION 1:8 TO 1:15

Figure 6.31 Standardised clinical portraiture settings, field of view and point of focus (PoF) (blue cross-line reticle) for essential portrait portfolio (EPP) images #1, #2 and #3.

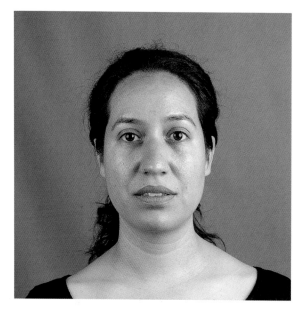

Figure 6.32 Essential portrait portfolio (EPP) image #1.

Figure 6.33 Essential portrait portfolio (EPP) image #2.

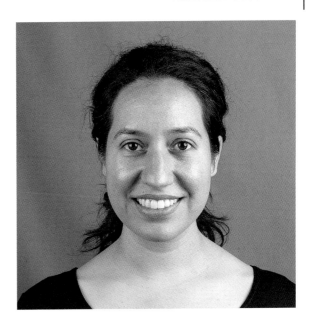

Figure 6.34 Essential portrait portfolio (EPP) image #3.

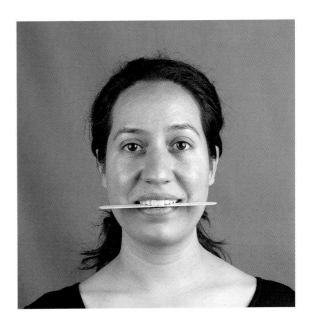

line, at the midpoint between the tragus and lateral canthus of the eye (Figures 6.35–6.37). Finally, for oblique views, EPP Images #6 and #7 the contralateral eye and its upper and lower eyelashes are visible, and the PoF is on the ala-tragus line at the intersection of the lateral canthus (Figures 6.38–6.40).

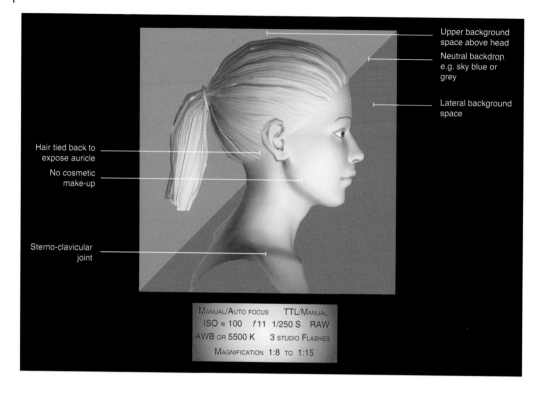

Figure 6.35 Standardised clinical portraiture settings, field of view and point of focus (PoF) (blue cross-line reticle) for essential portrait portfolio (EPP) images #4 and #5.

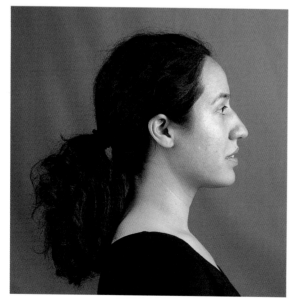

Figure 6.36 Essential portrait portfolio (EPP) image #4.

Figure 6.37 Essential portrait portfolio (EPP) image #5.

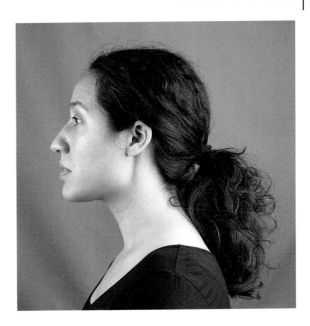

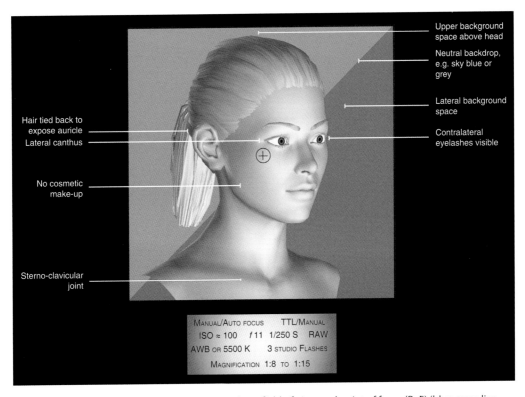

Upper background space above head

Neutral backdrop, e.g. sky blue or grey

Lateral background space

Contralateral eyelashes visible

Hair tied back to expose auricle

Lateral canthus

No cosmetic make-up

Sterno-clavicular joint

MANUAL/AUTO FOCUS   TTL/MANUAL
ISO ≈ 100   ƒ 11   1/250 S   RAW
AWB OR 5500 K   3 STUDIO FLASHES
MAGNIFICATION 1:8 TO 1:15

Figure 6.38 Standardised clinical portraiture settings, field of view and point of focus (PoF) (blue cross-line reticle) for essential portrait portfolio (EPP) Images #6 and 7.

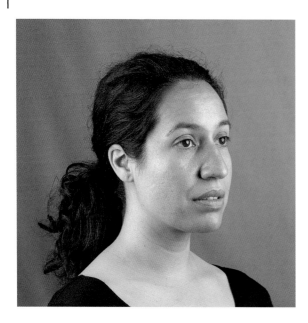

Figure 6.39 Essential portrait portfolio (EPP) image #6.

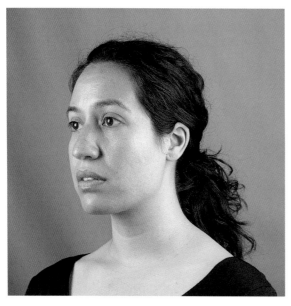

Figure 6.40 Essential portrait portfolio (EPP) image #7.

Optional Clinical Portraits

The first four optional clinical portraits are a repetition of the EPP #4 to #7 (profile and oblique views), but during a relaxed smile instead of inter-labial separation:

1) Profile right side – relaxed smile
2) Profile left side – relaxed smile
3) Oblique right side – relaxed smile
4) Oblique left side – relaxed smile

The above images are taken with identical settings, angle of view and PoF described for EPP images #4 to #7 (Figures 6.41 and 6.42).

Figure 6.41 Optional essential portrait portfolio (EEP) image #1 (profile right side relaxed smile).

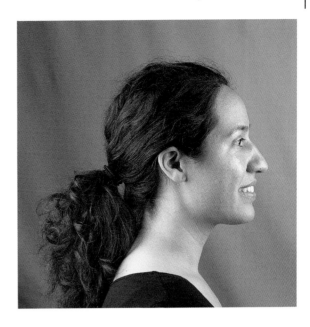

Figure 6.42 Optional essential portrait portfolio (EEP) image #4 (oblique left side relaxed smile).

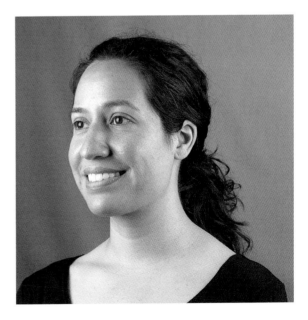

Depending on the discipline and/or type of therapy being undertaken, there may be additional specific facial views that are required for analysis, diagnosis, treatment planning, or reviewing and monitoring inter-treatment stages. Hence, it is impossible to show every type of clinical portrait in addition to the optional views mentioned above. However, the specialities that require particular facial images from different angles of view are orthodontics, aesthetic dentistry, cranio-maxillo-facial and aesthetic/cosmetic surgery. These extra images taken from specific angles of view allow assessment of skull deformities such as dysgnathia, cleft lip and palate, palsies, or acute traumas of the face, e.g. due to brawls or road traffic accidents. The set-up described for EPP can be used for any additional clinical portraits by varying the angle and position of the patient's head or camera, e.g. submental vertical view, supracranial oblique view,

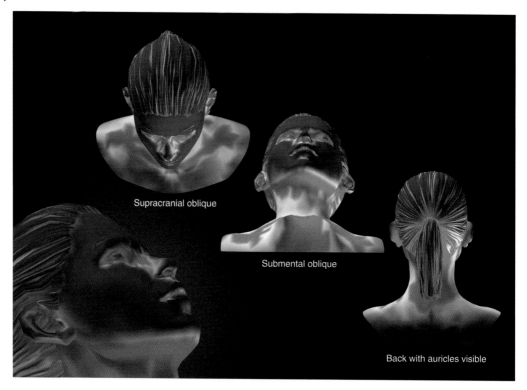

Figure 6.43 Examples of some views for specific modalities or discipline.

back view auricles visible, profile or frontal views with the chin pointing upwards, backwards, or downwards (Figure 6.43). Further images may be taken during different facial expressions such as frowning, grimace or various gazes of the eyes including squinting, glaring or shut (Schaff et al. 2006). Photographing children presents a challenge and is tedious and frustrating since patients are fidgety, and often agitated in the 'foreign' dental environment. The best practice is placing toddlers on the parent's lap so that they feel more comfortable, and create auditory or visual distractions as diversions form the task at hand. Also, setting the camera to auto-focus may circumvent blurred images, but not a guarantee as the focusing mechanism tries to negotiate a child's perpetual movements.

Non-clinical Portraiture Set-up

For non-clinical portraiture, the photographer needs to think with his or her eyes for creating tableaus that have visual panache (Figure 6.44). An impassioned portrait is created by unleashing the imagination and conveying the depth of the soul. This is entering into the realms of art and creativity, a subject that is sought rather than taught. However, for the sake of completion, a few non-clinical portraits, together with their set-ups, are presented below to tantalise the senses and stimulate the imagination.

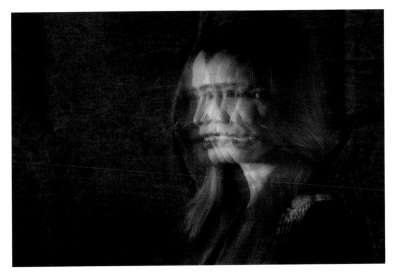

Figure 6.44 Non-clinical portraiture is limited only by the imagination.

Generic Studio Portrait

The generic studio portrait is typified by a coloured dappled background using an established set-up with three flashes. The key flash has a soft box to produce soft light, which is placed above and to the right or left side for classical Rembrandt lighting. A second fill light with a honeycomb grid for harder light is placed on the opposite side behind the subject to act as an edge (accent or rim) light. The background is illuminated separately with the third flash, which has a white bowl reflector to achieve substantial figure-to-ground separation between the subject and background. The intensity (power) and distance of the three flashes is tweaked for achieving the correct exposure (Figures 6.45 and 6.46). This set-up is ideal for business and formal portraits, as well as job applications or promotional purposes.

Flattering Portrait

A simple, but effective set-up yields spectacular results. In the following portrait, only a single flash is used as the key light above and behind the model, whilst a silver reflector acts as a fill light to bounce light onto the face. The effect is a faltering portrait that floods the subject with a burst of soft light, ironing out wrinkles and blemishes. The arrangement is reminiscent of shooting outdoors, with bright sunlight above and behind the subject with a judicially placed reflector to illuminate the face with a 'glow' of light. The set-up is also conductive for photographing the lips and teeth, since the light from the reflector can be manipulated to 'shine' on the smile. An optional black backdrop can be utilised, but is unusually superfluous since the reflected light from the fill light is insufficient to illuminate unwanted background objects (Figures 6.47 and 6.48).

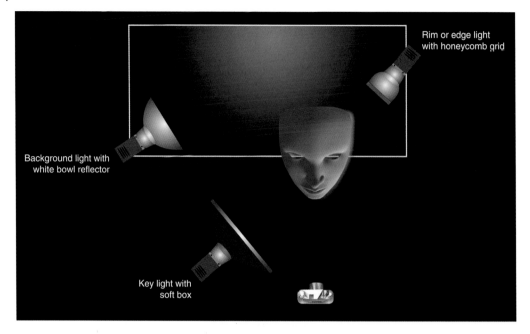

Figure 6.45 Generic studio portrait set-up using three flashes.

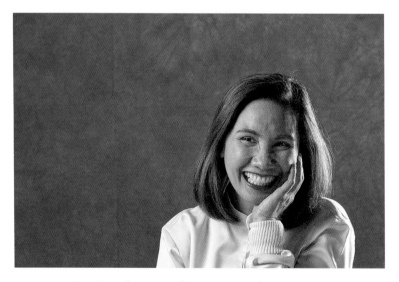

Figure 6.46 Generic studio portrait: f 11, 1/125 seconds.

Profile Portrait

The easiest method to emphasise a facial profile is illuminating the face head-on, whilst throwing the remainder of the head into partial darkness. The set-up consists of two flashes, the key light with a honeycomb grid produces relatively hard light, whilst a softer fill light of reduced intensity is used to illuminate the hair and cast a diffuse shadow of the face onto a cloth backdrop. The ensuing shadow further accentuates the brightly lit facial profile (Figures 6.49 and 6.50).

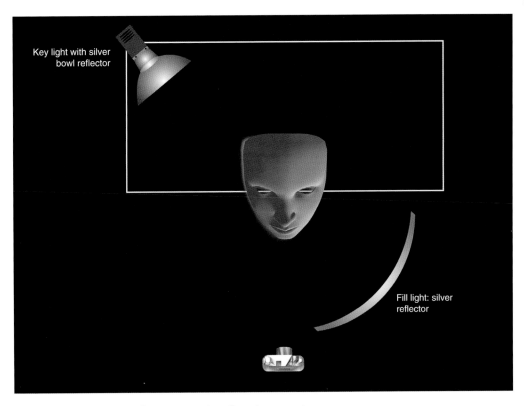

Figure 6.47   A simple but effective set-up for a flattering portrait.

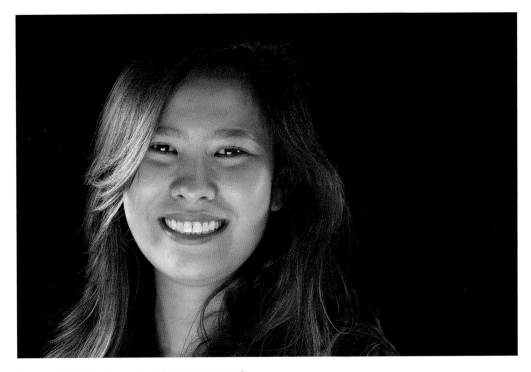

Figure 6.48   Flattering portrait: *f* 16, 1/125 seconds.

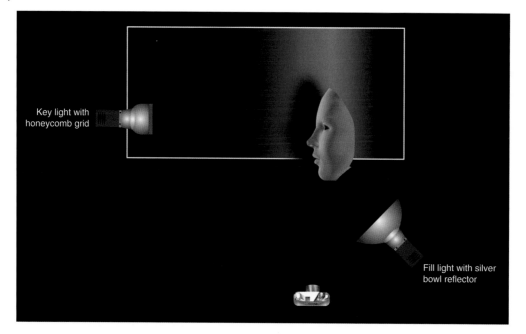

Figure 6.49 Profile portrait with head-on illumination by the key light, and a shadow cast by a fill light onto the background.

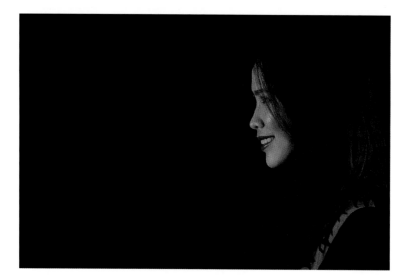

Figure 6.50 Profile portrait: *f* 8, 1/125 seconds.

Coloured Gel Portrait

Besides utilising coloured backdrops, another method for adding colour is placing a filter or gel over the flash head. Gels are available in several colours and offer a quick and convenient method for colouring light directed to specific parts of the face. In this set-up, a blue gel is used for the rim flash positioned just behind the subject to backlight the hair. The hair on the contralateral side is not illuminated to add colour contrast with the opposite side and the maroon background. The key light is relatively hard, located to the front left side of the

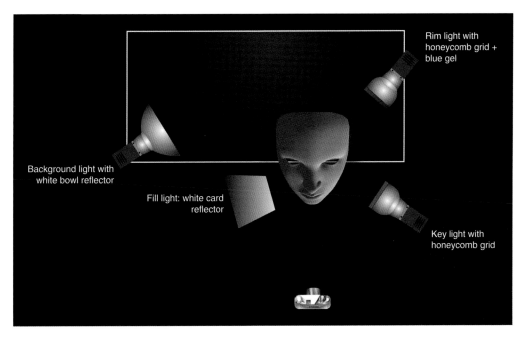

Figure 6.51 Coloured gel portrait set-up using two honeycomb grid attachments, one with blue gel as a rim or hair light.

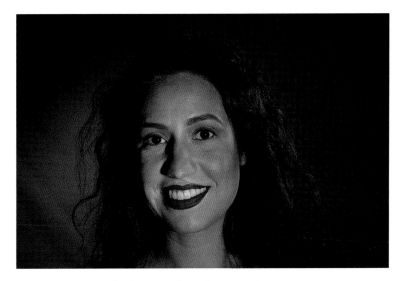

Figure 6.52 Coloured gel portrait: ƒ9.5, 1/125 seconds.

model, a white card on the right side as the fill light to fill in shadows, and a third flash illuminates the cloth backdrop (Figures 6.51 and 6.52).

Classical Smile Line Portrait

Although all non-clinical portraits potentially have high marketing value, dental marketing relies heavily on the lower third of the face or the smile, which is stereotypical for promoting a dental clinic or practice. The set-up for the classical smile line portrait is another take on the profile portrait (shown above) using a single key light placed above the subject instead of head-on. The model has a celestial gaze, that is emphasised by the overhead illumination. The relaxed smile beautifully conveys the parallelism of the maxillary incisal plane to the curvature of the mandibular lip. The overhead light is muted with a soft box and Velcro grid so that the face is awash with diffuse soft light that adds a pensive, heavenly quality to the composition. A second light is placed behind to illuminate the background and a white card reflector bounces light from the overhead soft box to illuminate the neck and chin (Figures 6.53 and 6.54).

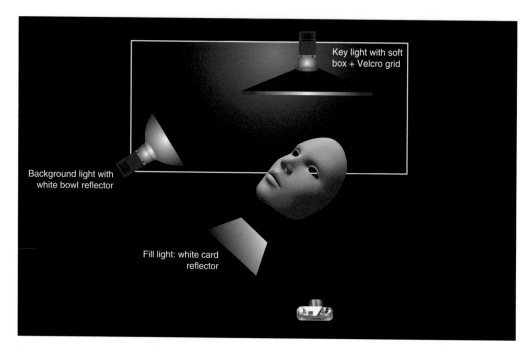

Figure 6.53 Smile line profile portrait with an overhead diffuse key light.

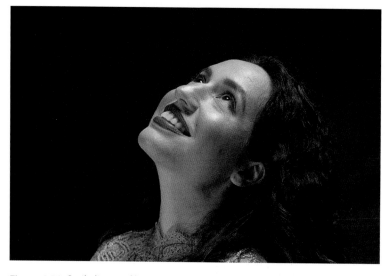

Figure 6.54 Smile line profile portrait: *f* 9.5, 1/125 seconds.

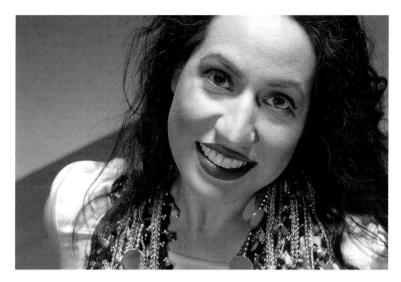

Figure 6.55 Smile line frontal portrait: *f* 9.5, 1/125 seconds.

Clinical vs. Non-clinical Portraiture

Finally, the last image aptly illustrates the difference between clinical and non-clinical portraiture. The set-up is similar to the previous image, but the overhead light illuminates both the model and background. The model is looking directly towards the camera, and again, notice the pleasing smile line characterised by the coincidence of the incisal edges of the maxillary teeth with the curvature of the lower lip (Figure 6.55).

A side-by-side compassion of Figures 6.33 and 6.55 clearly demonstrates the different visual impact of each image; the former depicts clinical reality, whilst the latter is a dopamine releasing portrayal of the same individual.

References

Ahmad, I. (2009a). Digital dental photography. Part 7: extra-oral set-ups. *Br. Dent. J.* 207 (3): 103–110.

Ahmad, I. (2009b). Digital dental photography. Part 5: lighting. *Br. Dent. J.* 207 (1): 13–18.

Bazos, P. and Magne, M. (2013). Demystifying the digital dental photography workflow. The big picture: facial documentation with high visual impact photography. *J. Cosmet. Dent.* 29 (1): 82–88.

Ettorre, G., Weber, M., Schaaf, H. et al. (2006). Standards for digital photography in cranio-maxillo-facial surgery – part I: basic views and guidelines. *J. Craniomaxillofac. Surg.* 34: 65–73.

Glazer, B. (2009). Portrait Photography in Prosthodontics. http://www.oralhealthgroup.com/features/portrait-photography-in-prosthodontics (accessed 23 May 2019).

Jung, C.G. (1969[1933]). *Archetypes and the Collective Unconscious.* Collected Works of C.G. Jung, Volume 9 (Part 1). Princeton, NJ: Princeton University Press.

Cambridge in Colour (2005–2017). Portraiture lighting. www.cambridgeincolour.com (accessed 23 May 2019).

Schaff, H., Streckbein, P., Ettorre, G. et al. (2006). Standards for digital photography in cranio-maxillo-facial surgery – part II: additional picture sets and avoiding common mistakes. *J. Cranio-Maxillofac. Surg.* 34: 366–377.

7

Bench Images

This module, more than any other in this book, allows the photographer to unleash creativity and free the imagination for producing pictures that have unique mood and composition, where an object or product can be shot from any angle, with any light source, and with any background (Figure 7.1). The so-called bench image is basically still life macrophotography, and allows the photographer complete control over subject matter and lighting, with few rules or limitations to express his or her vision in vibrant ways (Figures 7.2 and 7.3). Since the objects are 'still', the permutations for positioning are endless. Furthermore, similar to a painting, a still life photograph can tantalise the mind with a surreal 'hidden' meaning or message.

Uses of Bench Images

Dental bench images document a variety of dental items for communicating with fellow professional colleagues as well as patients. The most frequently photographed dental items are plaster casts or 3D-printed models of the maxillary and mandibular arches, diagnostic wax-ups, thermoplastic or 3D-printed surgical guides, transparent vacuum stents for intra-oral mock-up and chair-side temporisation, crowns, veneers, inalys/onlays, bridges and removable partial, full or implant-supported prostheses. Bench images can simply be for documentation, or analysis, treatment planning, research and teaching clinical and laboratory techniques (Ahmad 2009) – Figures 7.4.

In addition, many treatment modalities, such as orthodontics, require mandatory photographs of models for pre-operative records, treatment progress, post-operative outcomes and monitoring. Also, photographic communication facilitates second opinions form specialists, or approval from patients before finalising treatment plans. This may include assessing mounted casts on semi- or fully adjustable articulators for assessing lateral excursions, anterior guidance, raising the VDO (vertical dimension of occlusion), smile design and diagnostic wax-ups of proposed aesthetic and functional rehabilitation (Figures 7.5–7.8). Visual documentation also facilitates communication between patient/ceramist/clinical, such as scrutinising flaws in impressions before fabricating indirect restorations, which saves time and money and avoids clinical embarrassment in front of patients if the restoration fails to fit. A pre-operative plaster cast is also indispensable for reminding the patient of the starting point of dental therapy, its progress and final result. In addition, the dental technician can inspect and record porosity, fractures and fluorescence properties of ceramic restorations before delivery to the clinician.

Implant planning also benefits from photodocumentation, especially for multidisciplinary prosthetically driven treatment planning by liaising with oral surgeons, periodontists, prosthodontists and dental technicians for arriving at a feasible and predictable treatment plan. This

Essentials of Dental Photography, First Edition. Irfan Ahmad.
© 2020 John Wiley & Sons Ltd. Published 2020 by John Wiley & Sons Ltd.

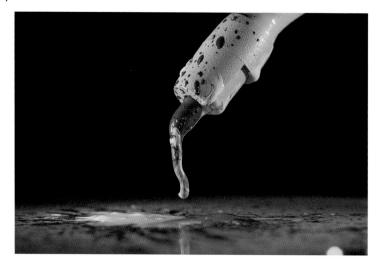

Figure 7.1 Bench shots are ideal for creating promotional images, when an object can be photographed from any angle, with any light, to convey the intended message to an audience.

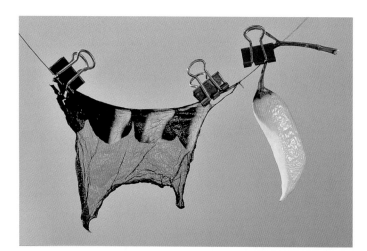

Figures 7.2 and 7.3 The creativity potential of bench images is limitless.

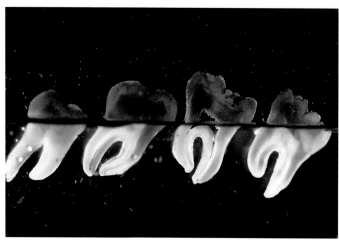

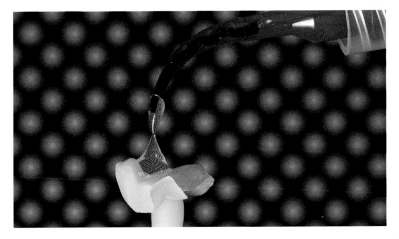

Figure 7.4 Stylised bench images are ideal for teaching techniques, e.g. ceramic etching of the intaglio surface of an inlay with hydrofluoric acid.

Figure 7.5 Pre-operative cast of a patient with altered passive eruption with short clinical crown lengths. The existing measurements are marked on the teeth, and with the proposed gingival zeniths after aesthetic crown lengthening. The marked areas at the incisal edges indicate the anticipated reduction necessary for achieving the correct width/length ratio of the teeth.

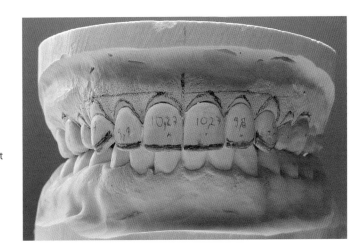

Figure 7.6 The proposed aesthetic crown lengthening and incisal edge reduction for rehabilitating pink and white aesthetics.

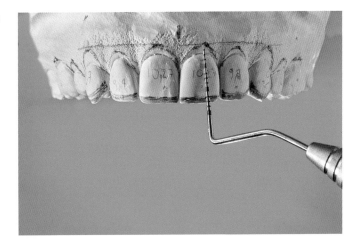

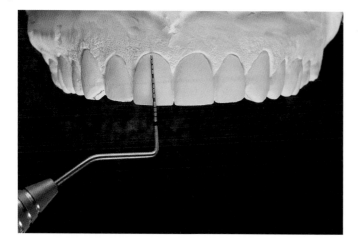

Figure 7.7 Plaster cast of the diagnostic wax-up showing the proposed crown lengths after perio-plastic surgical and restorative procedures.

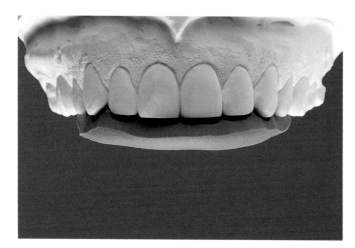

Figure 7.8 Plaster cast of the diagnostic wax-up cast with silicone index for guiding incisal edge reduction.

involves gaining input from specialists about 3D-printed surgical guides (designed using intra-oral and radiographic CBCT scans) or implant placement with concomitant soft and hard tissue augmentation (Figures 7.9–7.11). Finally, a clinical technique is often easier to explain and teach with a sequence of bench images, particularly for treatments involving posterior teeth (Figures 7.12–7.18). Similarly, a series of bench photographs are ideal for showing step-by-step laboratory techniques such as porcelain layering of ceramic crowns.

Backgrounds and Supports

The basic items required for bench images are a support to place the items to be photographed on and a suitable background. A backdrop is desirable for bench images to add interest to the composition and create figure-ground separation. A background and support can either be a single entity for a seamless transition between the foreground and background, or a bench to place the items and a separate background. Whichever option is chosen, the amount of background is crucial to a composition; too much background gives a sense of isolation and alienation, while too little signifies clutter and claustrophobia.

Several configurations are available for backgrounds/supports for bench images. The first is purchasing a professional still life table or macro studio that serves the dual purpose of

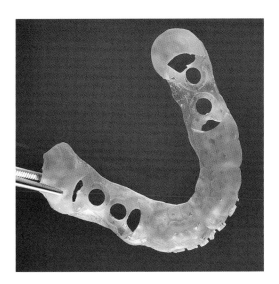

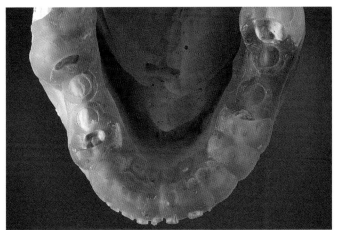

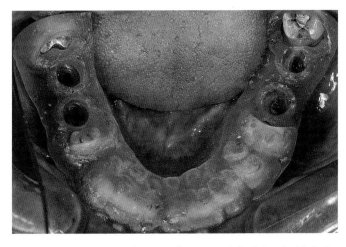

Figures 7.9–7.11 A second opinion from a specialist is invaluable before proceeding with treatment, e.g. a flapless procedure for implant placement using a 3D-printed surgical guide.

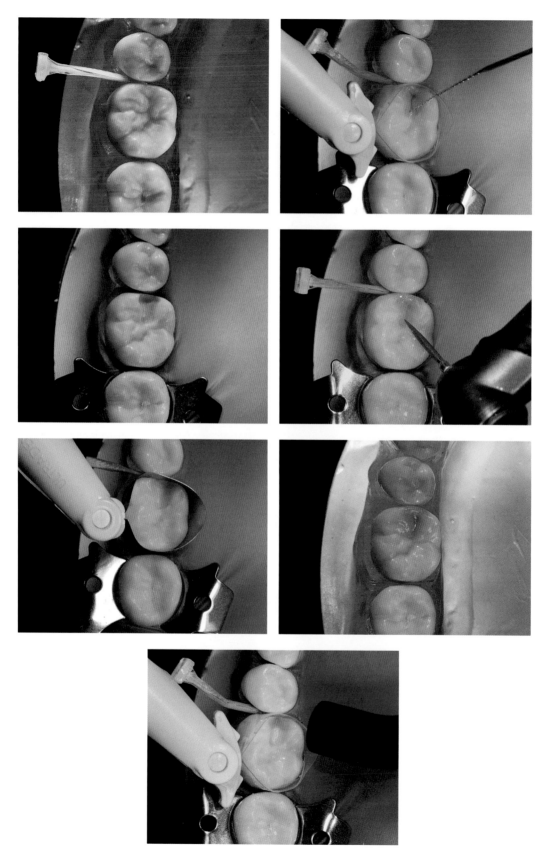

Figures 7.12–7.18 It is often easier to take a series of bench images with a consistent field of view for documenting a technique for didactic teaching, e.g. preparing and restoring a Class II cavity.

supporting the item(s) and acting as a background.[1] The table is readily adjusted to any height, the background changed to any colour and numerous flashes attached by brackets, clips and poles at any angle (Figure 7.19). The obvious advantage is that the photographic session is expedited with finesse, and the set-up is reusable for consistent and standardised images. This apparatus is also ideal for photographing a series of images showing a step-by-step technique. The drawbacks are that a macro studio contraption requires considerable space for the table, props and lighting, not to mention the additional financial outlay.

The second option is an improvised set-up, which is frugal, and somewhat tedious and time-consuming, but comes at a fraction of the cost. The essential items are a background which can either be suspended coloured cloths, cards, translucent Perspex* or a piece of black painted wood. If a piece of wood is used, various interchangeable coloured cards cut to size can be temporarily stuck onto the wood with reusable putty adhesive such as Blu-Tack* or Velcro*. The other items are reflective cards for fill-in reflectors, including a bench reflector of aluminium (kitchen) foil placed underneath the item to eliminate projection shadows. This set-up requires very little space, easily placed on worktops in a clinic or dental laboratory (Figure 7.20). The drawback is difficulty in obtaining standardised images, as most of the items are collated ad hoc. However, with a little patience this is overcome by marking positions of the background, lights and item to be photographed for consistent reproductions. Nevertheless, both professional and improvised set-ups yield equally satisfactory results, and the choice ultimately depends on available space, finances and perseverance.

For either set-up, it is preferable to mount the camera on a tripod and trigger it via a remote shutter release. This is advantageous for several reasons. First, it frees the hands for adjusting angles and positions of objects and playing with light. Second, it prevents camera shake if using continuous low-level illumination with long exposures, and third, for standardised images ensures the same framing (field of view), which is necessary for a series of shots documenting a particular technique.

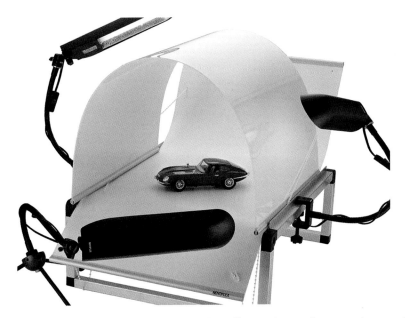

Figure 7.19 Professional still life table with ancillary equipment for macrophotography (MagicStudio, Novoflex, Germany).

---

1 https://www.novoflex.de/en/products-637/desktop-studio-magic-studio/magicstudio.html

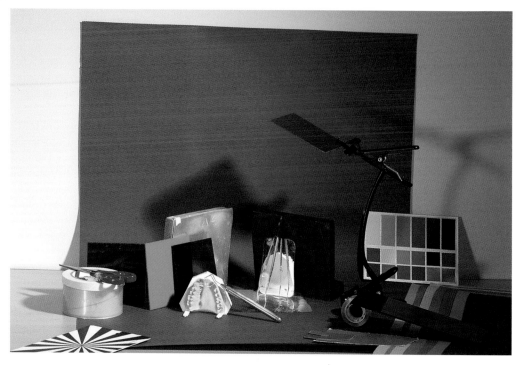

Figure 7.20 Improvised set-up for bench images, consisting of various coloured backgrounds, reflectors, mirror, Perspex sheets, clamps, grey card, etc., which can be tailored as necessary for a specific photograph.

The most frequently photographed objects are dental casts (models), which are usually mono-chromatic, bland and visually boring. Several techniques are employed for adding interest to the composition for attracting the attention of the viewer. The main item that adds interest is creative lighting (discussed below), which can make or break a picture. Another approach is adding col-our. This could be in the form of coloured lighting by covering flashes with gels, UV (ultra-violet) lamps, focused coloured beams of light (fibre-optic halogen, LED or lasers) or interesting col-oured and textured backdrops for enhancing colour contrast between the object and the back-ground. A further approach for enhancing figure-ground separation is selectively focusing on a specific items(s) or part of an item and throwing the surroundings out of focus (Figure 7.21).

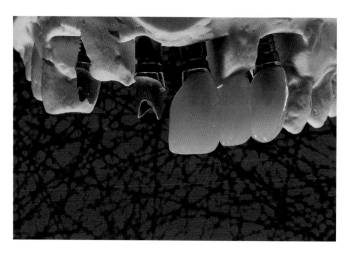

Figure 7.21 Selective focusing is an effective method for highlighting protagonist parts (enhancing figure-ground separation) while throwing the surroundings out of focus.

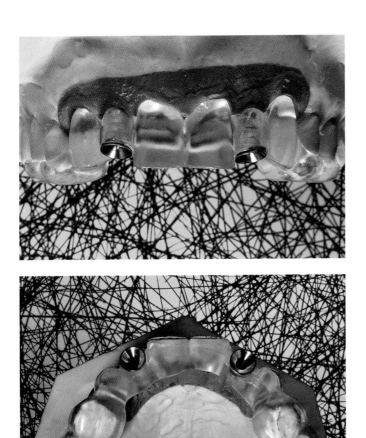

Figures 7.22 and 7.23 Although these two images using creative lighting have high visual impact, the entangled background distracts from the main item of interest, which is the surgical guide for placing two implants at the maxillary lateral incisor sites.

The choice of backgrounds is bewildering and daunting, but generally, light objects warrant darker backgrounds and vice versa for dark objects. The choice of colour also affects how an image is perceived, vivid colours are dynamic and create drama, whilst pale hues are placid, and convey serenity. It is also important that the background colour or texture is appropriate for a given object and harmonises with it. If the background is incongruous with the main subject, visual tension ensues causing rejection. Also, backgrounds should add interest, but at the same time not distract or overpower the main subject/object of interest (Figures 7.22 and 7.23).

Lighting

There are several choices of light sources for bench images, either flashes or continuous light. The flash options are studio flashes used for portraiture (Module 6) or twin bilateral compact flashes used for intra-oral views (Module 5). Ring flashes are not recommended as the light output produces flat, dull images. Since the objects to be photographed are relatively small, studio flashes are cumbersome, time-consuming to set up, and perhaps an overkill. The compact flashes are easily manoeuvred, but with a few provisos. First, compact flashes should be detachable so they can be hand-held, and second, the trigger mechanism is wireless to facilitate positioning at any angle without having to worry about trailing or tangling cables that interfere with the composition or are visible in the picture. Furthermore, if an improvised set-up is used, compact flashes are an ideal accompaniment, requiring little space and easy to manipulate. Another point to remember is that instead of splashing out on several flashes, still life photography offers the option of judicially using reflectors and mirrors to bounce light, which is both effective and economical.

Continuous light sources include incandescent or halogen Anglepoise® table lamps, fluorescent tubes, fibre-optic cables, HMI (hydrargyrum medium-arc iodide) or UV lamps (black lights). A continuous light source has the benefit of seeing the visual effect of shadows and highlights before taking a picture. However, the potential drawback with continuous light sources is that the camera must be mounted on a tripod if long exposures are anticipated, white balance must be carefully calibrated to avoid colour casts and the high cost if using HMI illumination. Other types of lights include fibre-optic cables that focus light to various size spots for special effects.

The basic principles of lighting discussed in Module 3, and for portraiture in Module 6, are also applicable for bench images. Directional lighting creates depth with shadows and highlights, emphasising texture and surface detail, whilst uniform illumination results in flat, two-dimensional bland images. One of the endearing aspects of bench photography is that time is not a concern, and the photographer is liberated by the constraints of clinical photography. Objects and lighting can be changed endlessly until the desired effect is attained. However, in a busy dental practice, this luxury may not be affordable for everyone, and therefore, it is prudent to have a set-up that is perpetually ready and accessible for expediting a bench image photographic session.

The position of the lights determines which parts of the object(s) are highlighted. Also, the flash ratio is discretional, but should be asymmetrical for achieving three-dimensional imagery. A single detachable flash is ideal for unidirectional illumination from various angles, such as from one side, above, below, behind or any angle in between. Placing flashes head-on creates a similar effect to a ring flash, and therefore should be avoided. When photographing a dental cast, either with or without restorations/appliances, placing the flash to one side emphasises surface texture, gingival architecture, gingival stippling, incisal embrasures and facial topography and lines angles (Figure 7.24). A flash placed below or above (depending on whether the maxillary or mandibular teeth are being photographed) highlights the free gingival margins, crown finish lines, incisal lobes and incisal edge chips or wear facets (Figure 7.25). Placing a flash behind transilluminates wax-ups or ceramic restorations revealing translucencies and characterisations of ceramic layering including mamelons and incisal halos, emphasises incisal edge morphology, and accentuation finish lines for detecting undercuts in tooth preparations (Figures 7.26 and 7.27). Finally, a bench reflector, e.g. aluminium foil, placed below models is ideal for filling in shadows from the key light on the lingual/palatal aspects of the teeth (Figure 7.28).

Bench Image Set-ups

Unlike standardised set-ups for extra-oral, intra-oral (EDP) and clinical portraiture (EPP) portfolios, it is difficult, or even impossible, to standardise bench images. Hence, the set-up for bench images is unique for a specific modality or discipline, and the intended purpose of the image, i.e. for clinical documentation or marketing and promotion. Also, the allocated space in a clinic or institution determines the type of set-up, which may be rudimentary or

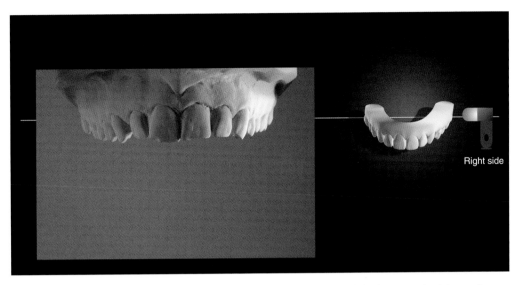

Figure 7.24 A single flash placed to one side creates distinct highlights and shadows, emphasising surface detail.

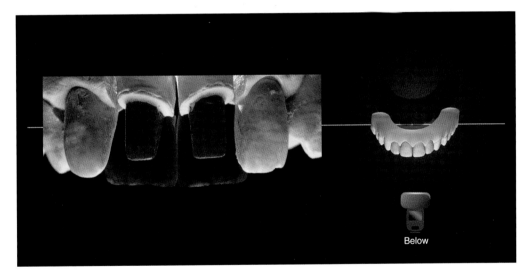

Figure 7.25 A single flash placed below (for maxillary teeth) is ideal for visualising crown preparation finish lines, free gingival margins and incisal lobes.

grandiose. Figure 7.29 shows the schematic for a generic bench image set-up, consisting of key light, fill light and reflectors, which can be reflective cards (white, silver, gold), foil, or an intra-oral or face mirror. A separate flash illuminates the backdrops, which are either cloth, paper, Perspex or bespoke scenery to complement the main object(s). A bench reflector, if required, is placed below the object to fill shadows. Alternately, a seamless surface (cloth, paper, plastic) can support the object as well as acting as a backdrop. Moreover, the generic set-up is a guide, which can be tailored by adding or omitting ancillary equipment/items for achieving the desired photographic effect.

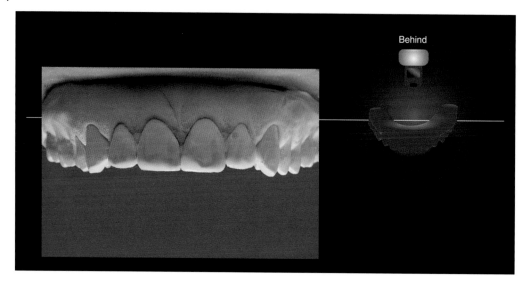

Figure 7.26 A single flash placed behind a dental cast highlights translucencies of diagnostic wax-ups.

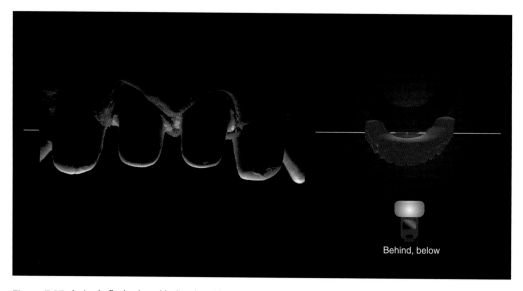

Figure 7.27 A single flash placed behind and below creates silhouettes of the teeth, which is particularly useful for detecting undercuts in tooth preparations.

Equipment Settings

The equipment settings are determined by the intended use of the images. If consistency and repeatability is paramount, the set-up is devised with constant settings and positions all concerned items. This is achieved by marking the position of the object and photographic equipment and any accessory items with a pen or adhesive masking tape. In addition, the flashes are supported by brackets and not hand-held, and all camera and flash settings are noted, or a user preset is created in the camera menu that can be recalled for a specific type of image. Table 7.1 summarises settings and guidelines for bench image.

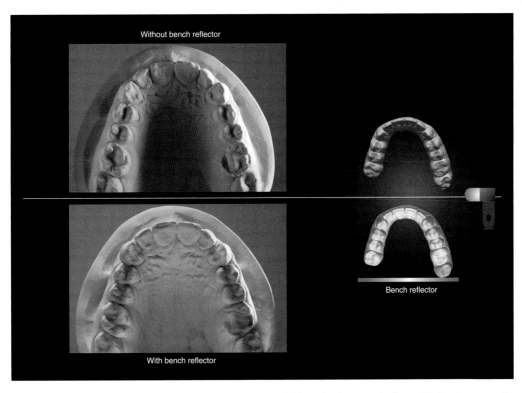

Without bench reflector
Bench reflector
With bench reflector

Figure 7.28 A bench reflector placed underneath the model fills in shadows on the lingual/palatal aspects of the teeth.

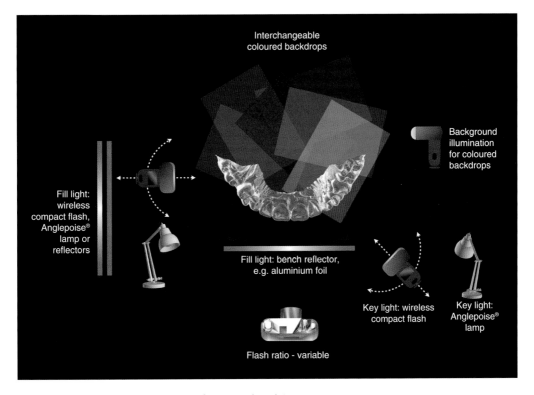

Figure 7.29 Schematic representation of a generic bench image set-up.

Table 7.1 Settings and guidelines for bench image set-ups.

Item	Setting/description	Notes
Focus	Manual or auto-focus	
Exposure metering	Manual or TTL	Manual: histogram or take a few test shots to ascertain correct exposure
ISO	50–200	
Aperture	Any, depending on the the desired effect. For standardised images use $f22$	For selective focusing on a specific part of an object(s), $f4$ is a good starting point
Shutter speed	1/125 s or 1/250 s	Flash synchronisation speed depends on a specific camera brand
Image data format (file format)	RAW or DNG	
White balance	Automatic or manual	Manual: numerical value input, or take a reference image with an 18% neutral density grey card
Flash/continuous light	Flash: detachable, wireless flashes (single or bilateral)	Single flash: alter distance or intensity for correct exposure
	Continues light sources: halogen, fluorescent, LED, laser, HMI, UV	Bilateral flashes: adjust fill light: key light ratio to 1 : 2. If images are too bright or too dark, alter intensity of flashes, or move flashes closer or further away until correct exposure is achieved
		Continuous light: use slow shutter speeds, ensure camera is tripod-mounted
Magnification factor	1 : 1 to 1 : 3 (depends on size of object(s))	Only relevant for full-frame sensors, or set predefined focusing distance on lens, or see below for field of view
Point of focus (PoF)	Variable, depending on object(s) and desired effect	Hand-held cameras: for predefined magnification or focusing distance, move camera backwards and forwards until focus is obtained
		Tripod-mounted camera: for predefined magnification or focusing distance use macro stage for focusing
		If using auto-focus, ensue that lens axis is centred on point of focus
Field of view (composition)	Use rule of thirds, leading lines, diagonal and converging lines, visual weight, balance, Golden Proportion, dominance, figure-ground	Experiment by breaking rules for unique and interesting images
Background	Black or any colour depending on desired effect	Velvet cloth, e.g. black, cards, translucent Perspex, plastic, or textured/coloured backdrops

The examples below illustrate some examples of set-ups for bench images, which can be tailored for specific needs.

Dental Casts (Models) with Black Background

The first set-up is useful for photographing plaster casts or 3D-printed models, e.g. before, during and after orthodontic treatment, or for any modality that requires documentation of models for analysis, treatment planning and monitoring. A black background is chosen to complement the relatively insipid models, whilst equipment settings and positions are noted for ensuring consistency. The black backdrop can be black velvet cloth, card or a painted wood block.

The object to be photographed is placed in front or on top of the background with a bench reflector (e.g. aluminium foil) underneath to fill in shadows on the lingual or palatal aspects of the arch. The recommended lighting is either continuous light from an Anglepoise lamp, twin bilateral flash configuration (similar for taking intra-oral pictures), which should be mounted on bracket below the camera. Instead of using two flashes, a single flash and a reflector judicially placed on the opposite produces the same result. Ring flashes are contraindicated as they render a dull image devoid of shadows and highlights that and obliterates fine detail. A continuous light source offers the advantage of visualising the lighting effect before taking the picture, but the drawback is that a slower shutter speed is required due to the relatively low-level light output. (Figures 7.30 and 7.31).

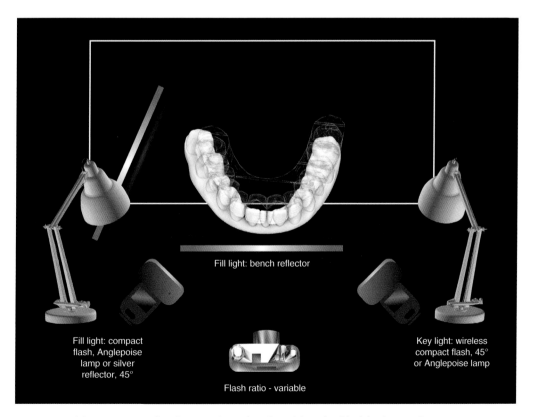

Fill light: bench reflector

Fill light: compact flash, Anglepoise lamp or silver reflector, 45°

Flash ratio - variable

Key light: wireless compact flash, 45° or Anglepoise lamp

Figure 7.30 Schematic set-up for photographing dental models with a black background.

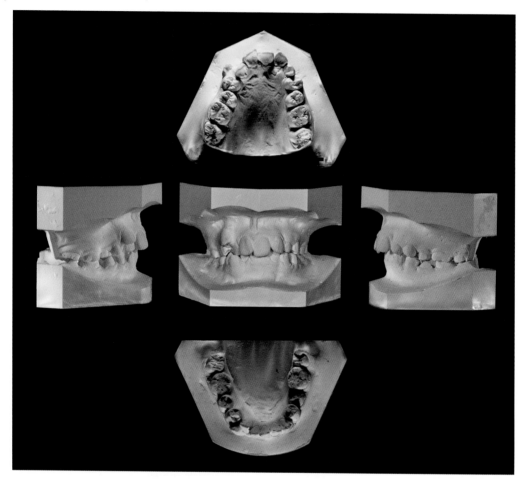

Figure 7.31 Plaster casts photographed with the set-up shown in Figure 7.30.

Dental Cast with Coloured Background

Colour adds interest to a composition, especially for achromatic objects. However, colour should be used carefully. If the object itself is colourful, a black or white background is more appropriate, rather than a coloured background that causes visual chaos. Conversely, monochromatic items benefit from a textured or colourful backgrounds by counterbalancing bland objects. This bench set-up uses a lilac background with the key flash positioned above. An overhead light is ideal for highlighting the incisal edges, and clearly visualising tooth surface loss (TSL) or tooth wear. Since a coloured backdrop is placed behind the object, background illumination is required to avoid projection shadows, which also creates visual separation of the object from its surroundings, giving an enhanced figure-ground appearance (Figures 7.32–7.34).

Implant Supported Temporary Crown with Red Background

Photographing individual items such as artificial restorations usually require various angles of view to capture different aspects of the prosthesis. This is accomplished by placing the item on the bench and then altering its position to capture various views. Alternately, small items are best held in

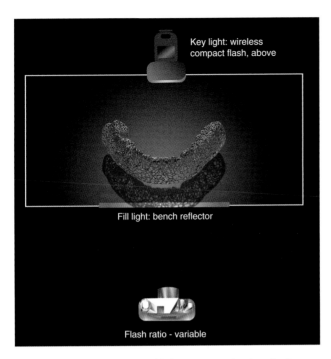

Key light: wireless compact flash, above

Fill light: bench reflector

Flash ratio - variable

Figure 7.32 A single overhead light causes projection shadows onto a coloured background, which is avoided by…

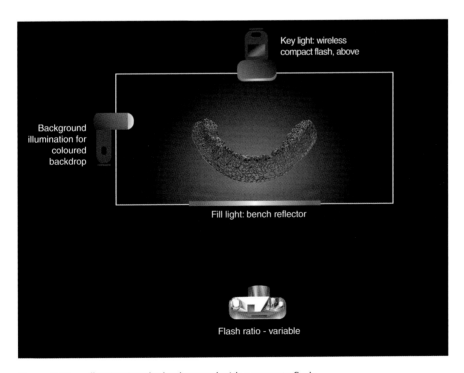

Key light: wireless compact flash, above

Background illumination for coloured backdrop

Fill light: bench reflector

Flash ratio - variable

Figure 7.33 …illuminating the background with a separate flash.

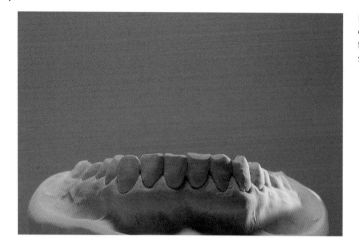

Figure 7.34 Mandibular plaster cast showing incisal edge wear facets, photographed with the set-up shown in Figure 7.33.

tweezers or Spencer Wells forceps and turned around to show different aspects of the restoration. In this case implant supported temporary crown was secured with an implant screwdriver, which was grasped with dental tweezers. Several angles were photographed using the following set-up. Highly reflective stainless steel items rely on specular reflections to highlight their shiny surfaces. Therefore, several flashes, combined with shiny silver reflectors, are used to maximise specular surface reflections. Two flashes are needed, one overhead and the second to one side, whilst the reflectors are placed underneath and to the contralateral side to bounce light back onto the metal surfaces. The red background is lit separately with a third flash (Figures 7.35 and 7.36).

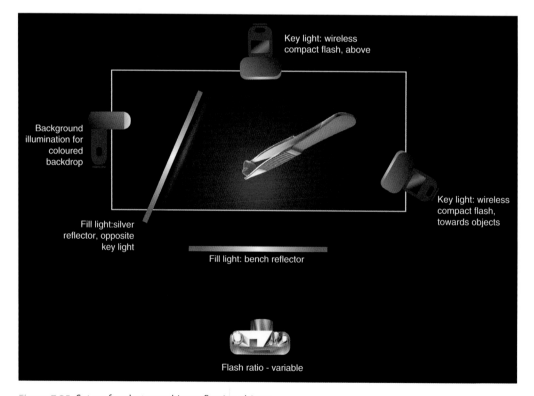

Figure 7.35 Set-up for photographing reflective objects.

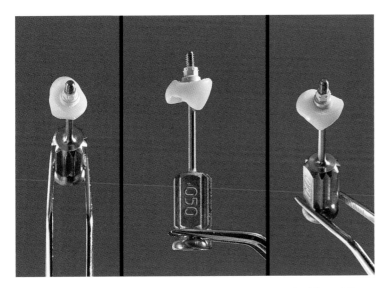

Figure 7.36 Implant supported temporary crown photographed from different angles of view using the set-up shown in Figure 7.35.

Perspex Backgrounds

Another method for creating dynamic images with colour is using translucent Perspex sheets. Perspex sheets are available in various colours from art and craft or hobbyist suppliers, who can cut the sheets to the appropriate dimensions depending on the size of the object to be photographed. The sheet acts as a background and a key flash is placed behind the Perspex to create a spectacular glow of colour. For solid objects the effect is a silhouette, whilst for translucent items such as vacuum stents or surgical guides, the effect is a semi-silhouette that highlights intricate details. The flashes are positioned carefully to be perpendicular to the lens axis to avoid projections shadows (Figure 7.37). In addition, the coloured glow can be manipulated to produce either uniform illumination, or a vignetting effect, that is centralised or located at the top, bottom, right, left, or anywhere on the background with a seamless transition, depending on the position and distance of the rear flash (Figure 7.38). The set-up for this composition is shown in Figure 7.39 and the resulting image in Figure 7.40.

If a silhouette effect is not required, the item can be directly illuminated by another key light with a fill light to fill in the shadows. This approach combines the coloured glow background of the Perspex sheet as well as correctly illuminating the main item(s). The second key light is placed to one side so as not to point the light directly onto the item, as this causes unwanted reflections in the Perspex sheet. The set-up is shown in Figure 7.41 and the resulting photograph in Figure 7.42 shows the same surgical guide as in Figure 7.40, captured in a different light. Another example using this set-up is shown in Figure 7.43.

A variation of the above set-up is using two Perspex sheets with different opacities (or colours), which creates an abrupt transition of colour. In addition to the key flash located behind the sheets, another key flash is placed below to highlight the crown preparation finish lines or incisal edges of artificial restorations. To complete the set-up, two silver reflections on both sides of the 3D-printed models act as fill lights to illuminate the sides of the model (Figures 7.44–7.46).

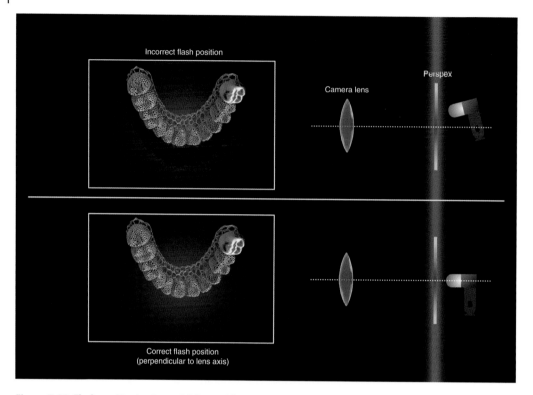

Figure 7.37 Flash positioning is crucial for avoiding unwanted projection shadows.

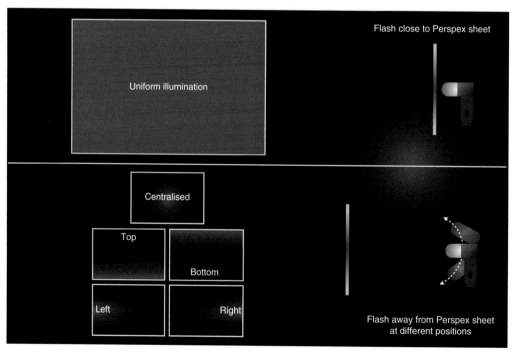

Figure 7.38 The location and type of coloured glow depends on the distance and location of the rear flash.

Figure 7.39 Set-up for Perspex background with a single key light flash.

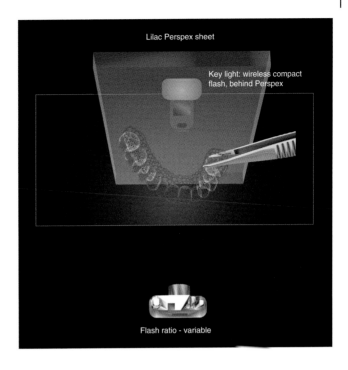

Figure 7.40 3D-printed surgical guide for implants photographed using the set-up shown in Figure 7.39.

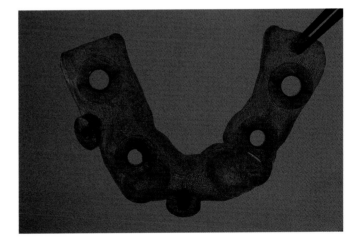

Bokeh Composition

Bokeh is the manner in which a lens captures out of focus, or blurs, point light sources. The shape of the Bokeh is an inherent property of the lens and is determined by the shape and degree of opening of the aperture diaphragm. The shape of the polygon Bokeh is created by the diaphragm leaves, e.g. pentagon or heptagon, but can also be a perfect circle. The effect adds a magical twinkle appearance in the background as blurred dots of lights, whilst the subject is sharply focused in the foreground. The set-up consists of a foil placed behind the object, with a key flash above and behind to transilluminate the translucent/transparent object, while

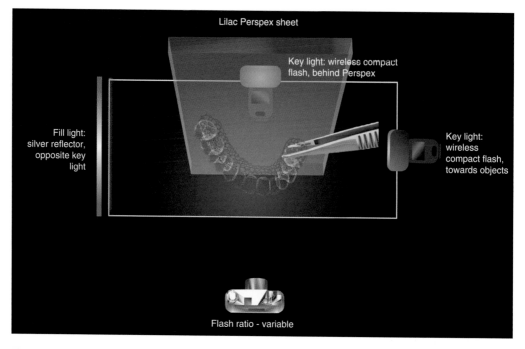

Lilac Perspex sheet

Key light: wireless compact
flash, behind Perspex

Fill light:
silver reflector,
opposite key
light

Key light:
wireless
compact flash,
towards objects

Flash ratio - variable

Figure 7.41 Set-up for Perspex background with a key light flash behind the Perspex and another key light and fill light to directly illuminate the 3D-printed surgical guide.

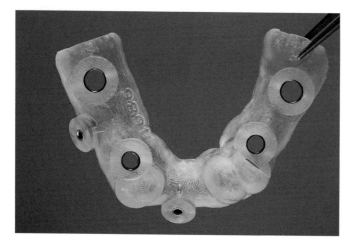

Figure 7.42 3D-printed surgical guide for implants photographed using the set-up shown in Figure 7.41.

another flash is angled to create point specula reflections off the foil surface. The distance between the foil and flash is varied until the desired bokeh is obtained (Figures 7.47–7.48).

Stroboscopic Effect

The stroboscopic effect is a method of freezing movement of an object or subject as it traverses across the frame, analogous to stop-motion images. It is useful for illustrating moment, or simply creating a stylish image for captivating an audience. This is a creative effect involving as

Figure 7.43 3D-printed maxillary model with a thermoformed transparent guide for aesthetic crown lengthening of the maxillary anterior sextant using the set-up shown in Figure 7.41.

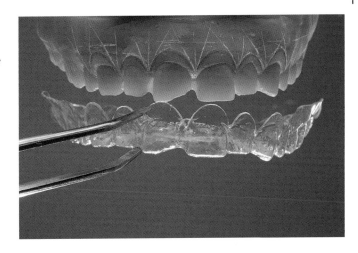

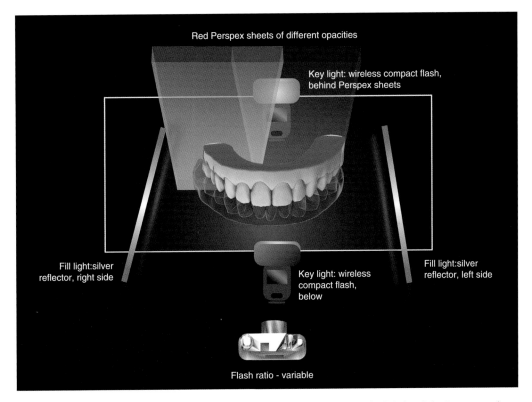

Figure 7.44 Set-up with two Perspex sheets of different opacities, a key light flash behind the Perspex and another below, plus two silver reflectors as fill lights.

many as 40 flash burst/second, far greater than taking successive multiple shots that are limited to usually 10 frames/second.

The effect is possible with both studio and compact flashes by selecting the 'Strobo' mode in the menu. Most contemporary flashes offer this option as standard, but lower spec flashes may not have this facility. There are three variables to consider: the power or duration of output, the number of flashes and the frequency of the flashes (flashes/second), expressed in Hertz (Hz).

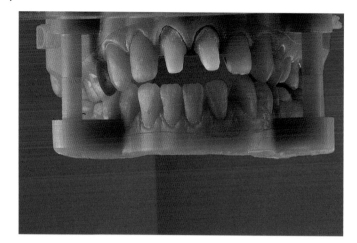

Figure 7.45 3D-printed models highlighting the crown preparation margins on the maxillary central incisors using the set-up shown in Figure 7.44.

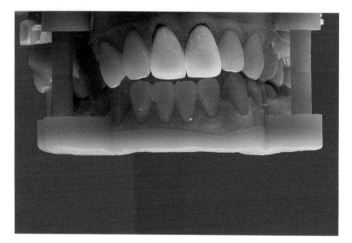

Figure 7.46 3D-printed models highlighting the incisal edges of the e-max* all-ceramic crowns on the maxillary central incisors using the set-up shown in Figure 7.44.

The intensity or output of a flash is determined by its duration – a faster duration means less power, but a greater number of flashes that can be fired per second, i.e. a faster burst rate. The three variables are interlinked, and a little experimentation is required to achieve optimal results. For example, if the power (duration) is reduced to 1/128, frequency set at 20 Hz and number of flash count set to 10, the shutter speed is calculated as follows:

$$\text{Shutter speed} = \text{number of flashes} / \text{frequency} \, (\text{Hz})$$

In the illustration above, this would mean a shutter speed of 0.5 second. However, the exposure is also influenced by the ISO and *f*-stop, which need to be adjusted accordingly. Once the flash(es) and camera are configured, the set-up is fairly straightforward. The key flash is placed on one side and fill-in reflectors on the opposite side and bottom or top of the object. A black background is ideal, preferably in a darkened room to avoid blurring of motion due to stray ambient light. Also, it is essential to mount the camera on a tripod to prevent camera shake. Figure 7.49 shows the set-up for a stroboscopic effect and examples of three images are shown in Figures 7.50–7.52.

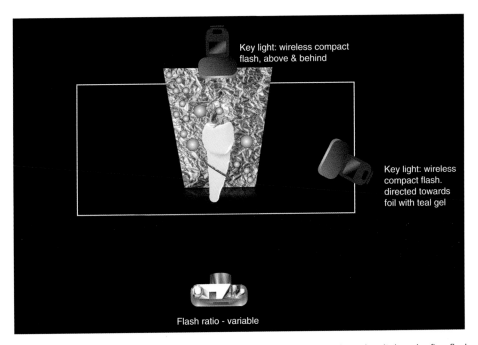

Key light: wireless compact flash, above & behind

Key light: wireless compact flash. directed towards foil with teal gel

Flash ratio - variable

Figure 7.47 Set-up for a Bokeh composition with a foil background and two key lights, the first flash placed above and behind, and a second flash directed towards the foil.

Figure 7.48 Bokeh composition: fractured ceramic crown on fractured tooth photographed with the set-up shown in Figure 7.47.

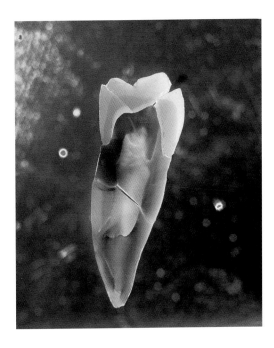

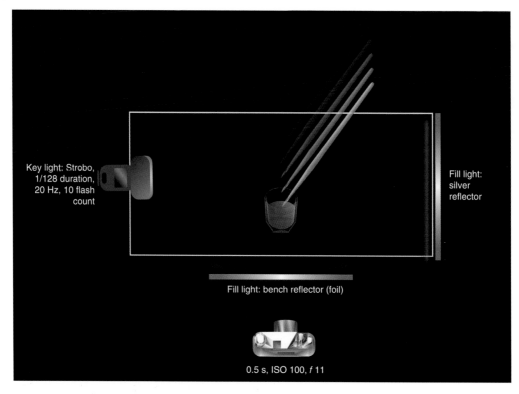

Key light: Strobo,
1/128 duration,
20 Hz, 10 flash
count

Fill light:
silver
reflector

Fill light: bench reflector (foil)

0.5 s, ISO 100, *f* 11

Figure 7.49 Stroboscopic effect set-up.

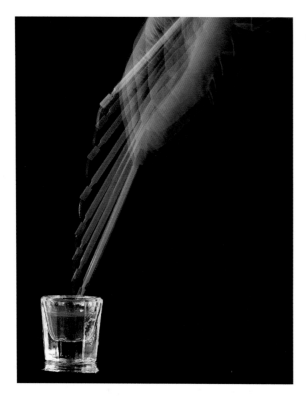

Figure 7.50 Stroboscopic effect with the set-up described in Figure 7.49 showing a brush being dipped into a plaque disclosing liquid in a dappen dish.

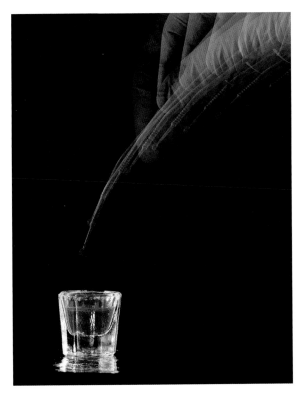

Figure 7.51 Stroboscopic effect with the set-up described in Figure 7.49 showing a micro-brush being dipped into a plaque disclosing liquid in a dappen dish.

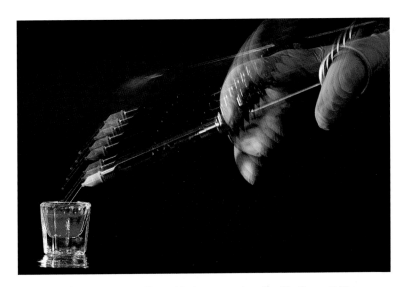

Figure 7.52 Stroboscopic effect with the set-up described in Figure 7.49.

Reference

Ahmad, I. (2009). Digital dental photography. Part 7: extra-oral set-ups. *Br. Dent. J.* 207 (3): 103–110.

8

Special Applications

The special applications presented in this module are advanced principles for maximising the full potential of digital dental photography. These include taking additional images for elucidating certain features, or analysing images for effective communicating with patients and fellow colleagues. Whilst the essential dental portfolio (EDP), essential portrait portfolio (EPP) and optional images discussed in previous modules are sufficient for most modalities, some procedures require specific types of imagery for multi-diagnosis and facilitating collaborative care. Also, the topics covered in this module are more demanding than routine dental photography, require extra equipment and specialised training to become fully conversant with these techniques.

Detailed Analysis of Hard and Soft Tissues

A good standard of practice for dental photodocumentation is the obligatory nine EDP, combined with the seven EPP, plus selective optional images depending on the needs of the given speciality. However, these standardised images may not 'tell the whole story', and additional photographs are necessary to complete the story. Therefore, the photographic set-ups need to be modified for capturing salient features for detailed evaluation. This involves minor recalibration of camera and light settings, but the main difference is the positioning of the patient and photographic equipment for visualising pertinent points of interest.

The major problem with analysing dentine and enamel is that natural teeth have an anisotropic structure. The outer enamel layer is highly reflective, encouraging specular reflections that obscure the underlying characterisations within the teeth. However, specular reflections (glare) off the surface are ideal for assessing micro and macromorphology, texture and lustre of the outer enamel layer. In order to visualise tooth characterisations, light needs to pass through the tooth rather than be reflected off its surface. Hence, it is difficult to simultaneously visualise texture and characterisations, and two different types of illumination are necessary for discerning each of these entities. This usually entails taking two separate pictures with different lighting for the right and left sides of an arch; one side to visualise texture, and the other side to visualise characterisation of the enamel and dentine strata.

In order to encourage specular reflections, a single unidirectional flash (key light) is placed on one side, and a reflector on the opposite side to bounce light back to fill in the shadows. The key light is muted by a diffuser to attenuate its harsh output. The reflectors can either be a silver or white card, the former produces a cooler light, while the latter reflects a more neutral light. On the key light side, the light is essentially hard and unidirectional that encourages specular reflections, while on the contralateral reflector side the light is diffuse and softer that facilitates

Essentials of Dental Photography, First Edition. Irfan Ahmad.
© 2020 John Wiley & Sons Ltd. Published 2020 by John Wiley & Sons Ltd.

transmission through the tooth. In addition, changing the position of the key light and reflectors alters the locations of the highlights and shadows, allowing subtle nuances of the dentogingival elements to be visualised (Figure 8.1). Furthermore, the highlights and shadows produced with this set-up create images that are three dimensional for conveying depth, and full of detail for analysing dentogingival anatomy. On the key light side the following are clearly discernible, the macro and micromorphology of enamel, including facial undulations (Figure 8.2), incisal lobes, incise edge wear, chips (Figure 8.3), fractures, perikymata (Figure 8.4), surface

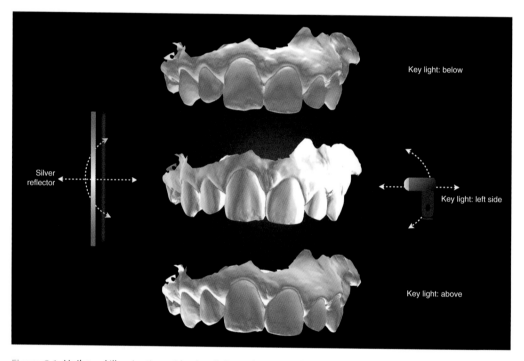

Figure 8.1 Unilateral illumination with a key light and a silver reflector on the contralateral side to diminish, but not eliminate shadows. Alerting the positions of the key light and reflector changes the location of highlights and shadows.

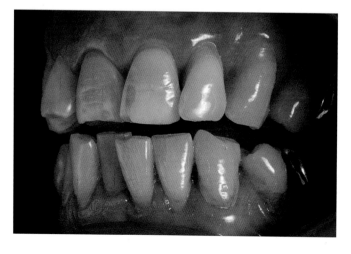

Figure 8.2 Macromorphology: facial undulations.

Figure 8.3 Serrated incisal edge tooth wear.

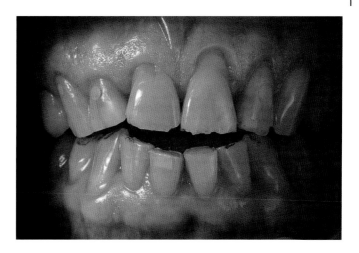

Figure 8.4 Perikymata and incisal edge lobes.

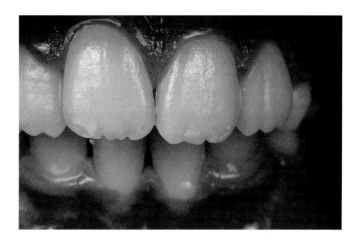

irregularities as well as texture and lustre. In addition, the specular reflections also emphasise soft tissue topography such as peaks and troughs of the gingival architecture, presence or absence of gingival stippling, gingival clefts, frenal attachments, demarkation of the free gingival margins, and assessment of periodontal biotypes (thick, thin) and periodontal bioforms (flat, normal, scalloped). Also, as unidirectional light stresses edges, defective filling or crown margins are more noticeable (Figures 8.5 and 8.6). Finally, the interproximal shadows are conducive for revealing gingival embrasures or 'black triangles' (Figure 8.7).

On the opposite reflector side, the light is transmitted through the tooth to reveal characterisations. The diffuse light is ideal for visualising incisal and interproximal translucencies, dentine mamelons, incisal halos, secondary or sclerotic dentine, islands of hypocalcification (Figure 8.8) and physiological or traumatic fracture lines (Figure 8.9). A black contraster placed behind the teeth further emphasises translucencies, but exposure compensation is required, especially if using TTL metering. Also, optical properties such as goniochromism of natural teeth and composite fillings are clearly visible. The latter is particularly relevant when matching composite shades to natural teeth so that the restorative material has a similar translucency parameter as dentine and enamel. This avoids conspicuous composite fillings, which may

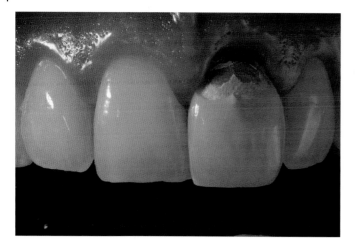

Figure 8.5 Delaminated veneering porcelain exposing the opaque and metal layers of a porcelain fused to metal crown on the left maxillary central incisor.

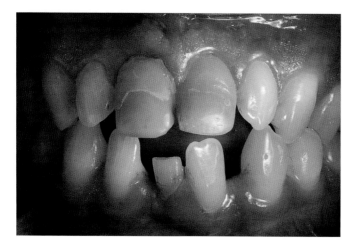

Figure 8.6 Directional lighting highlighting the defective restoration in the maxillary right central incisor that is impinging and inflaming the gingival margin.

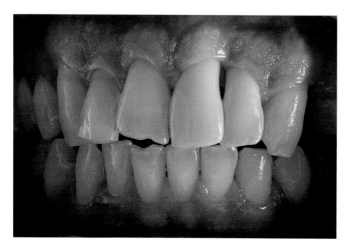

Figure 8.7 Selective lighting highlighting the pronounced gingival embrasure between the left maxillary central and lateral incisors.

Figure 8.8 Island of hypocalcification within the enamel layer.

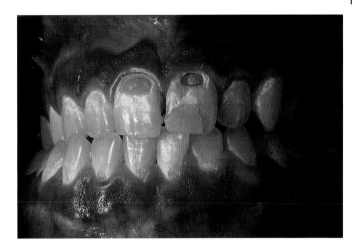

Figure 8.9 Diffuse light created by a silver reflector on the left side of the patient emphasises the characterisation within the left maxillary central incisor, including internal fracture lines, dentine striations and defective composite restorations.

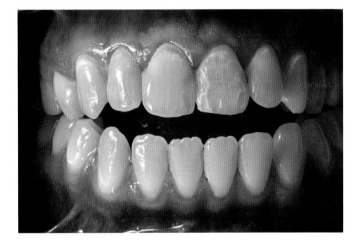

appear too opaque or too translucent, failing to blend with the surrounding tooth substate (Ryan et al. 2010).

The photographic set-up for achieving unidirectional lighting is a modified version of EDP Image #5 (Module 5), but with a higher flash ratio. The images can either be dento-facial, intra-oral of the entire arch, or a few teeth or areas of soft tissue that require scrutiny. The magnification ratio is variable ranging from 1 : 2 to 1 : 1, depending on the shape and size of the lips, arches and teeth, and therefore it is difficult to specify the exact positions of the patient, camera, key light and reflector. The best approach is to take a series of images until the desired features are captured either by altering the angles of the flash/reflector, the patient, the camera, or a combination of all three (Figure 8.10). A ring flash can be used if it has the facility to turn off the right or left flash tubes for achieving unidirectional lighting. However, compared to a detachable unilateral flash, a ring flash does not allow the flexibility in positioning as it is usually fixed onto the front of the lens. The salient guidelines for detailed analysis of hard and soft tissues images are summarised in Table 8.1.

In order to demonstrate detailed analysis of hard and soft tissues, the case study below shows replacement of defective composite restorations in the maxillary sextant. The photographic set-up uses a single compact flash as the key light on one side, which alternates from the right

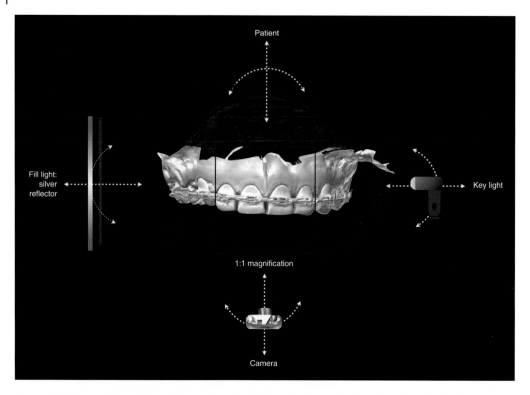

Figure 8.10 The position of the patient, camera, key light and reflector is altered until the desired features are captured. At a 1 : 1 magnification, the field of view is approximately the four maxillary incisors.

to left with a silver reflector on the opposite side. The set-up yields a flash ratio of the key light: silver reflector of approximately 1 : 4, but varies depending on the intensity of the light output and the angle and proximity of the reflector to the compact flash. A pre-operative reference shot is taken with uniform illumination using a ring flash (flash ratio of 1 : 1) that produces a flat, two-dimensional image (Figure 8.11). The subsequent images were taken using a key light and silver reflector (fill light), alternating the flash and reflector on the right and left sides. The side of the key light produces hard lighting, while the reflector side produces soft lighting (Figures 8.12 and 8.13). This set-up creates images that display depth and three-dimensional quality for clearer analysis. On the key light side the edges of defective filling margins, perikymata, enamel texture and gingival stippling are emphasised, while on the reflector side, characterisation within the teeth are more noticeable such as decay, translucencies and hypocalcification. (Figures 8.14 and 8.15). Also, altering the field of view by increasing the magnification factor to 1 : 1, altering the position of the patient's head, the camera, key light and reflector to various angles reveals subtle nuances that can be studied in detail (Figures 8.16 and 8.17). After replacing the defective restorations, the post-operative images are taken using a similar set-up to the pre-operative pictures to show salient features by altering illumination on the right and left sides (Figures 8.18–8.20).

Opalescence and Fluorescence

There are two further optical properties of teeth that require special lighting for visualisation: opalescence and fluorescence. Opalescence is the optical property of an object to appear bluish

Table 8.1 Settings and guidelines for detailed analysis images.

Item	Setting/description	Notes
Focus	Manual	
Exposure metering	TTL or manual	Manual: take a few test shots to ascertain correct exposure or use histogram
ISO	50–200	
Aperture	f22	
Shutter speed	1/125 s or 1/250 s	Flash synchronisation speed depends on a specific camera brand
Image data format (file format)	RAW or DNG	
White balance	Automatic or manual	Manual: numerical value input, or take a reference image with an 18% neutral density grey card
Flash	Single unilateral flash or ring flash on one side and a silver or white reflector on the opposite side. The flash ratio should be greater than 1 : 2	Unilateral flash: with diffuser, reduce intensity to 1/2 or 1/4 Ring flash: turn off right or left side flash tubes If images are too bright or too dark, alter intensity of flashes, or move flash closer or further away until correct exposure is achieved
Magnification factor	1:2 to 1 : 1	Only relevant for full-frame sensors, or set predefined focusing distance on lens
Point of focus (POF)	On selected teeth or point of interest	Hand-held cameras: for predefined magnification or focusing distance, move camera backwards and forwards until focus is obtained Tripod-mounted camera: for predefined magnification or focusing distance use macro stage for focusing
Field of view (composition)	Centre of frame	At 1 · 1 magnification with full frame sensor cameras, the field of view approximately frames the four maxillary incisors
Background	Black contraster or oral cavity	For black contraster with TTL metering: exposure compensation required by either increasing 1 f-stop (smaller aperture), or moving the light source further away

with reflected light and amber with transmitted light. Natural enamel possesses opalescence, rendering a bluish appearance with reflected light, and an amber glow with transmitted light, particularly at the incisal edges where the enamel layer is thickest. Many aesthetic dental restorative materials, such as ceramics and composites, also mimic this property for emulating natural enamel. The second optical property, fluorescence, is primarily a feature of dentine that confers vitality to a tooth. A metarmeric fluorescent artificial restoration often is conspicuous under ultra-violet (UV) illumination, which is prevalent in night clubs or discos. Also, restorations with a brighter shade usually have greater fluorescent emissions, whereas the opposite is true for darker shades.

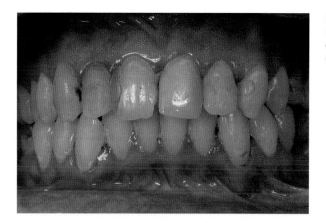

Figure 8.11 Uniform illumination using a ring flash with a 1 : 1 flash ratio that creates a flat, two-dimensional image (pre-operative status).

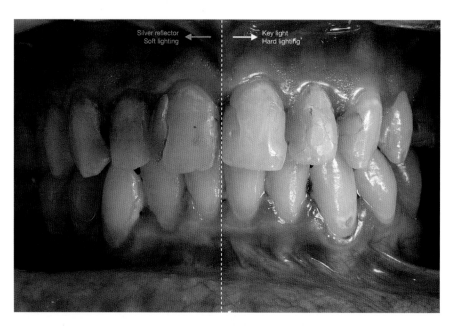

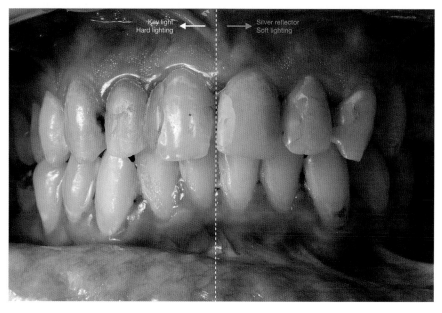

Figures 8.12 and 8.13 Hard and soft lighting with flash and silver reflector, respectively.

Figure 8.14 Hard (left side of patient) and soft lighting (right side of patient) – pre-operative image appears dynamic and three-dimensional, compared to Figure 8.11. The specular reflections are limited to the left side corresponding to the key light, while on the right side the diffuse light is created by a silver reflector.

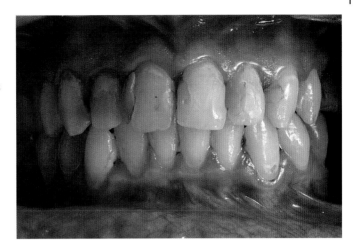

Figure 8.15 Hard (right side of patient) and soft lighting (left side of patient) – pre-operative image appears dynamic and three-dimensional, compared to Figure 8.11. The key light and silver reflector are reversed from right to left side of the patient, respectively.

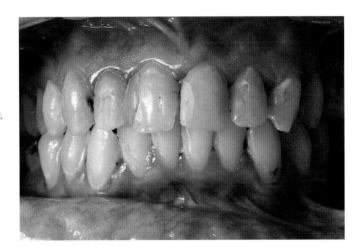

In order to photograph opalescence and fluorescence requires using specific continuous light sources that often have low intensity. Hence, a large aperture, or slow shutter speeds are necessary for ensuring sufficient illumination for correct exposure. Since a large aperture compromises depth of field (DoF), a slower shutter speed is the better option, but with the proviso that the camera is secured on a tripod and assuming the patient stays still to prevent blurred images. However, with bench images of still objects, longer shutter speeds are less problematic. For capturing intra-oral opalescence, a fibre-optic light is placed behind the incisal third of the tooth at various angles to record the amber glow or orange shinning from the enamel (Figures 8.21 and 8.22). For intra-oral fluorescent images, UV lamp(s) are judicially positioned so that they do not appear in the picture, and the patient and all dental personnel wear tinted safety glasses for protection from UV radiation. As well as recording fluorescence of dentine, UV illumination is also useful for detecting early carious lesions, ascertaining the depth of dental fluorosis lesions, extent of intrinsic staining, porosity in artificial restorations and visualising plaque biofilm accumulation with disclosing tablets or liquids (Figures 8.23 and 8.24).

The equipment required for generating fibre-optic and UV illumination is discussed below, followed by photographic set-ups for capturing opalescence and fluorescent of artificial restorations or extracted teeth.

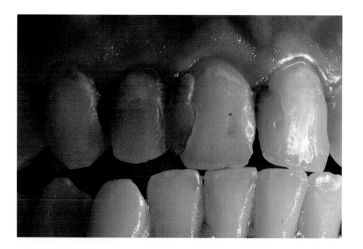

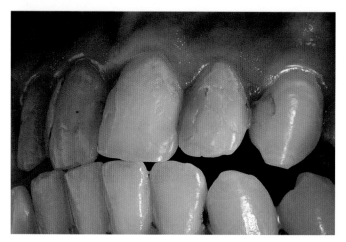

Figures 8.16 and 8.17 Increasing the magnification to 1 : 1 and altering the position of the patient, camera or lighting reveals further nuances of the dentogingival anatomy for a detailed analysis.

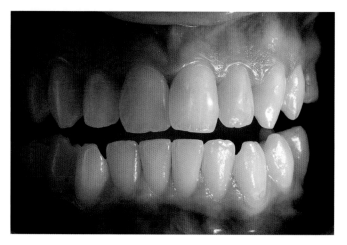

Figure 8.18 Hard (left side of patient) and soft lighting (right side of patient) – post-operative image showing replacement composite restorations. The specular reflections from hard lighting on the left emphasises the free gingival margins, gingival stippling, surface texture and lustre of enamel, incisal edges and perikymata. On the opposite side, soft lighting emphasises colour nuances within the teeth, hypocalcification islands and incisal translucencies. Also, notice the outline of the distal composite filling in the maxillary right central incisor which appears more translucent compared to the surrounding tooth substate. However, in the next image, the filling is almost inconspicuous as specular reflections conceal the filling outline. This phenomenon is termed goniochromism, i.e. the property of a material to appear different when the angle of view or illumination is altered.

Figure 8.19 Hard (right side of patient) and soft lighting (left side of patient) – post-operative image showing replacement of defective composite restorations. The key light and silver reflector are reversed from right to left side of the patient, respectively. Notice that the distal composite filling in the maxillary right central incisor is camouflaged by specular reflections.

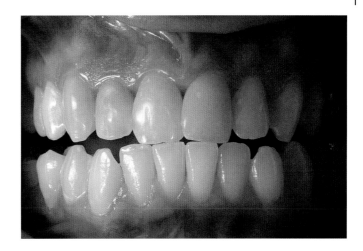

Figure 8.20 Magnified post-operative view with the key light on the right side of the patient. The specular reflections emphasise the free gingival margin, gingival architecture and stippling, facial undulations on the maxillary right central incisor, and perikymata on the mandibular teeth. On the left side of the patient (softer lighting), the incisal edge translucencies of the maxillary left central and lateral incisors are clearly visible (compare with image Figure 8.17).

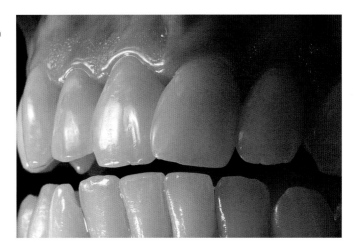

Figure 8.21 Intra-oral fibre-optic transillumination allows visualisation of enamel translucencies and incisal halos.

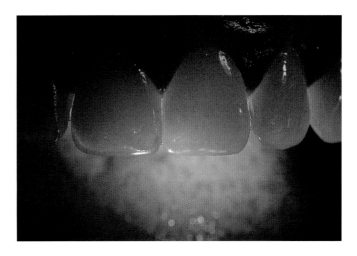

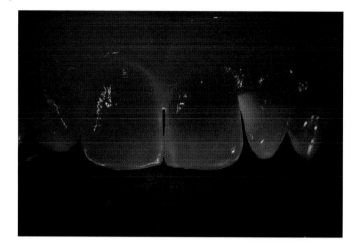

Figure 8.22 Changing the angle of intra-oral fibre-optic transillumination reveals the orange glow reminiscent of opalescence located at the incisal edges where the enamel layer is thickest.

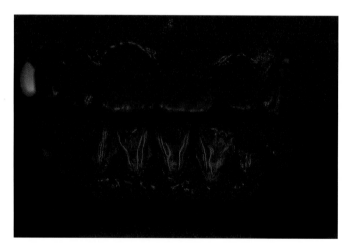

Figure 8.23 Ultra-violet (UV) illumination showing metarmeric fluorescence of artificial restorations that fail to optically integrate with the surrounding natural dentition.

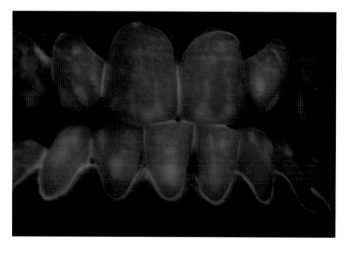

Figure 8.24 Ultra-violet (UV) illumination for visualising plaque biofilm after rinsing with a disclosing agent.

Fibre-Optic Illumination

Fibre-optic light sources are a special type of illumination for highlighting certain details, or for unique photographic effects. Fibre-optic light is delivered by flexible encased cables containing bundles of minute light transmitting fibres. The continuous light is generated by either halogen, LED or lasers, and the intensity is alterable by a rheostat, e.g. Kaiser Macrospot 1500 Fiber-Optic Lighting System (Kaiser, Germany) – Figure 8.25. The dental applications of fibre-optic illumination are intra-oral transillumination for showing dentine and enamel characterisation, carious lesion, enamel porosity or depth of fluorotic or hypocalcified lesions. The extra-oral uses include selectively illuminating certain parts of extracted teeth and artificial restorations, or discerning fine details of dental instruments. Furthermore, the orange glow of natural enamel at the incisal edges due to opalescence is clearly visualised with fibre-optic transillumination. A simple set-up is transilluminating all-ceramic units by placing a single fibre-optic light source behind and towards the camera, making sure that it is not visible in the picture. An optional second flash with a coloured gel illuminates the background to add interest by colour contrast with the main object (Figures 8.26 and 8.27).

UV Illumination

The ability of an object to emit light when illuminated with an UV light source is termed fluorescence. Fluorescence is an inherent property of dentin, and to a lesser extent enamel. Also, certain pathology such as pre-cancerous or early carious lesions are easier to detect with UV light. In the natural dentition, fluorescence confers vitality, and many restorative materials such as ceramics and resin-based composites emulate this feature (Ahmad and Chu 2003). In order to visualise fluorescence, the tooth or artificial restoration is illuminated by a UV lamp. Since most UV lamps emit low-intensity light, extended exposure times are necessary, and it is mandatory to mount the camera on a tripod to prevent camera shake and blurred images. Another precaution when using UV lamps is to wear tinted safety or dark sunglasses to protect the eyes from UV irradiation. Figure 8.28 shows the set-up using sectioned teeth illuminated by UV light to show fluorescence within a natural tooth (left), and an all-ceramic crown on a prepared tooth (right) – Figure 8.29.

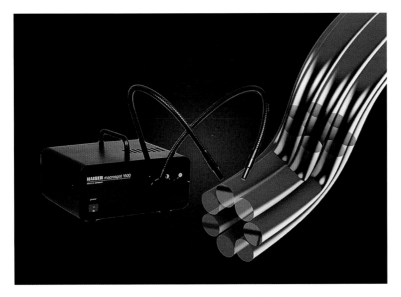

Figure 8.25 Fibre-optic unit with various sizes of flexible light transmitting cables (Kaiser, Germany).

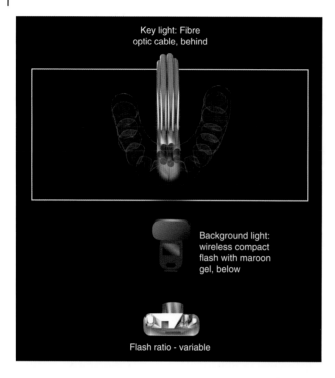

Figure 8.26 A simple set-up using fibre-optic illumination.

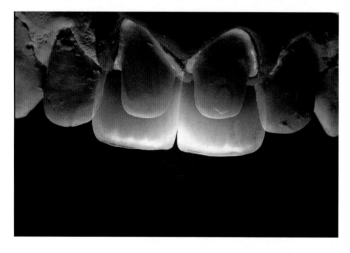

Figure 8.27 Transillumination is particularly useful for visualising incisal edge opalescence, translucency, staining and dentine mamelons in artificial restorations, photographed with the set-up shown in Figure 8.26.

Finally, fibre-optic lights can be coloured by filters, focused with lenses, and combined with flashes and UV lamps for creating visually stunning images: Figures 8.30–8.32 show some examples of creative effects using fibre-optic and UV illumination.

Colour Fidelity

An image that faithfully reproduces colour is prerequisite for any medical or dental use. This is particularly relevant for distinguishing between healthy and diseased tissues, and shade analysis of teeth for prosthodontic and restorative dentistry. The correct colour rendition of the soft

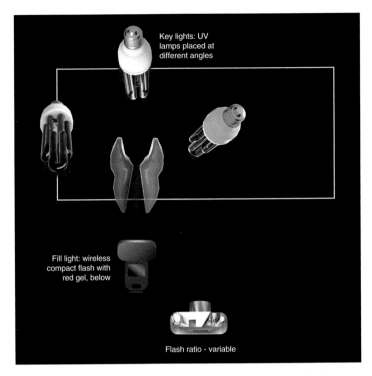

Key lights: UV lamps placed at different angles

Fill light: wireless compact flash with red gel, below

Flash ratio - variable

Figure 8.28 Set-up for ultra-violet (UV) illumination with a flash below covered with a red gel.

Figure 8.29 Ultra-violet (UV) illumination showing fluorescence of a natural tooth (left) and ceramic crown (right).

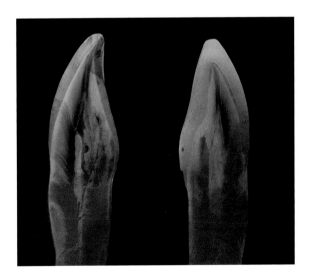

tissues is essential for disciplines such as oral medicine, periodontology, and oral surgery. A colour shift from pink to red to blue can signify health, inflammation or cyanosis, respectively. Also, the apparent shade of a tooth or teeth is useful for elucidating aetiology, differential diagnosis and treatment options. For example, discolouration of the entire dentition due to intrinsic staining may warrant tooth whitening, whereas isolated discolouration of a single tooth may signify trauma or haemolytic breakdown following root canal therapy. Dental images are also

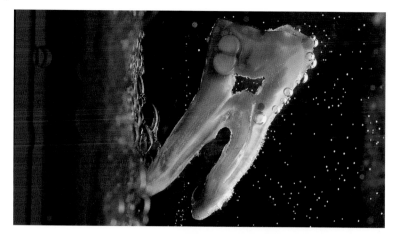

Figure 8.30 Exfoliation (fibre-optic + compact flash).

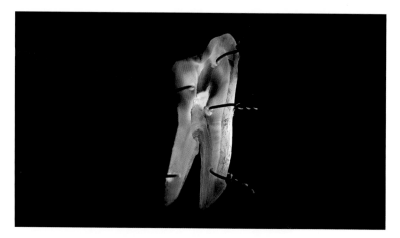

Figure 8.31 Barbed wire (fibre-optic + ultra-violet [UV]).

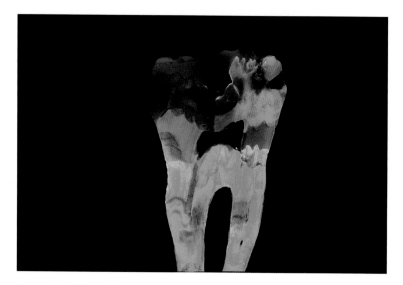

Figure 8.32 Waves (ultra-violet [UV]).

used for matching the shade of artificial restorations with adjacent teeth. Therefore, for diagnosis, comparison and communication, colour accuracy and colour consistency are mandatory. Although this appears straightforward, due to several variable factors, achieving colour fidelity in dental photography is not as easy as it seems.

The first item to consider is the object(s) being photographed, i.e. the teeth and surrounding soft tissues. The interaction of light with a tooth is complex, involving reflection, refraction, transmission as well as other optical characteristics such as fluorescence and opalescence mentioned above (Chu et al. 2004). The shade of a tooth is also affected by the degree of hydration, the colour temperature of the illumination (metamerism) – Figures 8.33 and 8.34, CRI (colour rendering index) rating of the light source and the angle of illumination (goniochromism). In addition, the tooth has three optical layers, consisting of the pulp, dentine and enamel, which all influence its perceived colour. The colour of the oral mucosa and gingival apparatus also shows considerable variations, influenced by systemic conditions such as anaemia and local factors such as melanin pigmentation or pathological changes.

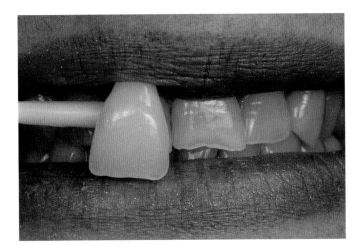

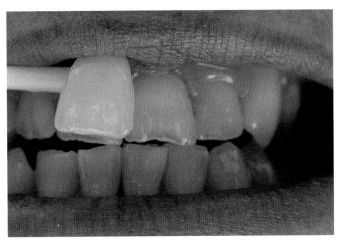

Figures 8.33 and 8.34 Meteramism: a shade tab may match under one type of illumination (5500 K), but mismatch when viewed with light having a different colour temperature (6500 K).

The second item to consider is the imaging chain that produces an image, consisting of the CPD triad: starting at the Capture stage (camera), moving on to Processing (software) and ending with the Display media (monitor, projector, printer) (Figure 8.35). At present, there is a lack of interconnectivity and consistency among systems for digital photography. Furthermore, at each stage of the imaging chain, the hardware and software from several manufacturers is used, often with different colour spaces and ICC (International Color Consortium) profiles (Badano et al. 2015), and therefore the apparent colour is device-dependent. This is compounded by the unique white balance algorithms of cameras from different manufacturers, with little or no standardisation. The quality or colour temperature and CRI rating of light is another issue, combined with flash diffusers that can alter the colour rendition beyond the visually perceivable threshold, ranging from ΔE 1.22 to ΔE 2.66 (Witzel et al. 1973; Paravina et al. 2015). Hence, devices at each stage of the digital workflow require calibration if colour consistency is to be a realistic possibility. At the capture stage, a reference grey card image (Hein and Zangl 2016) is indispensable for calibrating pictures for a particular lighting set-up. At the processing stage, it is important to ensure that the colour space in the software matches that of the camera, e.g. sRGB or Adobe RGB, and finally, each display device is periodically calibrated for colour consistency (see Module 9). A crucial point worth remembering is that excessive manipulation in imaging software not only degrades image quality, but also changes colour. For example, correcting a grossly under- or overexposed image will severely affect the colour rendition of the image, resulting in unwanted colour casts that reduce its diagnostic or comparison value (Snow 2006). Nevertheless, even with the above

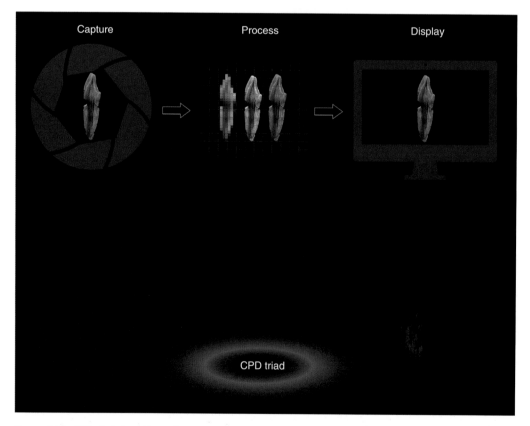

Figure 8.35 CPD triad: the colour of an image varies according to a particular medium or device, i.e. camera, software or monitor.

contingencies, the key issue is that digital photography offers relative, rather than absolute, colour assessment. However, for the majority of clinical documentation this limitation is acceptable for diagnosis and communication.

Shade Analysis

The advent and wide acceptance of digital cameras has opened up a new method for shade evaluation using dSLR cameras in conjunction with imaging software (Hein et al. 2017). This digital shade analysis allows an assessment of colour that can readily be used for selecting composite shades, or sharing the shade analysis information with dental technicians for fabricating indirect restorations (Lee et al. 2015).[1] Colour, similarly to dental occlusion, is shrouded in mystery: perplexing for the novice and challenging for the expert (Chu and Tarnow 2001). There are three methods for assessing tooth shade: visual, instrumental and photographic (Ahmad 2000). The visual is a comparative approach, using either prefabricated or custom-made shade tabs. Shade analysis for direct restorations can either be with shade tabs, or placing increments of various composite shades on the tooth to be restored for choosing the best match (Yap et al. 1995; da Costa et al. 2010) (Figures 8.36 and 8.37). For indirect restorations, the only option is shade tabs placed adjacent to the teeth for judging the colour. When photographing shade tabs, it is important that the tabs are positioned in the same optical axis as the teeth, and the light is positioned to avoid specular reflections that may alter the perceived colour (Llop 2009).

The second method for shade assessment is instrumental that directly measures the shade of the tooth using devices such as colorimeters or spectrophotometers (Ishikawa-Nagai et al. 2010; Yoshida et al. 2010), and outputs a numerical value according to the CIE L*a*b* colour co-ordinates (Paravina 2002). Examples include Crystaleye Spectrophotometer˙ and Vita EasyShade˙, which give acceptable and repeatable colour measurements (Odaira et al. 2011). Another instrumental method for shade evaluation is intra-oral scanners (IOS), which have built-in shade assessment tools for providing an instant read out of tooth shade according to either the Vita Classical˙, or Vita 3D˙ shade guides (Figure 8.38).

The third approach is photographic, involving taking a photograph of tabs from the chosen shade guide (e.g. Vita 3D or Vita Classical) in line with optical axis of the tooth, and a grey

Figure 8.36 Direct shade analysis for composite restorations can either be accomplished with a prefabricated shade guide, or placing increments of composite on the tooth to be restored. It is important to carry out shade assessment before isolating with rubber dam to ensure that the teeth are not dehydrated.

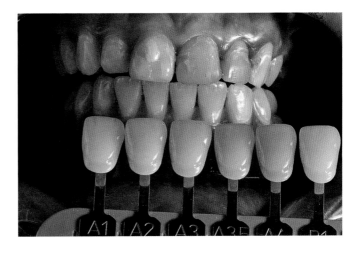

---

1 http://www.clearmatch.com/index.htm (accessed 6 April 2010).

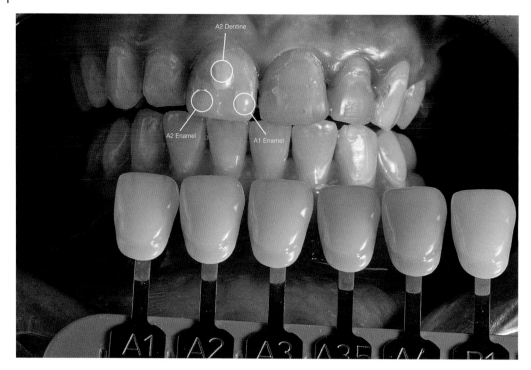

Figure 8.37 Composite increments placed directly on the right maxillary central incisor.

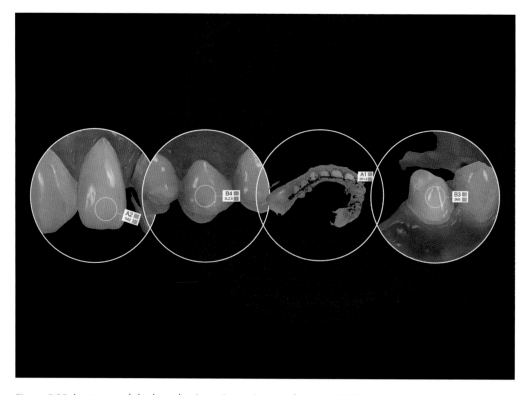

Figure 8.38 Instrumental shade evaluation using an intra-oral scanner (IOS).

card for colour calibration (Figure 8.39). The teeth are hydrated and not desiccated to prevent a colour shift. The image should be devoid of specular reflections, which is achieved by either using muted reflection set-up described above, or attaching a polarising filter onto the front of the lens that optically eliminates the enamel layer. Using a polarising filter requires exposure compensation by increasing the aperture by 1 *f*-stop, or moving the light source closer (Figure 8.40). Also, the flashes should not be positioned inferior or superior to the lens axis as the unwanted illumination of the background 'red' oral cavity conveys a reddish appearance of the teeth. This is particularly relevant for ring flashes mounted on the front of the lens. The image is then imported into the appropriate photo-editing software, and the white balance calibrated with the grey card. The next step is taking colour measurements at various sites of the tooth, e.g. incisal, middle third (body), and cervical aspects. At each site, the software calculates colour co-ordinates that are translated into shade tab equivalents of the chosen shade guide, and used for selecting appropriate shades of ceramic powders or composite increments (Khoo 2015; Oh et al. 2010). In order to concentrate on hue and chroma of the teeth and shade tabs, the background oral-cavity can be converted to black and white in the processing software. A formidable challenge is assessing the value (brightness and darkness) of a tooth, since the hue and chroma components of colour dominate a composition. To mitigate this influence,

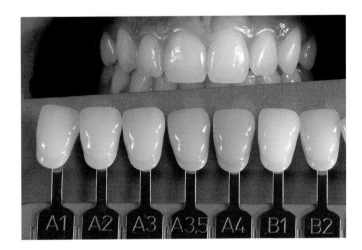

Figure 8.39 Vita Classical shade guide photographed with an 18% grey card in line with the optical axis of the maxillary teeth.

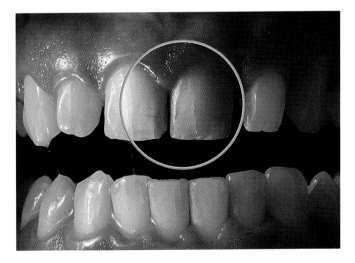

Figure 8.40 A polarising filter is useful for eliminating superficial specular reflections to allow analysis of the shade and characterisations within the enamel and underlying dentine layers.

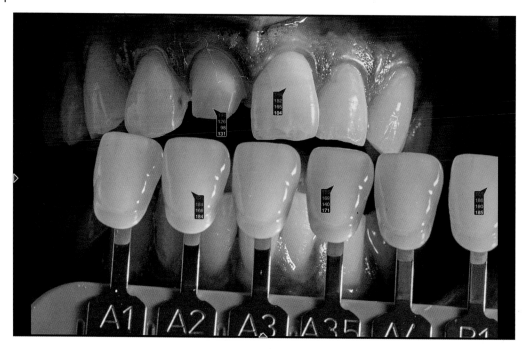

Figure 8.41 Photographic digital shade analysis: Comparative colour readouts (red, green, blue and value in white text) of the prepared abutment, contralateral maxillary left central incisor and shade tabs.

an achromatic image is necessary for judging value, especially at the incisal edges where the enamel layer is thickest. The easiest way for achieving this is in processing software by moving the saturation slider to zero for producing a black and white image.

The example below illustrates photographic digital shade analysis for matching the colour of a crown on the right maxillary central incisor to the contralateral left central incisor. Following tooth preparation, the tooth abutment is photographed with a Vita Classical shade guide, which is in line with the optical axis of the maxillary anterior sextant. After performing a colour calibration with a grey card, the images are evaluated with colour readouts at specific sites. The colour swatches have four numerical values, red numbers represent the red channel, the green numbers the green channel, the blue numbers the blue channel, and the white numbers the value or brightness on a greyscale from 0 to 255 (Figure 8.41). The best way to visualise shade is by chromatically isolating the teeth in imaging software. This is relatively easily using the colour editor by selecting the colour of the teeth and rendering the remainder of the image as black and white (Figure 8.42). From the edited image, it is apparent that the closest colour match of the maxillary left central incisor is the A2 shade tab (Figure 8.43). For assessing value, the hue and chroma of the teeth are digitally removed, leaving a black and white image of the teeth (Figure 8.44). This allows assessment of the value without being distracted by hue and chroma of the teeth. Although the shade (hue and chroma) of tooth #21 match only one tab, i.e. A2, its value matches two tabs, i.e. A2 and B1 (Figure 8.45).

Although digital shade analysis is not an absolute method for colour determination, it is nevertheless invaluable for analysing the chromatic nuances within teeth, which allows mapping geographical distribution of shades as a guide for artificial restorations. The starting point for chromatic mapping is taking an image that is devoid of specular reflections, either with judicial lighting, or using a polarising filter. After importing the image into imaging software, the

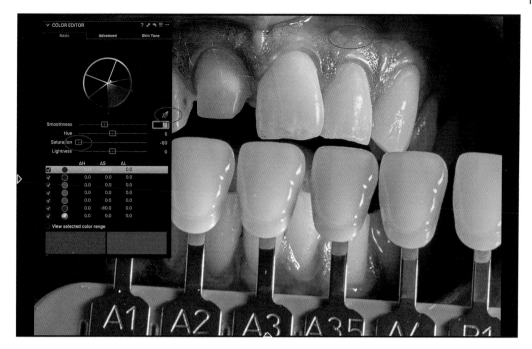

Figure 8.42 Photographic digital shade analysis: The teeth and tabs are chromatically isolated by the colour editor for evaluating hue and chroma.

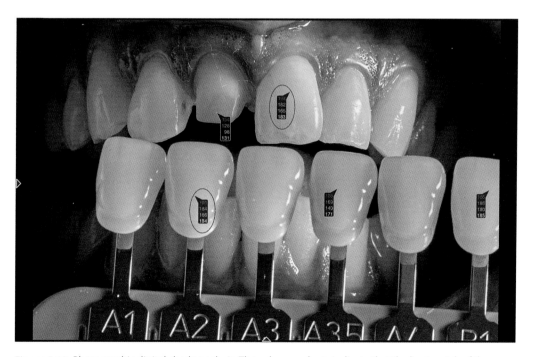

Figure 8.43 Photographic digital shade analysis: The colour readouts indicate that the best match of the contralateral maxillary left central incisor is the A2 shade tab (red circles).

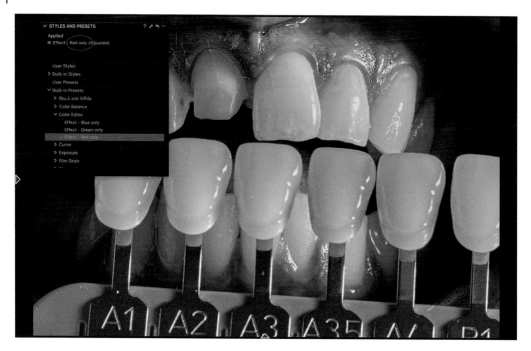

Figure 8.44 Photographic digital shade analysis: To assess value, hue and chroma of the teeth are digitally removed, leaving only a black and white image of the teeth and shade tabs.

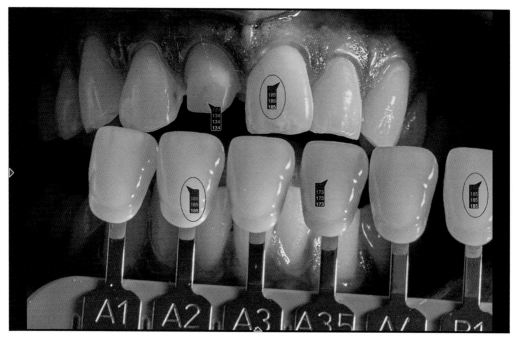

Figure 8.45 Photographic digital shade analysis: Notice that the value of tooth #21 matches the value of both A2 and B1 shade tabs (red circles, value = 185).

Figure 8.46 Chromatic mapping: pre-operative image showing acute fractures of the maxillary right central and lateral incisors.

Figure 8.46 Chromatic mapping: pre-operative image showing acute fractures of the maxillary right central and lateral incisors.

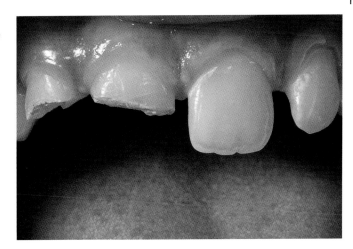

Figure 8.47 Chromatic mapping: the brightness is reduced and the contrast increased to visualise chromatic distribution and characterisations.

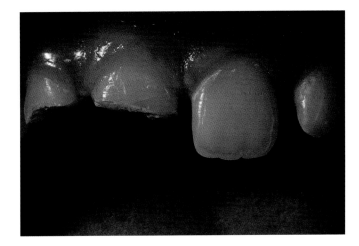

brightness is reduced and contrast increased, which not only emphasises 'hidden' tooth characterisations, but also the gradual colour transitions traversing from the cervical regions to the incisal edges (Salat et al. 2011). A drawing software is then used to map out the chromatic distribution, and annotate specific characterisations (Figures 8.46–8.49).

Scale Reference Markers

A scale reference marker is usually a graduated ruler or periodontal probe, which is included in the photograph for measuring dimensions of teeth or soft tissue anatomy. As the dimensions of images change during enlargement or reduction in processing software, a reference marker is a useful guide, irrespective of the relative scaling or magnification (Figures 8.50–8.53). This allows scaled measurements, which can be used for calculating the width/length ratio of teeth, distal width progression for smile design, size of incisal embrasures, anterior overjet and overbite (Figure 8.54), diastemata, occlusal clearance, vertical dimension of occlusion (VDO), degree of maxillary gingival exposure during smiling, tooth exposure during the habitual lip position and smiling, width of keratinised gingiva, degree of gingival scalloping, interdental

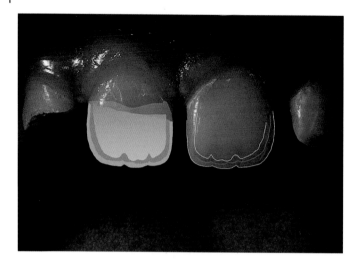

Figure 8.48 Chromatic mapping: a drawing software is used to chart a chromatic map, including characterisations such as dentine mamelons and incisal halos.

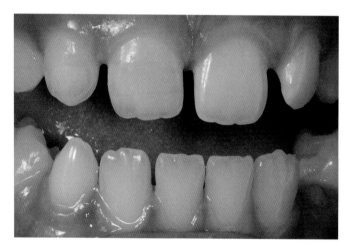

Figure 8.49 Chromatic mapping: post-operative result showing coronal restitution of fractures with direct resin-based composite incremental layering.

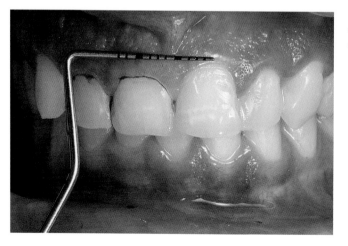

Figure 8.50 Existing uneven gingival zeniths around teeth #11 and #21.

Figure 8.51 Esthetic crown lengthening for correcting uneven gingival zeniths using a periodontal probe as a reference marker: initial clinical crown length of tooth #11 = 7.5 mm.

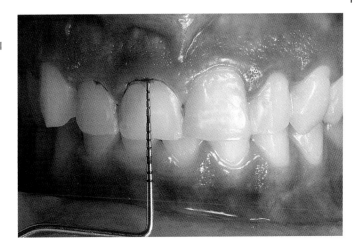

Figure 8.52 Symmetrical gingival zeniths around teeth #11 and #21 after crown lengthening.

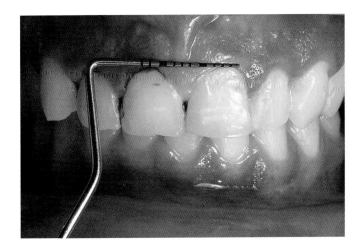

Figure 8.53 Post-operative result after one week healing.

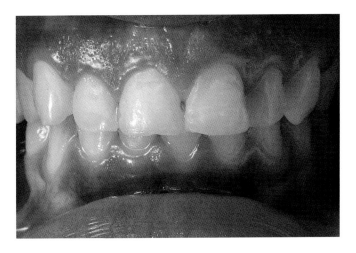

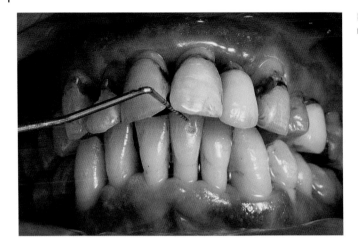

Figure 8.54 Periodontal probe measuring the anterior overjet.

papilla fill (Ahmad 2005) and the size of soft tissue pathological lesions. Finally, a proportional reference is also useful for scale calibration in smile design software, and for designing manual or virtual wax-ups, temporaries and definitive restorations.

Annotations

Starting a course of aesthetic treatment without taking pre-operative pictures is inviting trouble, no different to placing implants without a CBCT (cone beam computed tomography). This is particularly relevant if the proposed treatment is elective or purely for enhancing beauty. Also, aesthetics is fraught with subjectivity and idiosyncrasies, and if the outcome is not as anticipated, or fails to satisfy the patient, lack of photographic documentation is indefensible if litigation ensues. Therefore, anything that helps facilitate aesthetic treatment is a godsend.

A simple and effective method for aesthetic treatment planning is adding annotations to images that serve as a starting point for analysis. This involves using drawing software for adding text and reference lines of salient features on images taken from different perspectives. For example, most aesthetic treatments start with a diagnostic wax-up, and annotated instructions for the dental technician are invaluable for finalising the proposed aesthetic treatment plan. Also, most drawing software offer the facility to covert the annotated images into PDFs (Personal Document Files), which can be attached to e-mails for communication with patients, ceramists and specialist. The case study depicted in Figures 8.55–8.61 shows annotated instructions to the ceramist for altering the initial wax-up to satisfy patient's wishes.

Drawing software is available either as free or paid downloads. Most major software houses such as Adobe®, Apple®, Corel® and Microsoft® offer several packages that are user-friendly, with intuitive features that require little training. For dental purposes, a simple software that can add text, draw lines, curves and shapes is all that is required, and is often part of the pre-installed software that comes with all computers. Examples of popular drawing programmes include Adobe Illustrator, CorelDraw® or ACD Canvas™. Alternately, a Google® search for 'drawing software' offers a vast list to choose from.

Many key reference lines for aesthetic appraisal can be annotated on photographs including the inter-pupillary line, facial and dental midlines, Rickett's E-plane, naso-labial angle, gonial angle, commissure line, inclination of the incisal plane, smile line (maxillary incisal plane with

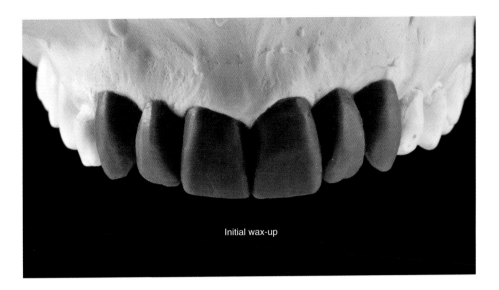

Initial wax-up

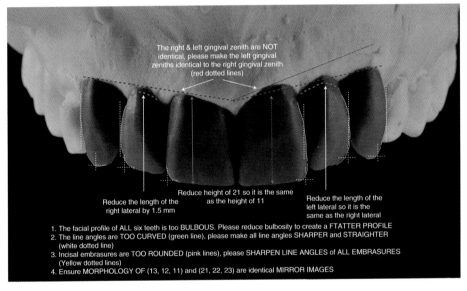

The right & left gingival zenith are NOT
identical, please make the left gingival
zeniths identical to the right gingival zenith
(red dotted lines)

Reduce the length of the
right lateral by 1.5 mm

Reduce height of 21 so it is the same
as the height of 11

Reduce the length of the
left lateral so it is the
same as the right lateral

1. The facial profile of ALL six teeth is too BULBOUS. Please reduce bulbosity to create a FTATTER PROFILE
2. The line angles are TOO CURVED (green line), please make all line angles SHARPER and STRAIGHTER
   (white dotted line)
3. Incisal embrasures are TOO ROUNDED (pink lines), please SHARPEN LINE ANGLES of ALL EMBRASURES
   (Yellow dotted lines)
4. Ensure MORPHOLOGY OF (13, 12, 11) and (21, 22, 23) are identical MIRROR IMAGES

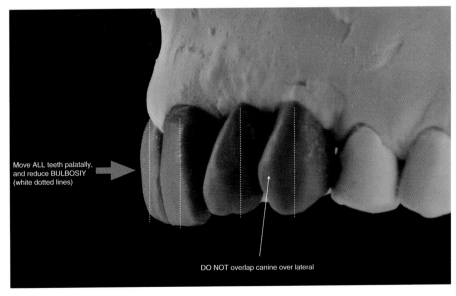

Move ALL teeth palatally,
and reduce BULBOSIY
(white dotted lines)

DO NOT overlap canine over lateral

Figures 8.55–8.61 Annotated instructions are invaluable for designing and finalising a diagnostic wax-up
before commencing a course of aesthetic treatment.

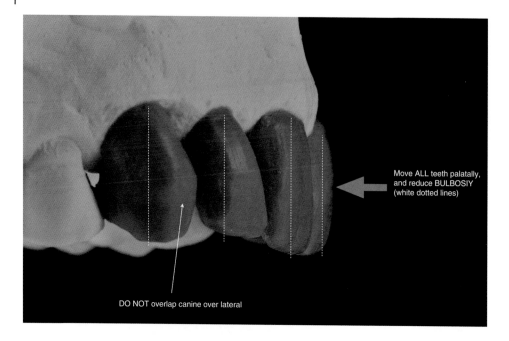

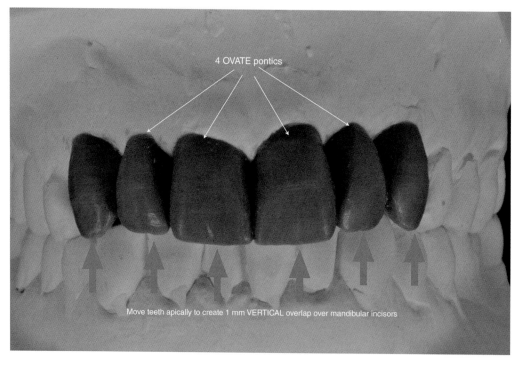

Figures 8.55–8.61 (Continued)

lower lip coincidence), axial inclination of teeth, mesial-distal width progression, gingival aesthetic line (GAL), gingival display at rest and smiling, and bilateral negative space. These, and other reference lines, are essential for a multidisciplinary co-treatment approach, and for communicating with patients about the present state of affairs, and whether the proposed aesthetic

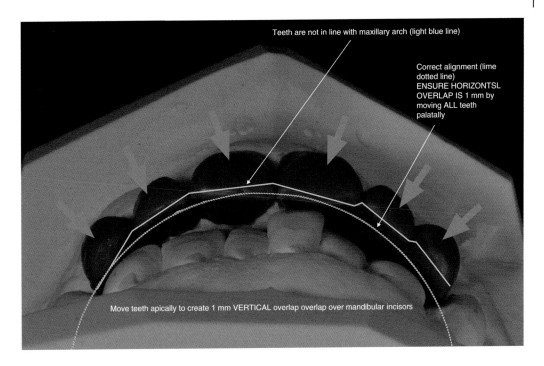

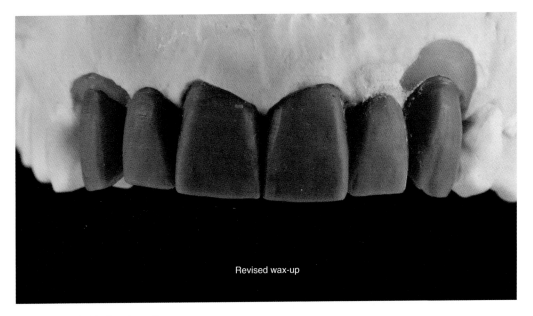

Figures 8.55–8.61 (Continued)

prescription is clinically feasible. Similar to aesthetic treatment, orthodontic therapy and cranio-maxillo-facial surgery also benefit from annotations by marking key reference lines such as the Frankfurt plane, ala-tragus plane (Camper's line), Rickett's E-plane, Steiner plane (angle of lower border of mandible Go-Gn), curves of Spee and Wilson and sphere of Monson, overjet and overbite, and molar and canine relationships.

As mentioned above, annotations are used for creating chromatic and characterisation distribution maps following a digital shade analysis. As well as outputting numerical values for shade, a digital shade analysis shows characterisation and chromatic distribution within a tooth. This information is used for creating maps using drawing software that serve as a guide for reproducing subtleties within composite incremental layers using effect tints and stains. Similarly, a chromatic map is useful as an annotated laboratory prescriptions for indirect restorations (Figures 8.62–8.66). Finally, annotations are ideal for conveying anomalies that

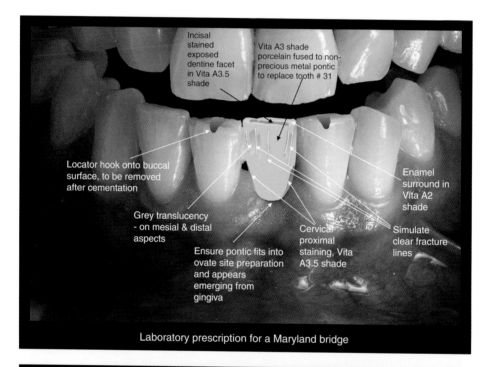

Laboratory prescription for a Maryland bridge

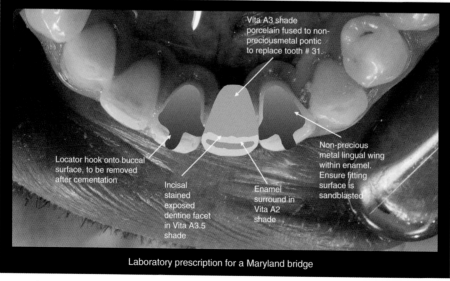

Laboratory prescription for a Maryland bridge

Figures 8.62–8.64 Annotated laboratory instruction for fabricating a Maryland bridge for replacing a missing mandibular incisor.

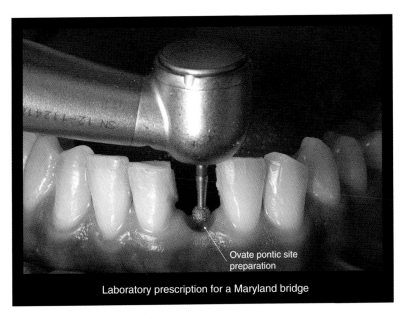

Ovate pontic site
preparation

Laboratory prescription for a Maryland bridge

Figures 8.62–8.64 (Continued)

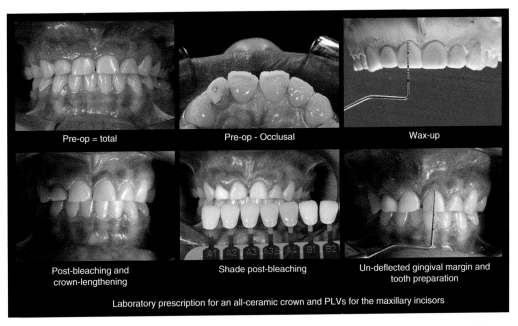

Pre-op = total

Pre-op - Occlusal

Wax-up

Post-bleaching and
crown-lengthening

Shade post-bleaching

Un-deflected gingival margin and
tooth preparation

Laboratory prescription for an all-ceramic crown and PLVs for the maxillary incisors

Figures 8.65 and 8.66 Annotated laboratory instruction for fabricating an all-ceramic crown and porcelain laminate veneers (PLVs) for the maxillary incisors.

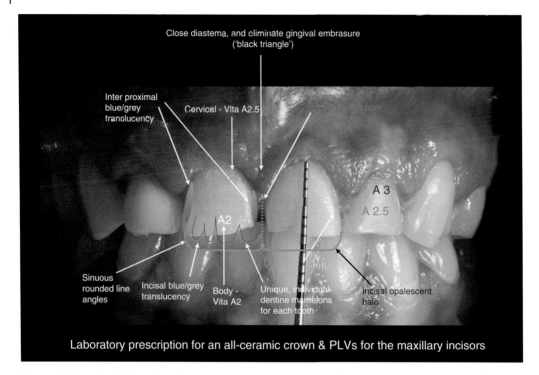

Close diastema, and eliminate gingival embrasure
('black triangle')

Inter proximal
blue/grey
translucency

Cervical - Vita A2.5

A 3

A 2.5

A2

Sinuous
rounded line
angles

Incisal blue/grey
translucency

Body -
Vita A2

Unique, individual
dentine mamelons
for each tooth

Incisal opalescent
halo

Laboratory prescription for an all-ceramic crown & PLVs for the maxillary incisors

Figures 8.65 and 8.66 (Continued)

require correction at the try-in stage before definitive cementation of indirect restorations (Figure 8.67).

Bleaching (Tooth Whitening)

Tooth whitening, either in-office or home bleaching, is an innocuous, minimally invasive procedure for dental aesthetic enhancement. However, careful documentation is essential for comparison to standard reference shade guides for assessing and monitoring the bleaching process (Figures 8.68 and 8.69).

Phonetics

The majority of aesthetic treatment involves altering the anterior teeth, which are predominantly responsible for speech. This is also true for orthodontics, where positioning of the anterior teeth should not interfere with speech. A detailed evaluation of phonetics is required, before and after treatment, for ensuring that any prescribed treatment has not, and will not, affect phonetics. A phonetic analysis involves asking the patient to iterate various sounds for determining existing speech impediments or preventing them afterwards. The 'm' 'Emma' or 'me' sound determines the amount of tooth display at the habitual or 'rest' position, which is Image #1 of the EDP. The extra images required are as follows. The 's' sound assesses the vertical dimension of speech; typically a 1–2 mm separation between

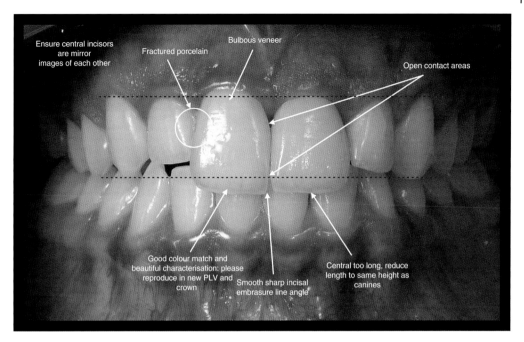

Ensure central incisors are mirror images of each other

Fractured porcelain

Bulbous veneer

Open contact areas

Good colour match and beautiful characterisation: please reproduce in new PLV and crown

Smooth sharp incisal embrasure line angle

Central too long, reduce length to same height as canines

Figure 8.67 Try-in-stage of a porcelain laminate veneer (PLV) on maxillary right central incisor and an all-ceramic crown on the maxillary left central incisor.

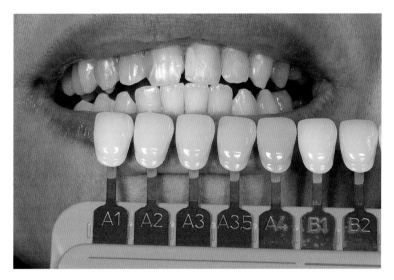

A1 A2 A3 A3.5 A4 B1 B2

Figure 8.68 Pre-bleaching with reference shade guide.

the maxillary and mandibular anterior teeth is necessary to avoid lisping (Figure 8.70). The 'f' or 'v' sounds determine the axial inclination of the maxillary central incisors, i.e. the buccal aspects of the maxillary incisors touch the mucosal rather than the cutaneous aspect of the mandibular lip (Figure 8.71). Other sounds including 'th' or words such as 'Mississippi' that do not require photographic documentation, but their audio clarity should be noted.

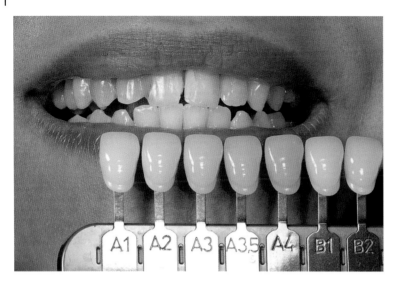

Figure 8.69 Nine weeks post-bleaching with reference shade guide.

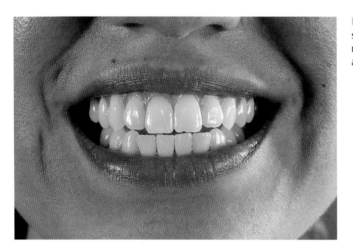

Figure 8.70 Phonetics: with the 's' sound, a 1–2 mm separation is noticeable between the maxillary and mandibular anterior teeth.

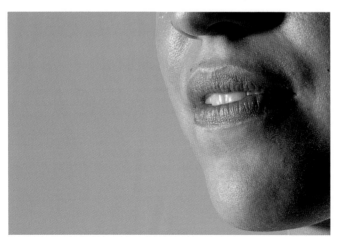

Figure 8.71 Phonetics: with the 'f' or 'v' sounds, the mucosal aspect of the mandibular lip partially covers the labial surfaces of the maxillary incisors.

Furthermore, the impact of proposed treatment on phonetics can be assessed during intra-oral mock-ups with either acrylic, or composite restorations that are copied from the diagnostic wax-up simulations. A mock-up also allows changes to be made by removing or adding flowable composite until phonetics are satisfactory, and the final tooth shape can then be copied for the definitive restorations.

Occlusal Analysis

An analysis of the occlusion is warranted for several dental disciplines. The photographic set-ups for these image is identical to that for EDP intra-oral images, but the patient is asked to position the teeth in various positions for reviewing maximum intercuspation (MI), centric relation, anterior guidance (protrusion) and lateral movements for canine guidance or group function (Figures 8.72–8.74). Also, intra-oral submental oblique views with the head retroclined

Figure 8.72 Occlusal analysis: maximum intercuspation (MI).

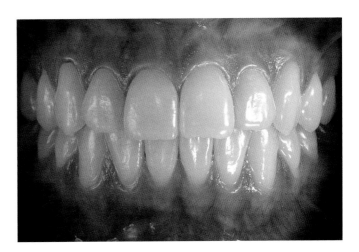

Figure 8.73 Occlusal analysis: protrusion.

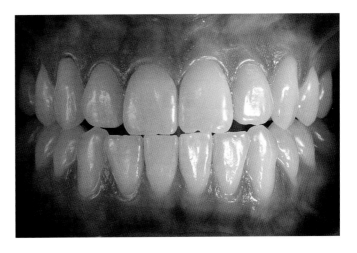

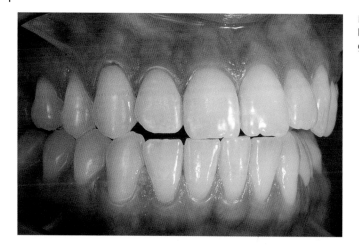

Figure 8.74 Occlusal analysis: lateral excursions (canine guidance/ group function).

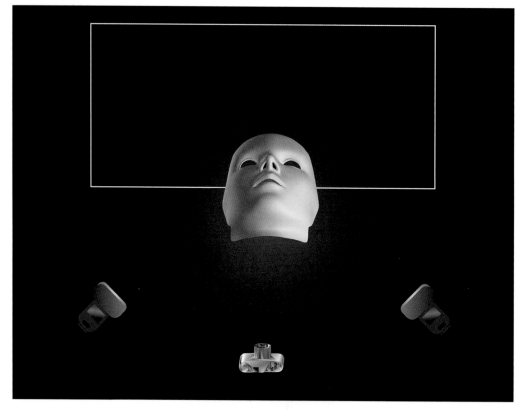

Figure 8.75 The intra-oral submental oblique view involves reclining the head, and positioning the camera inferiorly.

and the cameras positioned inferiorly, are useful for viewing the teeth from an inferior perspective (Figure 8.75). From this angle in MI, the Angle's anterior relationship is clearly visible, and with the teeth separated, allows clear visualisation of prepared crown margins of teeth in the maxillary anterior sextant (Figures 8.76–8.78).

Figure 8.76 The frontal view in maximum intercuspation (MI) does not allow assessment of the overjet.

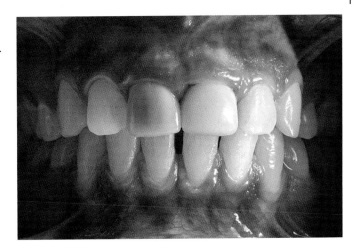

Figure 8.77 The same patient as in the previous figure with an intra-oral submental oblique view in maximum intercuspation (MI) allows visualisation of Angle's anterior relationship.

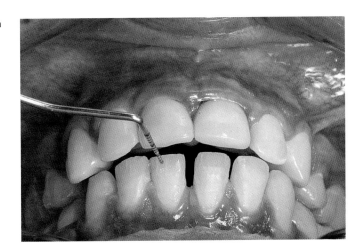

Figure 8.78 An intra-oral submental oblique view with the teeth separated allows tooth preparation finish lines of the maxillary teeth to be clearly discernible.

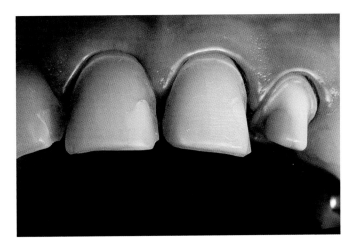

Treatment Sequences

Treatment sequencing involves documenting step-by-step clinical or laboratory techniques. Also, a sequence of images can demonstrate the use of particular instruments or materials for a restorative or surgical modality. A series of images should follow standardisation protocols ensuring that photographic settings, lighting and position of the object or subject are as identical as possible with the same magnification and field of view. These images can either be intra-oral, or bench shots. The former is trying and challenging for procedures such as surgical techniques, and a compromise if often inevitable. Conversely, bench images allow greater control for positioning and framing, so that each image in the series is more conformative. Whichever the method, a series of images is indispensable for teaching, publishing, marketing and dento-legal documentation. Figures 8.79–8.89 show a step-by-step perio-plastic surgical procedure for root coverage using a regenerative tissue matrix, AlloDerm.

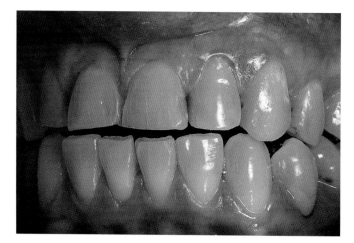

Figure 8.79 Pre-operative status showing gingival recession around maxillary left lateral incisor.

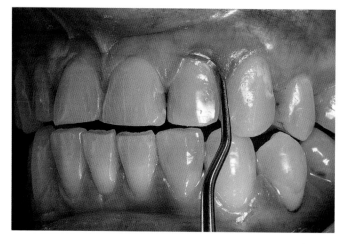

Figure 8.80 The root surface is planed with a curette…

Figure 8.81 …followed by conditioning with citric acid gel.

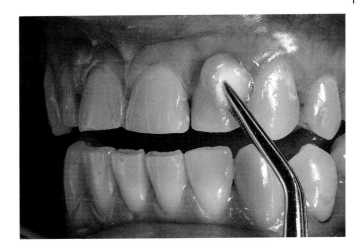

Figure 8.82 An intra-sulcular flap elevation around the lateral incisor is started on the mesial aspect and continued…

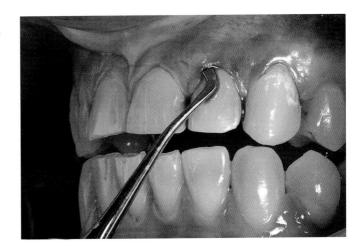

Figure 8.83 …to the mid-facial and distal aspects.

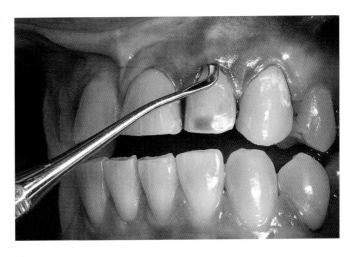

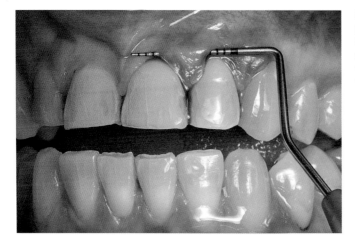

Figure 8.84 A periodontal probe passed under the closed flap (mesial aspect of lateral incisor) shows sufficient elevation of a full thickness flap without encroaching the interdental papilla.

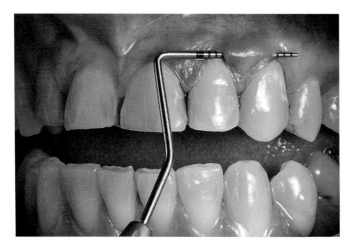

Figure 8.85 A periodontal probe passed under the closed flap (distal aspect of lateral incisor).

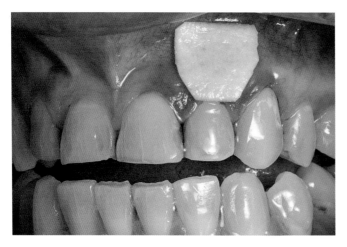

Figure 8.86 AlloDerm grafting material cut to the appropriate size…

Figure 8.87 …and eased under the elevated closed flap approaching from the sulcus

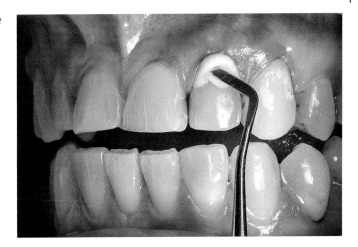

Figure 8.88 4/0 black silk sling suture to secure the graft and simultaneously position the flap in a coronal direction.

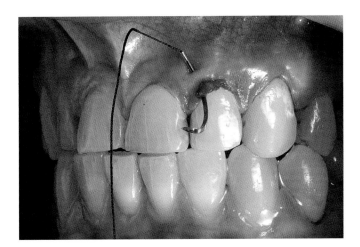

Figure 8.89 Completed perio-plastic root coverage surgical procedure.

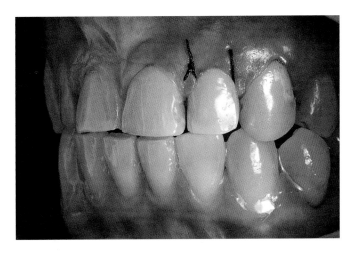

Endodontic Documentation

The use of an operating microscope for endodontic treatment is becoming increasing commonplace. Today, it is rare to encounter an endodontist specialist who does not use magnification for root canal therapy. The ability to visualise the minutest detail and explore additional or accessory canals has truly revolutionised endodontic therapy. Many reputable optical manufacturers such as Carl Zeiss* and Leica* have entered the arena, producing high-end, ergonomically designed operating microscopes. Taking photographs with operating microscopes is relatively simple, either with the built-in digital still or video camera, or attaching a dSLR with an appropriate adaptor. A beam splitter divides the light for the eyepiece and the camera so that ancillary illumination is usually superfluous. The image quality depends on the resolution of the camera sensor, as well as adequate illumination. Since space and access are limited, a dental mirror is ideal for taking reflected images, which can subsequently be laterally inverted (flipped) in editing software to correct orientation. The resulting images are useful for analysing canal morphology, detecting fractures and co-diagnosing with colleagues (Figure 8.90).

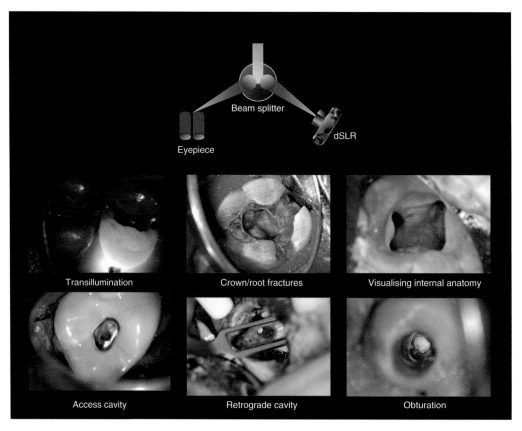

Figure 8.90 An operating microscope with beam splitter plus attached dSLR is ideal for photographing endodontic procedures (Source: clinical images courtesy of Dr. Faisal Alonaizan).

Focus Stacking

The ever-increasing processing power of computers and innovative software have popularised techniques such as focus stacking. Focus stacking is a method for increasing the DoF for landscape and macrophotography. Since DoF diminishes with increased magnification, having a method for apparently having all parts of an object or subject in focus is extremely advantageous for macro and microscopic analysis. The process involves taking a series of images at different points of focus (PoF), which are subsequently combined in dedicated focus staking software to create a single image with vastly increased DoF (Figure 8.91). The process is similar to HDR (high dynamic range) photography for increasing the dynamic range of an image.

Video

Nearly all cameras and smartphones have the capability to record video footage, and although it is not the remit of this manuscript to describe motion pictures, it is with mentioning that this facility opens up new horizons. If a picture is worth a thousand words, imagine the value of a video. It goes without saying that recording clinical or laboratory procedures is an adjunct for training and lecturing. However, similar to still photography, a learning curve should be anticipated, since the time and perseverance involved is substantial and challenging. Nevertheless, the option to make videos is worth contemplating, maybe not imminently, but perhaps at some future time.

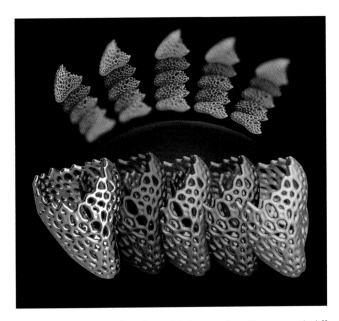

Figure 8.91 Focus stacking is combining a series of images with different points of focus (PoF) to form a composite image with increased depth of field (DoF).

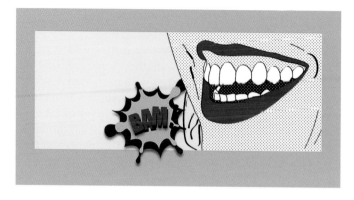

Figure 8.92 An artistic image in the style of Roy Lichtenstein.

Promotional and Artistic Imagery

Images for marketing, promotion and lecturing, accentuate clinical achievements and beautify patients. Hence, their intended use is to set the senses reeling for engaging the audience. Although having limited clinical significance, these images are indispensable for promoting a product or service. Therefore, the photographer has a certain degree of artistic licence for expressing his or her creativity by visually enhancing a particular product or treatment outcome that is enticing and attention seeking. Some examples of non-clinical portraits are shown in Module 6, and this book has copious examples of treatment sequences for many modalities. Finally, dental artistic images are conceived from within rather than learned by didactic teaching, and their ulterior motive is visual impact rather than clinical usefulness.

Artistic imagery requires an imaginative, and not necessarily a mescalinized individual, which is beyond the scope of this book (Huxley 1954) – Figure 8.92.

References

Ahmad, I. (2000). Three-dimensional shade analysis: perspectives of color. Part II. Practical. *Periodont. Esthet. Dent.* 12: 557–564.

Ahmad, I. (2005). *A Clinical Guide to Anterior Dental Aesthetics*. London: BDJ Books.

Ahmad, I. and Chu, S. (2003). Light dynamic properties of a synthetic low-fusing quartz glass-ceramic material. *Pract. Proc. Aesthet. Dent.* 15 (1): 49–56.

Badano, A., Revie, C., Casertano, A. et al. (2015). Consistency and standardization of color in medical imaging: a consensus report. *J. Digit. Imaging* 28: 41–52.

Chu, S., Devigus, A., and Mieleszko, A. (2004). *Fundamentals of Color: Shade Matching and Communication in Esthetic Dentistry*. Chicago, IL: Quintessence.

Chu, S.J. and Tarnow, D.P. (2001). Digital shade analysis and verification: a case report and discussion. *Pract. Proced. Esthet. Dent.* 13: 129–136.

da Costa, J., Fox, P., and Ferracane, J. (2010). Comparison of various resin composite shades and layering technique with a shade guide. *J. Esthet. Restor. Dent.* 22 (2): 114–124.

Hein, S., Tapia, J., and Bazos, P. (2017). eLABor_aid: a new approach to digital shade management. *Int. J. Esthet. Dent.* 12 (2): 186–202.

Hein, S. and Zangl, M. (2016). The use of a standardized gray reference card in dental photography to correct the effects of ve commonly used diffusers on the color of 40 extracted human teeth. *Int. J. Esthet. Dent.* 11: 246–259.

Huxley, A. (1954). *The Doors of Perception*. Chatto & Windus and Harper & Row.

Ishikawa-Nagai, S., Yoshida, A., Da Silva, J.D. et al. (2010). Spectrophotometric analysis of tooth color reproduction on anterior all-ceramic crowns. Part 1. Analysis and interpretation of tooth color. *J. Esthet. Restor. Dent.* 22: 42–52.

Khoo, T.S.J. (2015). A comparison between a photographic shade analysis system and conventional visual shade matching method. MS (Master of Science) thesis. University of Iowa. http://ir.uiowa.edu/etd/1860 (accessed 23 May 2019).

Lee, W.S., Kim, S.Y., Kim, J.H. et al. (2015). The effect of powder A2/powder A3 mixing ratio on color and translucency parameters of dental porcelain. *J. Adv. Prosthodont.* 7 (5): 400–405.

Llop, D.R. (2009). Technical analysis of clinical digital photographs. *J. Calif. Dent. Assoc.* 37 (3): 199–206.

Odaira, C., Itoh, S., and Ishibashi, K. (2011). Clinical evaluation of a dental color analysis system: the Crystaleye spectrophotometer. *J. Prosthodont. Res.* 55 (4): 199–205.

Oh, W.-S., Pogoncheff, J., and O'Brien, W.J. (2010). Digital computer matching of tooth color. *Materials* 3: 3694–3699.

Paravina, R.D. (2002). Evaluation of a newly developed shade – matching apparatus. *Int. J. Prosthodont.* 15: 528–534.

Paravina, R.D., Ghinea, R., Herrera, L.J. et al. (2015). Color difference thresholds in dentistry. *J. Esthet. Restor. Dent.* 27: S1–S9.

Ryan, A.-N., Tam, L.E., and McComb, D. (2010). Comparative translucency of esthetic composite resin restorative materials. *J. Can. Dent. Assoc.* 76: a84.

Salat, A., Deveto, W., and Manauta, J. (2011). Achieving a precise color chart with common computer software for excellence in anterior composite restorations. *Eur. J. Esthet. Dent.* 6: 280–296.

Snow, S.R. (2006). Dental photographic images: strategies for accreditation success. *Aesthet. AACD Monogr.* 3: 38–43.

Witzel, R.F., Burnham, R.W., and Onley, J.W. (1973). Threshold and suprathreshold perceptual color differences. *J. Opt. Soc. Am.* 63: 615–625.

Yap, A.U., Bhole, S., and Tan, K.B. (1995). Shade match of tooth-colored restorative materials based on a commercial shade guide. *Quintessence Int.* 26 (10): 697–702.

Yoshida, A., Miller, L., Da Silva, J.D. et al. (2010). Spectrophotometric analysis of tooth color reproduction on anterior all-ceramic crowns. Part 2. Color reproduction and its transfer from in vitro to in vivo. *J. Esthet. Restor. Dent.* 22: 53–63.

Section 3

Processing Images

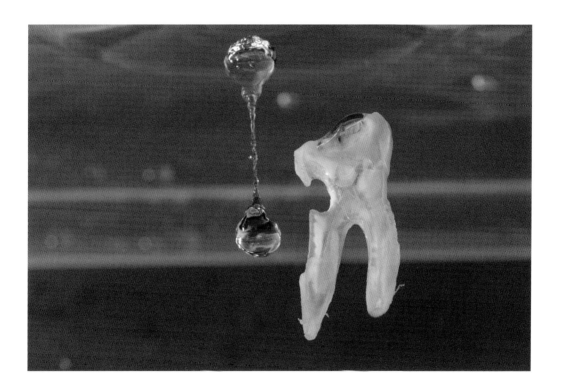

9

Processing Images

The penultimate stage of the CPD (Capture, Process, Display) imaging chain is processing or developing an image. This is analogous to film photography, which involved forwarding the exposed film for developing or processing in a darkroom. With digital photography, developing is performed with a computer using photo-editing or imaging software. At the outset, it is worth mentioning that while imaging software can correct many failings in technique, it cannot perform miracles (Ahmad 2009a). Also, there is no substitute for proper photographic technique, and if equipment settings and positioning are correct, only a few adjustments are required. Furthermore, any processing, no matter how insignificant, will ultimately deteriorate image quality. Therefore, before embarking on endless futile corrections, it is worth deciding whether it is fruitful to spend the time and effort, and not forgetting the frustration, trying to salvage an image, or whether it is easier to discard it and just take another one.

Monitor Calibration

Before importing images from the camera to a computer, it is essential that the display monitor is correctly, and periodically, calibrated. Calibrating a computer monitor ensures that images are viewed and edited with optimum colour fidelity, and any ensuing prints match as closely as possible to the image displayed on the monitor. In addition, proper calibration produces a more relaxing and comfortable viewing experience by reducing eye strain and fatigue. Also, editing images without calibration is not only counterproductive, but defeats the object of standardisation for comparison and photographic consistency.

There are several methods for calibrating a monitor, included built-in utilities within operating systems (Windows or Macintosh), web-based free or paid testing, or external hardware colorimeter devices. The first two methods are subjective, relying on the viewer's feedback for assessing variables such as gamma, brightness, contrast and colour balance settings. This is an expedient and economical method and adequate for the casual photographer who occasionally processes images. For the aficionados, a more precise and objective method involves using an external colorimeter device that is placed onto the monitor, e.g. Spyder5Elite (www.datacolor.com) (Ramsthaler et al. 2016). These devices are connected via a USB port, and the accompanying software guides the viewer through an automated calibration process (Figure 9.1). Although more expensive, this is a sure way for precise and accurate calibration for both viewing and editing dental images.

Essentials of Dental Photography, First Edition. Irfan Ahmad.
© 2020 John Wiley & Sons Ltd. Published 2020 by John Wiley & Sons Ltd.

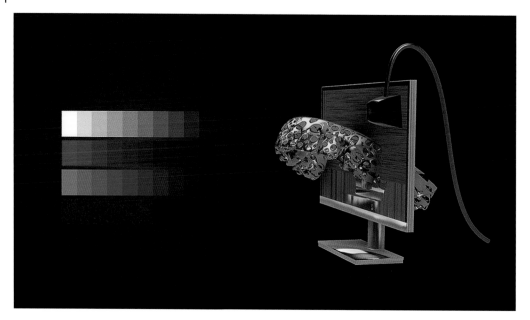

Figure 9.1 A colorimeter based monitor calibration device.

File Formats

There is only one virgin file format (RAW), i.e. the original image data that is captured with the digital camera. Once the image is opened in a photo-editing, imaging, drawing or publishing software, changes to the image occur, resulting in irretrievable loss of the original data. These changes include alterations to the bit depth, dynamic range and colour spaces. Therefore, before opening a RAW file in a software, it is prudent to back up the originals, preferably onto an external hard drive for safekeeping. This is not archiving the files, which is carried out after editing the images, but a precautionary measures to safeguard the original data files captured by the camera. The plethora of image file formats on the market is worthy of a PhD thesis. However, for dental applications, familiarity with only a few formats is required (Figure 9.2). At present, there is no single file format that serves all purposes, and therefore several formats are necessary depending on the intended use. There are two classes of image files, either uncompressed or compressed, and if compression is applied, it may be lossy or lossless. Furthermore, there is varying opinion as to which format is the ideal for image data storage, which leads to confusion and incompatibility. The first file format to consider is the proprietary RAW format, which is usually specific for a given brand of camera. This file contains the original unadulterated data, which can subsequently be converted into any file of choice. The three other ubiquitously accepted formats are TIFF (Tagged Image File Format), JPEG (Joint Photographic Experts Group) and PDF (Personal Document File). To this list can be added PNG (Portable Network Graphics) and EPS (Encapsulated PostScript), which are used for web-publishing and printing, respectively.

TIFF is the leading generic image file format offering lossless compression, but the size of these files is large and require substantial storage space on hard drives. Invented by the Aldus Corporation, and when opened in the LZW mode, named after its designers Lempel-Ziv and Welch, a TIFF file is as near as possible to the original RAW format. In addition, TIFF files can be imported into any imaging software for processing, and converted into other compressed file formats such as JPEGs. JPEGs are smaller size files at the expense of sacrificing quality by lossy compression. However, due to their smaller size, they are an ideal format for internet

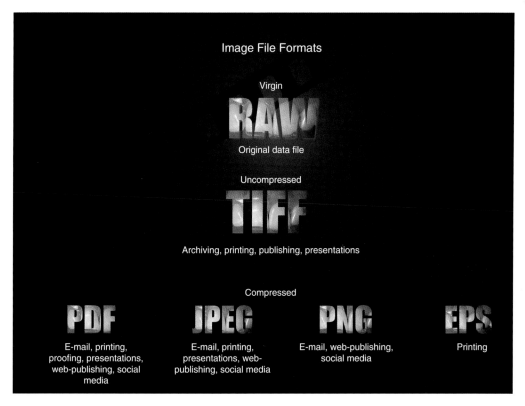

Figure 9.2 Image file formats for dental use.

communication such as attachments to e-mails. There are various varieties and qualities of JPEGs, ranging from Level 10 to Level 1; the higher the level, the greater the quality. Most cameras offer the option of capturing the initial image in JPEG format. While this offers advantages of taking more images before depleting the memory card storage capacity, the resulting images have inferior resolution, and cannot be converted later into the higher resolution TIFF format. The third file format is PDF, which also exhibits lossy compression with smaller file sizes compared to TIFF. The endearing feature of PDFs are that annotations can be added (see Module 8), which are invaluable for communicating various diagnostic detail, prescriptions to dental laboratories or proofing documents prior to printing. Due to their small size, PDFs can readily be attached with e-mails, and universally viewed by recipients with free downloads of Adobe® Acrobat software. The PNG file format offers small file sizes that are primarily intended for building websites. This format has essential features for creating and viewing websites with minimum upload times with reasonable quality. The EPS file format combines text and graphics, and is mainly used for publishing. Table 9.1 summarises some popular image file formats, their properties and intended uses.

Imaging Software

Although image processing is a complex procedure, it can broadly be categorised as editing or manipulation (Sandler and Murray 2002). This is analogous to writing a prose or narrative, where editing text involves corrections that allow the reader to more easily comprehend the message that is being conveyed, but not altering the message. On the other hand, manipulation

Table 9.1 Image file format properties and uses.

	RAW	Tagged Image File Format (TIFF)	Joint Photographic Experts Group (JPEG)	Personal Document File (PDF)
Colour mode (colour space)	RGB	RGB, CMYK, CIE L*a*b*	RGB, CMYK	RGB, CMYK
Colour (bit) depth	16 bit/channel	16 bit/channel	8 bit/channel	8 bit/channel
ICC profile	—	Yes	Yes	Yes
Compression	No	Optional	Yes	Yes
Alpha channel	No	Yes	No	No
Web-friendly	No	No	Yes	Yes
Uses	Archiving	Archiving, printing, publishing, presentations	E-mail, printing, presentations, web-publishing, social media	E-mail, printing, proofing, presentations, web-publishing, social media

RBG – red, green, blue.
CMYK – cyan, magenta, yellow, key (black).
CIE L*a*b* – Commission Internationale de l'éclairage colour co-ordinates.

alters the message or tells a different story to that of the original. Similarly, editing an image simply corrects technical issues without making alterations to the content of the image, i.e. the song remains the same. Conversely, image manipulation disguises or alters the image content, and therefore, its tune, to tell a different story. However, depending on disparate opinions, the line between editing and manipulation is often blurred, and some regard even the slightest alterations as forms of manipulation (Sheridan 2013).

The abundance of imaging software on the market is bewildering. There is innumerable choice aimed at every level of expertise, starting with the novice, enthusiast to the professional. The decision for selecting a particular product is influenced by three factors, cost, features, and the dedication of the user to utilise the full, or partial potential a software has to offer. These entities are interlinked and inseparable, and each factor determines the ultimate choice. Before recommending an imaging software for dental photography, a brief discussion about various products is necessary so that the purchaser is aware of what is available in terms of price, features and learning curves before making an informed decision.

All imaging software are not created equally, many are freely downloadable as open-source versions, which are readily accessible and instantaneous. Furthermore, all computers and cameras come with preloaded editing software such as Apple® Photos or Microsoft® Photos, or camera-specific packages, which are ready to use once the equipment is registered on the manufacturer's website. It is important to realise that whichever software is chosen, all are capable of accomplishing basic tasks such as altering colour temperature, exposure, orientation, cropping and dust removal with relative ease. However, these basic packages do not offer sophisticated features necessary for creativity and productivity.

The first item to consider is cost. The contenders for free software are the preloaded computer or camera specific programmes. The latter are usually basic packages that allow essential alterations mentioned above. Among the most popular free downloads are open-source products such as GIMP, Pixlr or Google Photos. The next bracket is the under US$ 100, which include Movavi Photo Editor, Corel AfterShot Pro, Pixelmator, Serif Affinity Photo and Adobe Photoshop Elements. The last category is the above US$ 100 price tag, such as Adobe Creative

Cloud, which includes Lightroom and Photoshop, ACDSee and Capture One. There are two options for purchasing photo-editing software, the first is outright purchase with periodic updates at a fraction of the initial outlay. The second option is a monthly subscription that can add up to over US$ 1000 per annum, depending on selected plug-ins for specific tasks or special effects. The advantage of subscription based software is that it is perpetually updated without having to purchase periodic updates, but the down-side is that the subscription is also perpetual, and one never actually owns the product.

The second item to consider is the number of features offered by the software, which varies considerably depending on the product. Besides price, the number of features or tools are crucial for choosing a product that suits the particular needs of the photographer. Below are some items worth considering before making a decision:

- System requirements – although obvious, it is prudent to check that the system requirements of the software are compatible with the computer specifications, e.g. the amount of disc space required, memory and graphics card
- Cross-platform capability – whether the software works exclusively on Windows® or Apple Mac®, or both operating systems
- Tethering or compact flash card reader – instead of using a flash card reader to transfer images from the camera to a computer, many software offer support for selected cameras (as many as 400 different cameras) to transfer images via a USB cable directly to a computer hard drive. In addition, some software has a live tethering feature that allows instant capture of the image directly into the software on the computer, and therefore bypassing storage onto a flash card
- Basic functions – most imaging software is capable of basic editing tasks such as correcting white balance, exposure, orientation, cropping, 'red eye' or dust artefacts removal, etc. However, it is beneficial to have the facility to make these adjustments both globally as well as locally, i.e. limited to certain parts of an image. Also, the editing should be non-destructive for maintaining image quality
- Image manipulation – these are features that alter the image by adding, removing, boosting or subduing parts of an image that the photographer feels are irrelevant, or the alterations will enhance the image for artistic or dramatic effects. This involve using filters, pre-set styles, LUTs (lookup tables), layers and masking tools for manipulating all, or part of an image. Many of these special effects are useful for creating images for marketing or promotion, but unwarranted for clinical fidelity
- 16-bit depth editing – some software, such as Photoshop Elements, limits some features to only an 8-bit file. However, since 16-bit editing allows greater processing without image degradation, it is advantageous to choose a software that permits 16-bit mode editing
- Web-based or hard-drive-based – particular software can only be used online for editing images without having to install them onto a computer hard drive. This is beneficial if hard drive space is limited, especially as graphic intensive software requires considerable disc storage capacity
- Cloud integration – another method for saving hard disc storage space is saving images on a virtual hard drive or digital cloud. The disadvantage is that uninterrupted and high-speed access to the internet is prerequisite for retrieving the images. In addition, cloud storage presents a potential security compromise, which is paramount for medically sensitive information such as photographs of patients
- Touch screen operation – this option is useful if using tablets or hybrid laptop-tablets for processing images
- Cataloguing – many imaging software are only capable of processing images, which must then be exported outside the software for storage. However, other programmes offer browser

and storage facilities within the software itself for easy access and retrievability. Cataloguing involves using keywords to tag images, for instance retrieving images of a specific treatment for showing patients before and after results. However, some practices or institutions may find cataloguing superfluous if they use practice management systems that allow images to be stored directly with the patient's dental records. Alternately, some clinics may prefer to archive images separately as a precaution that in the event the management software crashes, retrieving images is safeguarded, rather than having to wait for costly and protracted IT repairs

- File support – while most software support TIFF and JPEG file formats, not all support camera-specific RAW formats. If images are captured in proprietary RAW file format, it is worth checking if the software supports a particular camera brand and model. Another useful feature is the ability to output the edited files to the CMYK colour space, which is used for printing and publishing

- Output features – after editing or manipulations, it is helpful to have built-in export presets, or recipes, which facilitate outputting or exporting images for different purposes, e.g. archiving, printing or web-publishing

- Templates, plug-ins – these are usually third-party add-ons that facilitate specific tasks, including one-click preset fixes for editing, exporting, pre-formatted templates for brochures, calendars, flyers, greeting cards, or business stationary, to name a few. Another useful plug-in is LUTs, which alters the colour profile of an image to another predefined colour profile. This is beneficial for standardising a series of images so that colour rendition is identical for all images in particular portfolio

- Drawing tools – annotating images is helpful by adding lines, shapes and text for communicating with patients, colleagues or dental technicians. Many imaging software incorporate built-in drawing tool palettes for facilitating this process. However, some photographers may prefer to export the images after editing into a dedicated drawing software that they are familiar with

- Presentation apps – it is often beneficial to show patients a series of images depicting treatment sequences for education or treatment acceptance. This is usually accomplished with dedicated presentation software such as PowerPoint™ or Keynote.™ However, having apps build into a photo-editing software for creating mini presentations is advantageous and expedient

- Web and social media integration – newer software has the option of directly creating images that can be instantly shared on social media for e-marketing by e-mails or e-brochures. This offers convenience, but the caveat for confidentiality is paramount

- Soft proofing – this is a feature that allows the user to preview the printed version of the image before forwarding it to a printing device or printing house, ensuring that the printed image matches as close as possible to what is seen on the display monitor

- Automated back-up – is a particularly useful feature that facilitates backing-up images either to internal or external hard drives, or cloud storage, but respecting guidelines according to the HIPAA law (Health Insurance Portability and Accountability Act of 1996)[1]

- Training and technical support – is a must for novices, even for simple tasks such as correcting white balance or exposure. The established software houses excel in offering video tutorials, webinars, training, FAQ, guides, forums, and 24/7 online support that is indispensable for beginners, or even seasoned experts who stumble on software glitches or bugs requiring professional input for resolution

---

1 https://www.hhs.gov/hipaa/for-professionals/privacy/laws-regulations/index.html

• The final point to consider before choosing a software is the learning curve for negotiating the graphic user interface (GUI) of a programme. While most software interfaces appear similar, the ease of use can be challenging, and require professional training. Hence, a compromise is necessary; more features translate to a steeper learning curve, whereas less features translate to a vertical learning curve. If time is of the essence, it is better to select a software with an intuitive and simple interface having basic features that can be mastered within a relatively short space of time. This is where a polished commercial product wins hands down, compared to an open-source development product that may be trial and error for achieving the desired goals. Furthermore, if a problem is encountered with freebies, the user is often left stranded to struggle with insurmountable issues

To conclude, the ultimate choice of imaging software is unique to every photographer depending on cost, features and ease of use (Figure 9.3). At this juncture, the clinician or dental technician needs to decide whether photographic documentation is limited solely for dental use, a quasi-passion, or aiming to be creative and/or achieving professional heights? If the answer is solely for dental purposes, then any simple photo-editing software with basic functions will suffice, e.g. Apple Photos, Microsoft Photos, Google® Photos, etc. These software packages are free, have intuitive interfaces, a vertical learning curve, with many one-click preset options, easy to use and serve the majority of dental needs. For the intermediate or enthusiastic level, the choices are GIMP, Movavi Photo Editor, Corel® AfterShot Pro, Pixelmator, Serif Affinity Photo, IrfanView and Adobe Photoshop Elements. These programmes are more time-intensive to master, but offer many creative and preset features unavailable in basic versions. Lastly, if the intention is to be more creative, spend unlimited time learning new features, and jump to a professional level, the software of choice is Adobe Creative Cloud, ACDSee or Capture One. Photoshop (part of Adobe Creative Cloud) is undoubtedly the industry standard,

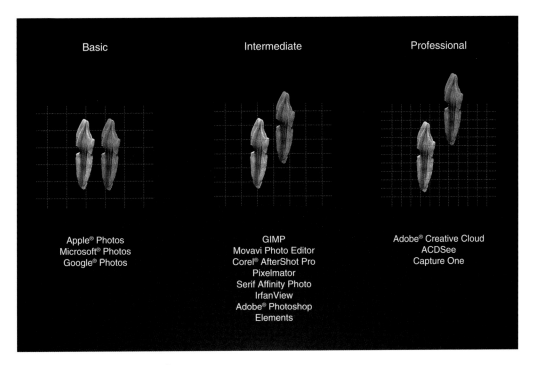

Figure 9.3 Choice of imaging software.

offering both image editing and manipulation, and creativity limited only by the imagination; if you can't do it in Photoshop, it probably can't be done. ACD Systems offer several software for processing, a powerful drawing and painting programme, plus a cataloguing image management system. Capture One is essentially an image editing software, with extensive presets, LUTs, a few manipulation effects plus comprehensive cataloguing facilities. The philosophy behind this software is processing images, without compromise, to their maximum potential, i.e. image quality, and only image quality, is the order of the day. Capture One (current version 12) is made by Phase One®, a company that manufactures high-end digital cameras. The software interface is geared for the professional, with intuitive menus and unique features that bring out the best in any image. Furthermore, the software is backed by helpful technical support, video tutorials, forums and blogs for expediting the leaning process.

Image Processing

Image processing begins with in-camera processing, during and after an image is taken. The camera software performs many processing tasks such as calculating exposure, white balance, file format conversion and other functions according to settings input by the user. For example, if JPEG or TIFF files are selected, processing the white balance and file conversion is performed inside the camera, and no further adjustments are required. However, for dental or professional photography, it is advisable to use RAW file formats, which require processing outside the camera by using imaging software (Snow 2013). The interface of most imaging software is very similar, consisting of a main viewer, browser, cascading menu options, fixed or floating tool-bars, and tabs, which can be customised according to personal preferences. In addition, default and personalised keyboard shortcuts help access functions with relative ease and speed.

As mentioned above, processing standardised dental pictures should be concerned only with image editing, rather than image manipulation. The pertinent questions are:

> What requires editing?
> What is ethically permissible?
> What is technically beneficial?
> What is technically detrimental?

As dental images are dento-legal records, alterations should be restricted to technical issues that allow the observer to 'read' the image more clearly, not unlike correcting typographical errors in text. In addition, limiting the amount of alterations also preserves image quality, which is essential for maintaining consistency. Hence, for clinical fidelity, image editing is ethically permissible, and indeed beneficial. On the other hand, stringent restrictions do not apply to images intended for marketing purposes, and therefore, manipulations for enhancing appeal and attention are acceptable.

While there is no substitute for good photographic technique at the capture stage, nearly all images require some form of retouching to polish the final result, no different to polishing a diamond for maximising its optical properties. These adjustments are part of the post-processing workflow that is performed sequentially starting with colour spaces, white balance, exposure, orientation and cropping, removing artefacts (dust particles), local adjustments (layers) and, lastly, sharpening. Although this is a truncated list of tasks that are not applicable for every image, but nevertheless, represents the salient adjustments that are essential for image editing. There are many other corrections that can be performed such as noise reduction, lens correction, moiré, colour and curves edits, applying LUTs, perspective changes, conversion of colour space to CMYK for printing and so on. However, these tasks are reserved for more experienced photographers, and usually superfluous for routine dental photography.

The last aspect to consider before making adjustments is choosing the most appropriate file format for editing or manipulation. The tolerance level of a file depends on its bit depth. In order for the human eye to perceive a smooth continuum from black to white, a bit depth of 8 is necessary, i.e. 256 shades of grey ($2^8 = 256$) (Figure 9.4). Therefore, to produce colour images, each of the three colour channels, red green, and blue (RGB), must have a bit depth of 8, which translates to 16.7 million colours (256 red × 256 green × 256 blue = 16.7 million) – (Figure 9.5). This is far greater than the human eye, which can discriminate around 10 million colours. Hence, in theory, an 8 bit/channel is more than adequate for colour perception. However, each edit and manipulation progressively reduces the bit depth, and extensive adjustments result in a bit depth that is below the visual perception of colour. Therefore, starting with a higher bit depth of 16 bit/channel with 65 536 brightness levels/channel, compared to 256 brightness levels/channel for 8-bit depth, allows greater flexibility and leverage for ensuring that the final bit depth is sufficient for visual perception. This is the reason that processing should be carried out using RAW files, or image captures with a higher bit depth, allowing greater manoeuvrability or 'editing headroom' without causing image posterisation (Ahmad 2009b).[2] Posterisation occurs when the tonal range of an image exceeds its bit depth, causing visible colour banding reminiscent of bill board posters. The reason why this occurs with posters is because the printing process uses only a few coloured inks, that are unable to reproduce seamless and subtle colour transitions. Posterisation of an image literally means 'tonal spaces' and is evident when the histogram is jagged with pronounced banding and spaces representing missing bits of information, or there is a colour space mismatch between the camera hardware and processing software (Figures 9.6–9.8).

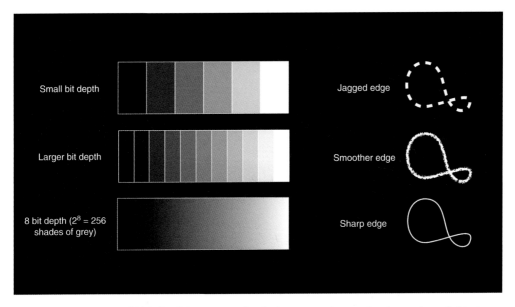

Figure 9.4 A minimum of 8 bit depth is necessary for the human eye to perceive sharp edges of objects or a seamless transition from black to white.

---

2 http://laurashoe.com/2011/08/09/8-versus-16-bit-what-does-it-really-mean

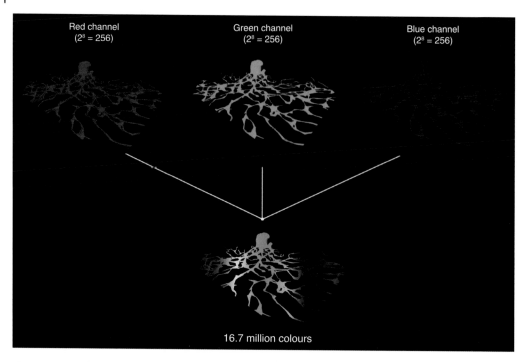

Figure 9.5 An 8 bit/channel is capable of producing 16.7 million colours by stimulating retina cells sensitive to the red, green, and blue (RGB) channels.

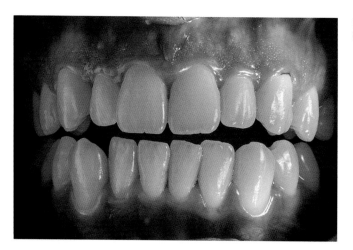

Figure 9.6 Posterisation: original image.

Colour Spaces

Colour spaces or colour profiles are illustrations of colour models, and the area they represent is called a gamut. A colour space of a device determines the amount of colour it can record (camera or scanner), display (monitor) or output (printer) (Devigus and Paul 2006). Every device has a specific colour space, with little standardisation between different manufacturers. However, the three widely accepted colour spaces are sRGB (standard red, green, blue), Adobe RGB and CMYK (cyan, magenta, yellow and key or black). Furthermore, discussions are in progress to create a medical RGB (mRGB) for standardising colour for medical and dental photography

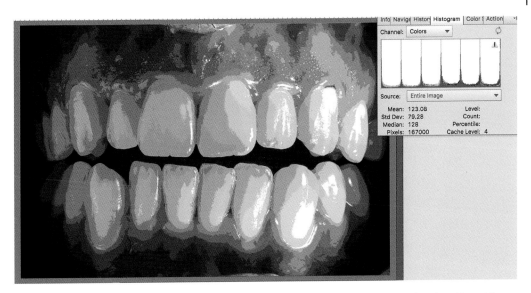

Figure 9.7 Posterisation: colour histogram showing a spiky appearance representing colour banding without seamless transition between missing colours.

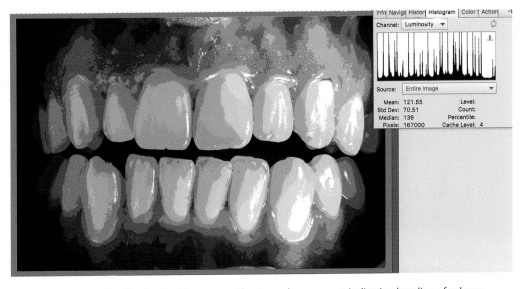

Figure 9.8 Posterisation: luminosity histogram with a jagged appearance indicating banding of colours.

(Badano et al. 2015). The sRGB can be regarded as a generic colour space, and although it has many variations, most camera and computer manufacturers have adopted it as a default. The proprietary Adobe RGB is a larger colour space, but requires a greater bit depth to take advantage of its bigger gamut. The CMYK is the smallest space and is primarily used for printing (Figure 9.9). When importing images from the camera to a computer, most imaging software automatically ensures that the colour space is appropriately matched. However, it is worth checking to avoid a mismatch between the colour space of the camera and the imaging software. Also, the colour space can readily be changed, for example from sRGB to Adobe RGB, to take advantage of a larger colour gamut when editing in 16-bit mode (Figure 9.10).

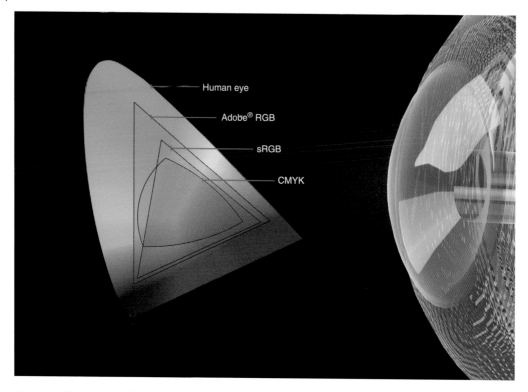

Figure 9.9 Comparison of various colour spaces.

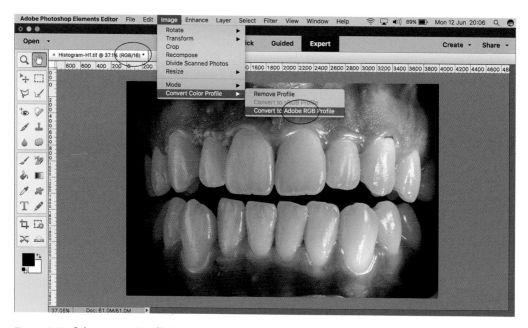

Figure 9.10 Colour spaces (profiles) can easily be changed in imaging software to take advantage of a larger gamut when editing in 16-bit mode (blue circles).

White Balance

The next item to check is the white balance. If the WB was set on the camera, no further calibrations should be necessary. However, if an 18% neutral density grey card was used for setting the white balance, which is probably the most accurate method for ensuring colour accuracy and consistency, calibration within the software is required. The reference image with the grey card is located and the 'neutral grey' or 'white balance' tool selected, depicted by a pipette. The computer mouse cursor is then clicked on the grey card in the image to calibrate the white balance. This setting is then saved and recalled for correcting the white balance of subsequent images in the same session (see Figures 3.25–3.28 in Module 3). Also, the reference image can be included with images from the same session for transmission via the internet, so that the recipient can calibrate the images on different monitor displays for ensuring colour consistency.

Exposure

After setting the white balance, the exposure needs to be evaluated. Imaging software offer a variety of adjustments for altering the exposure including increasing or decreasing the *f*-stop (exposure), contrast, brightness, brilliance, saturation, highlights, shadows, to name a few. Whilst these variables alter the exposure instantaneously, the process is ad hoc and whimsical. A more systematic and methodical approach is using the histogram. The histogram is one of the most misunderstood tools of digital photography, even though it offers precise control over many variables. As well as displaying exposure, the histogram is also used for determining colour distribution, contrast and dynamic range of an image.

The histogram is a graphical representation of the darkest, brightest and midtones in an image. The *x*-axis represents the tonal range, (256 graduations for an 8-bit depth image), while the *y*-axis is the amount of these tones distributed within an image (Nordberg and Sluder 2013). The darkest areas are the shadows on the left side of the *x*-axis, midtones in the middle, and the brightest areas are the highlights on the right side (Figure 9.11).The histogram is the equivalent of a light meter, and is found on the LCD screens of cameras, and in virtually all image processing software. There are many types of histograms such as total RGB (colour overlay) (Figure 9.12), individual red, green and blue channels (Figures 9.13–9.15), and luminosity (or luminance) (Figure 9.16). Each type displays different information, but the most widely used is the total RGB version. The histogram is an 8-bit function, regardless of the characteristics of the image being analysed, and shows 256 shades of grey. However, when editing in 16-bit mode, a histogram cannot show 65 536 values due to its small physical size on the screen, and is still represented as a 256 scale.

There is no ideal histogram, and its peaks and troughs are influenced by the subject matter of the photograph. For example, a black object has peaks confined to the left side (low key image), while a white object has peaks located on the right side (high key image). If the shadows are too dark, or the highlights too bright, the areas are said to be clipped, where detail is lost. Clipping is viewed by turning on the exposure warnings for highlights and shadows (Figure 9.17). Some detail may be retrievable by exposure correction, but if the clipped areas are extreme, detail is completely lost, irrespective of the amount of exposure compensation. As a general guide, the histogram of a correctly exposed picture (without excessively dark or bright [reflective] objects), has the majority of peaks concentrated in the midtone range with a few peaks in the shadows and highlight regions. This balanced, or average, exposure represents a numerical value of 128 (halfway between 0 and 255), and is used for calibrating most camera metering systems (Figure 9.18). The specific areas of highlights, midtones and shadows in any part of an

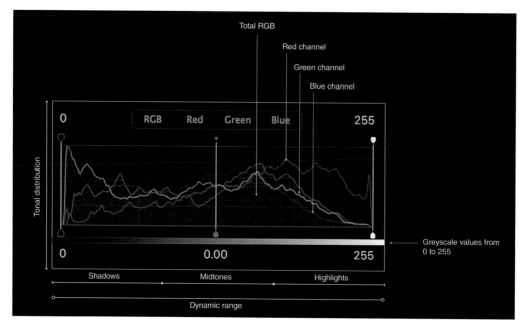

Figure 9.11 Schematic representation of a histogram.

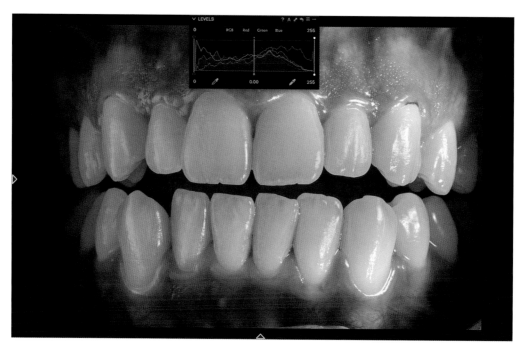

Figure 9.12 Histogram: total red, green, and blue (RGB).

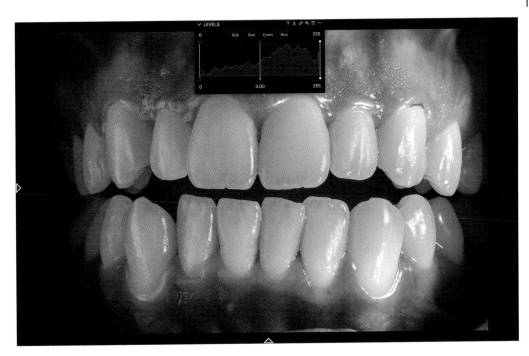

Figure 9.13 Histogram: individual red channel.

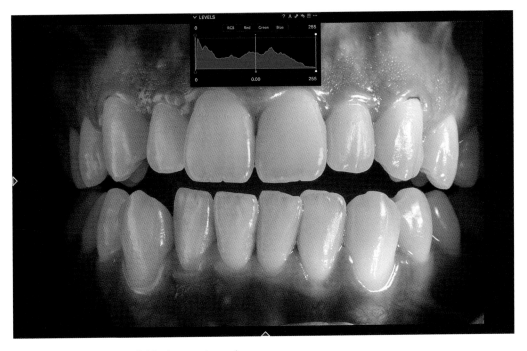

Figure 9.14 Histogram: individual green channel.

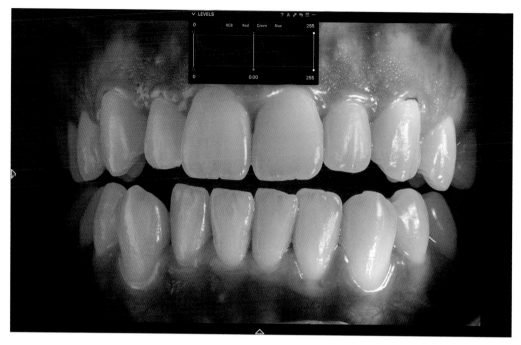

Figure 9.15 Histogram: individual blue channel.

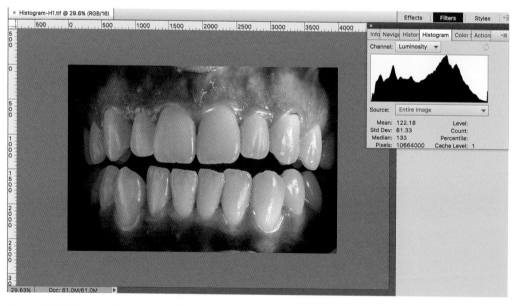

Figure 9.16 Histogram: luminosity or luminance.

image can be displayed on a histogram by hovering the mouse pointer over the image (Figure 9.19).

The crucial issue is the extent to which exposure can be altered without affecting resolution or introducing unwanted colour casts. This depends on the initial bit depth of the image, and the amount of correction necessary. If an image is over or underexposed, it may be 'pushed' (exposure

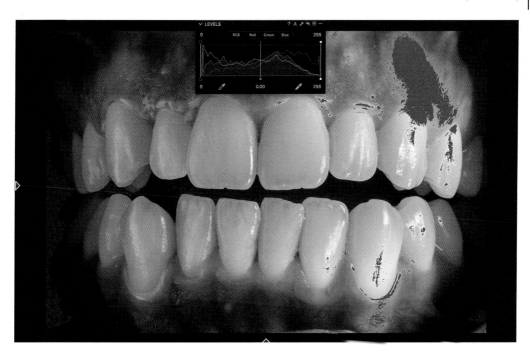

Figure 9.17 Clipping: red areas represent overexposed highlights, while blue areas signify underexposed shadows.

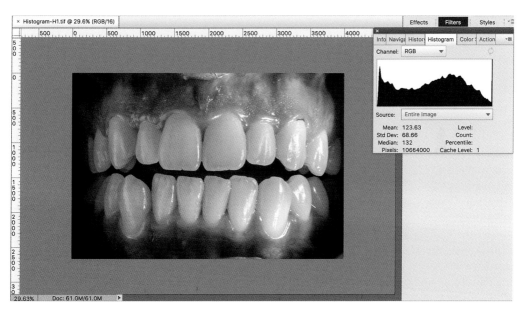

Figure 9.18 Average metering is the aim of most cameras for ensuring 'correct' exposure, represented by a large midtone region, with a few peaks in the shadow and highlight regions.

compensation) in editing software, by increasing or decreasing the level of brightness or darkness. But to what extent can it be 'pushed' without compromising quality? As a rule-of-thumb, an 8-bit overexposed or underexposed image can withstand a 1 f-stop exposure compensation without a noticeable deterioration in quality, while a 16-bit image allows greater latitude. The easiest

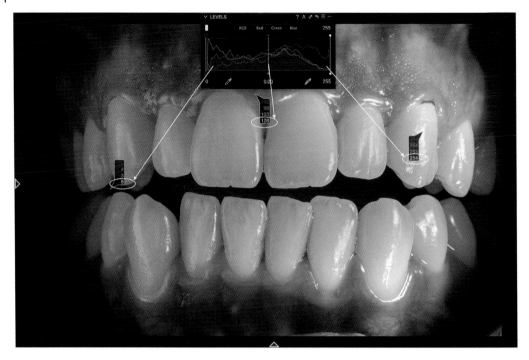

Figure 9.19 The tonal range of an image can be ascertained by hovering the mouse pointer to various sites of an image. The white text in the colour swathes indicate the shadows (5), midtones (128) and highlights (254).

method for correcting exposure is turning on the exposure warning to display over and underexposure areas. The exposure, contrast, brightness, brilliance, saturation, highlights or shadows are adjusted until the correction is acceptable. Care should be exercised not to completely eliminate areas of highlights and/or shadows to avoid a bland, flat image (Figures 9.20–9.23). However, if extreme exposure corrections are necessary, it is better, if possible, to take another picture rather than risking severe degradation in image quality (Figures 9.24–9.27).

The second element that a histogram is useful for is assessing the contrast of an image. This is determined by the aggregation or segregation of the peaks in a histogram. For a low contrast image, the peaks are clustered together, while for a high contrast image, the peaks are spread out (Figures 9.28–9.30). A hight contrast image, within limits, is vibrant, punchy and attracts attention. Conversely, a low contrast picture is dull, lacklustre and perceived as boring.

Another use of a histogram is ascertaining the dynamic range (DR). DR is a hardware property of the camera sensor, and indicates total tonal range from the darkest to the brightest, expressed as the number of *f*-stops that a sensor is capable of recording. The human eye can discern a DR of around 24 *f*-stops,[3] while most digital devices, in theory, are capable of recording an infinite amount of DR. However, it is the amount of usable DR that is important, and depends on bit depth of the imaging chip or sensor in a camera. The DR of digital cameras vary enormously, ranging from 4 to 15 *f*-stops (Figure 9.31). A large DR is ideal for display devices such as monitors or projectors, but the DR of printed media is limited to around 4 to 5 *f*-stops, and therefore suffers from detail loss by several *f*-stop[4] (see Figure 3.24 in Module 3). This is the reason why a picture that appears full of vitality on a computer monitor, is often insipid when printed. However, having a large DR spread over a small bit depth is futile and results in image

3 http://www.cambridgeincolour.com/tutorials/dynamic-range.htm
4 https://petapixel.com/2015/05/26/film-vs-digital-a-comparison-of-the-advantages-and-disadvantages

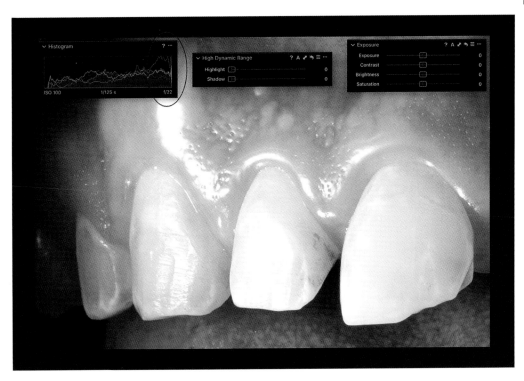

Figure 9.20 Initial image with excessive highlights (depicted by peaks on the right side of the histogram), which are obscuring surface detail of the maxillary right incisors and canine.

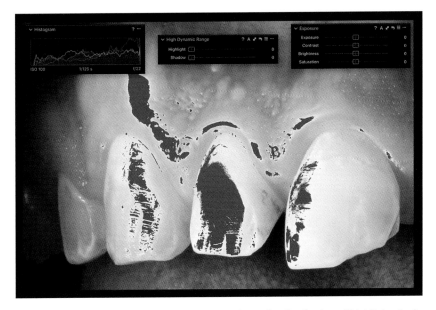

Figure 9.21 Turning on the exposure warnings shows the distribution of highlights (red areas).

posterisation, since the smaller bit depth cannot accommodate a large DR. There are two methods for circumventing this limitation, the first is using camera that has a 16-bit sensor, or using high dynamic range (HDR) photography, often referred to as image hallucination. HDR photography is a software process of 'stitching' together multiple bracketed exposure images

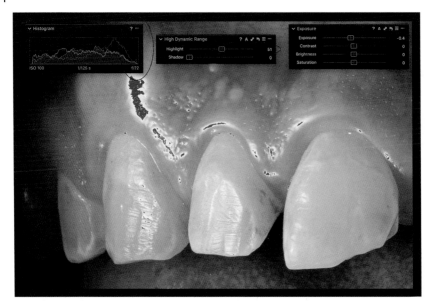

Figure 9.22 Adjusting the exposure reduces the highlights and the peaks on the right side of the histogram, which allow visualisation of the surface texture on the maxillary right incisors and canine. Notice that some of the highlight areas are intentionally left intact to maintain vitality and a three-dimensional quality of the image.

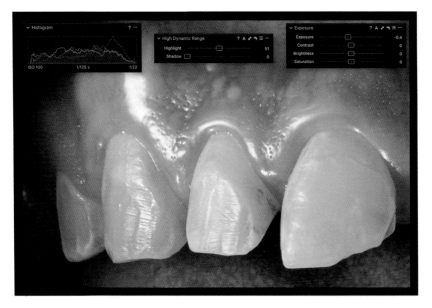

Figure 9.23 Adjusted image with exposure warnings turned off (compare with Figure 9.20).

for increasing the DR of an image.[5] This involves taking several pictures with different exposures that the imaging software converts into 32-bit open-ended brightness files. The files are then digitally merged into a single image for achieving a higher DR.

---

5 http://www.stuckincustoms.com/hdr-photography

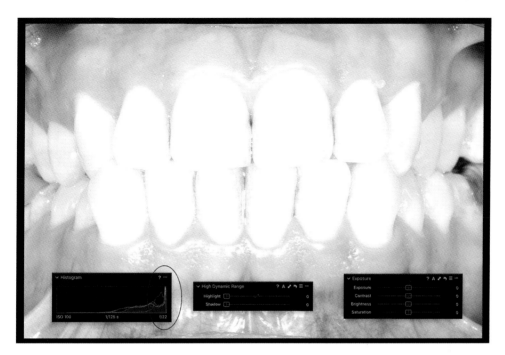

Figure 9.24 Initial grossly overexposure image. Notice the peaks isolated to the right side of the histogram.

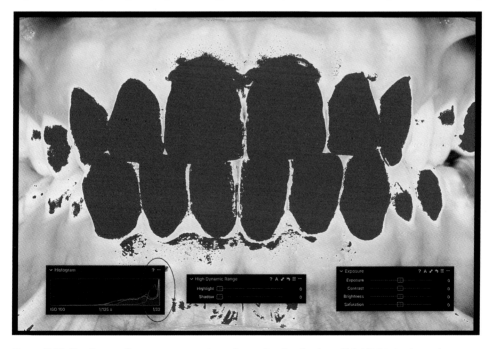

Figure 9.25 Turning on the exposure warnings shows the distribution of highlights (red areas).

Orientation, Scaling and Cropping

After correcting the exposure, the next stage is orientating and scaling the image in preparation for cropping. Orientation involves straightening the image so that it is parallel to the horizon. A frequent mistake is pseudo-aligning the incisal or occlusal plane so that it appears horizontal

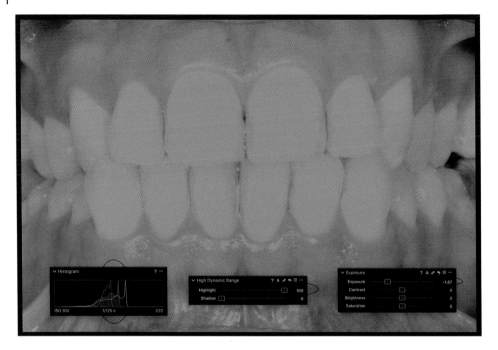

Figure 9.26 After drastically reducing the highlights by exposure compensation, the image quality deteriorates with a green colour cast. Although the peaks on the histograms are now located in the midtones region, the image is still overexposed.

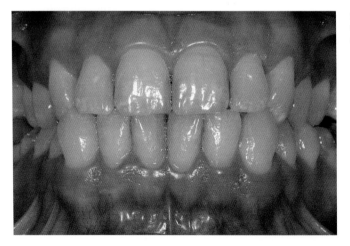

Figure 9.27 Another image taken with correct exposure (compare with Figure 9.24).

in intra-oral images. The correct alignment of the incisal plane is judged from the dento-facial or full face perspective with the head positioned correctly in the horizontal plane (see EPP Image #3: Fontal view – biting wooden spatula in Module 6). If the incisal plane is canted in this view, it should not be falsely re-aligned in the intra-oral views. However, most images require minor tweaks to orientate them correctly. It is best practice to turn on the vertical and horizontal grid lines option in the software for aiding orientation.

The next process is scaling. If the image was taken with pre-set magnification or a predefined focusing distance set on the lens, no further scaling is required. This ensures standard images

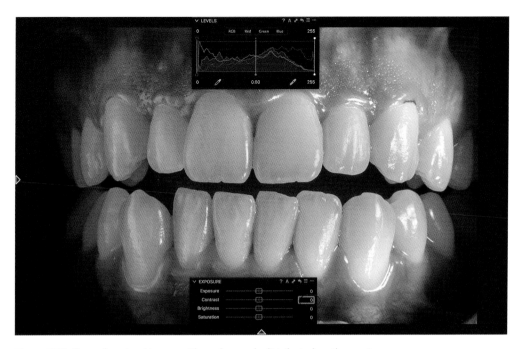

Figure 9.28 Normal contrast image with peaks evenly distributed on the *x*-axis.

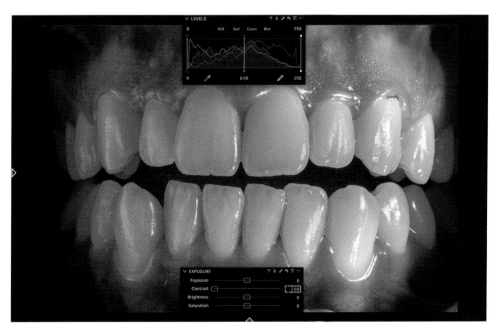

Figure 9.29 Low contrast image with peaks clustered together on the *x*-axis.

for inter- and intra-patient comparison. However, if the image was framed with a larger view, extraneous objects such as cheek retractors or mirrors will require cropping. Also, intra-oral images taken with mirrors need to be rotated and laterally inverted (flipped) – (Figures 9.32–9.38). In some circumstances it is necessary to crop or enlarge part of an image to show particular

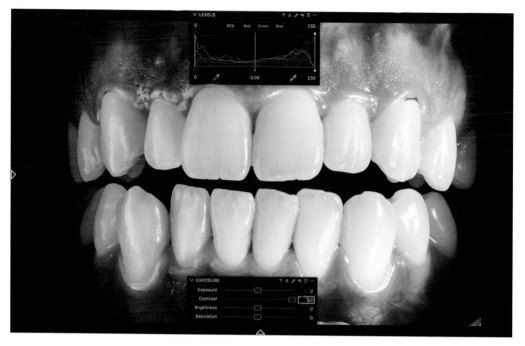

Figure 9.30 Hight contrast image with peaks spread out on the *x*-axis.

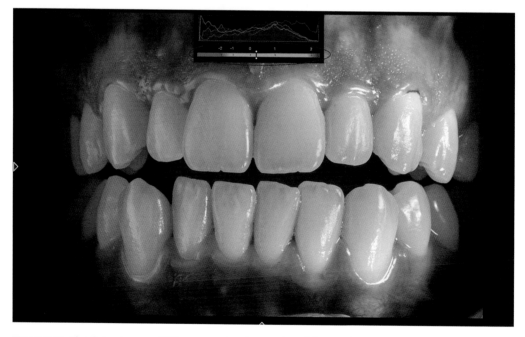

Figure 9.31 The dynamic range (DR), expressed as the number of *f*-stops, determines the amount of detail that a camera sensor can record from the darkest to the lightest part of an image.

Figure 9.32 Original image.

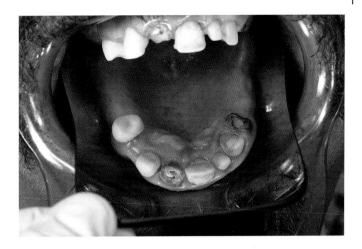

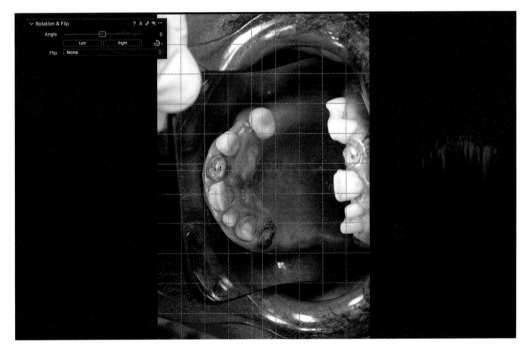

Figure 9.33 Rotate right 90°.

points of interest. The technical terminology for enlarging is interpolation, which is a mathematical algorithm process used by imaging software. Interpolation literally means stretching the image by inserting empty pixels (with no detail) to the desired enlargement. There are several types of interpolation formulae, but the important issue is that enlarging is not limitless, and should be judicially performed to prevent pixellation, which negates the initial scaling objective (Figure 9.39).

Some cropping is usually necessary if images have been re-aligned, and consists of two parts: aspect ratio and the physical size of the image. The aspect ratio ensures that the width/height of a series of images is constant, irrespective of their physical size. The aspect ratio can either be set on the camera or in the imaging software, and can either be portrait, or landscape. For

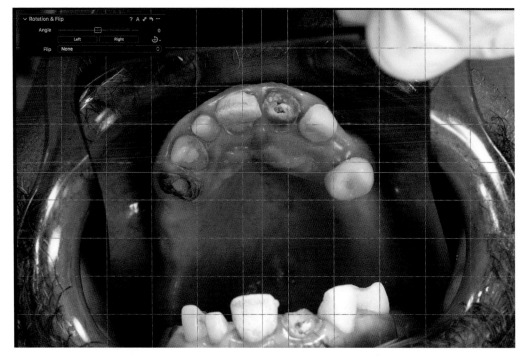

Figure 9.34 Rotate right 90°.

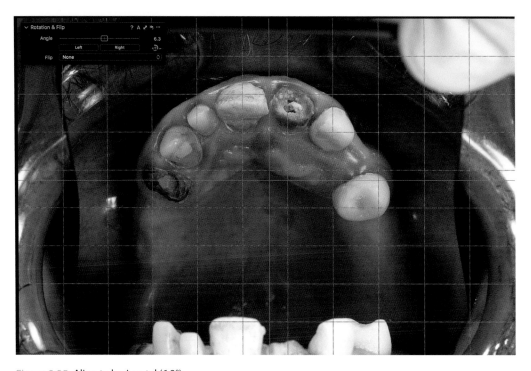

Figure 9.35 Align to horizontal (6.3°).

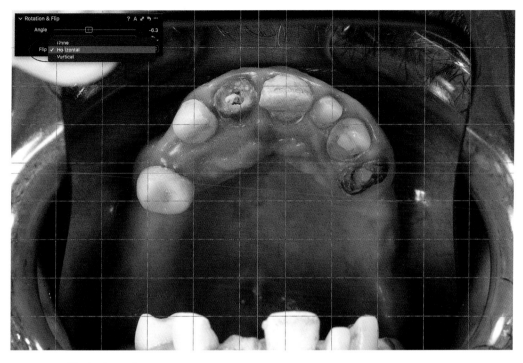

Figure 9.36 Flip horizontally.

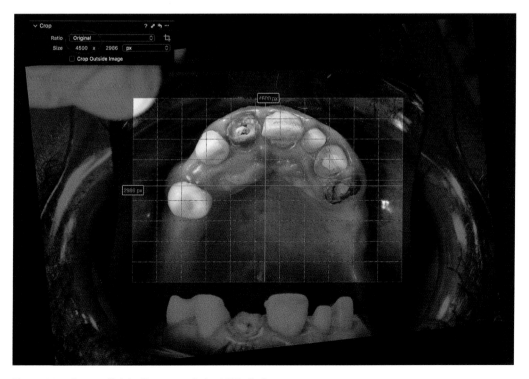

Figure 9.37 Crop to 'Original' aspect ratio by 4500 pixels.

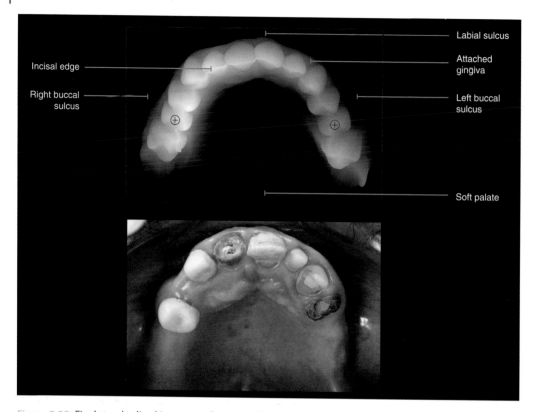

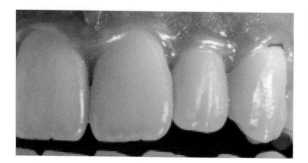

Figure 9.38 Final standardised image comforting to EDP image #8.

Figure 9.39 Excessively enlarging an image causes unwanted pixillation.

ensuring consistency, the aspect ratio can be left unchanged (original) corresponding to the camera sensor, or changed manually in the software for specific ratios such as square, 2 : 3, 5 : 7, 16 : 9, etc., (Figures 9.40–9.43). Imaging software also offer an unconstrained option for freely cropping the image to an unattributed ratio. However, this results in images with different widths and heights that compromise standardisation. The second point to consider is the physical size of the image. Once again, to ensure uniformity, all images should be the same size. This is achieved, concurrently with cropping, by numerically inputting the size of the image using the preferred units, e.g. pixels (px), inches (in), mm, or cm (Figures 9.44–9.46).

As well as ensuring the correct aspect ratio and size, cropping is also invaluable for composing an image so that it conforms to chosen composition rules, and standardising fields of view mentioned in Module 4. Ideally, a picture should be composed at the capture stage to minimise editing. However, obtaining a proper field of view for dental images is challenging. The field of view

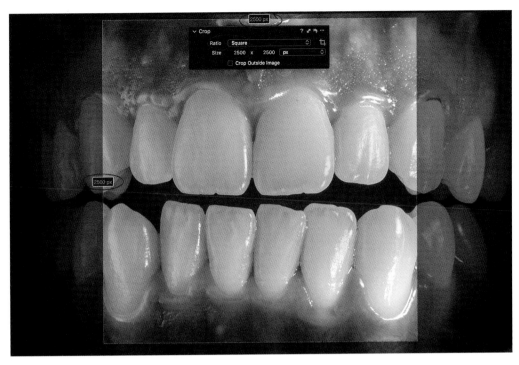

Figure 9.40 Aspect ratio – square (notice that the width is constant at 2500 pixels for all the examples below, but the height of the image varies according to the aspect ratio).

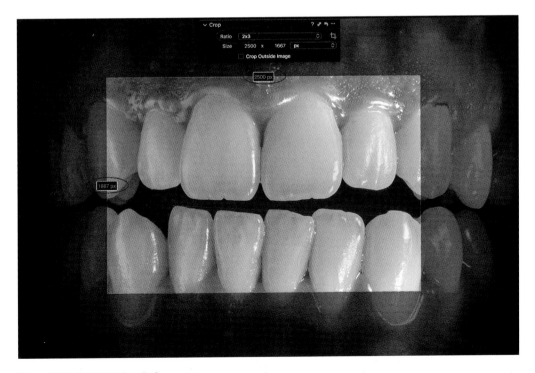

Figure 9.41 Aspect ratio – 2 : 3.

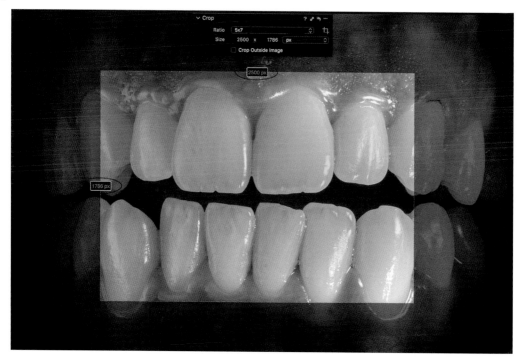

Figure 9.42 Aspect ratio – 5 : 7.

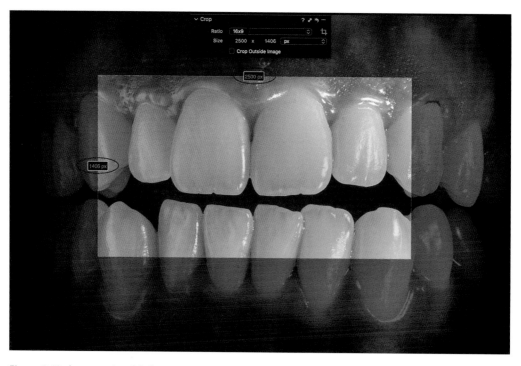

Figure 9.43 Aspect ratio – 16 : 9.

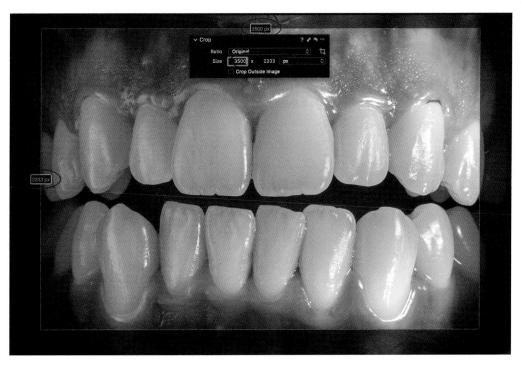

Figure 9.44 The size of an image can be numerically input using the number of pixels, e.g. 3500×2333 (determined by aspect ratio)…

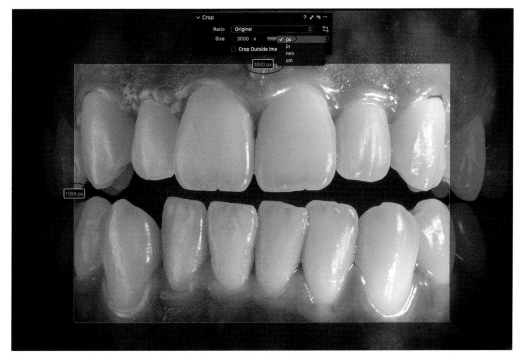

Figure 9.45 …or 3000×1999 pixels, etc.

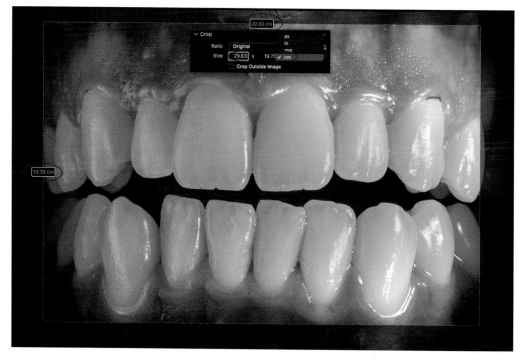

Figure 9.46 The size of an image can also be numerically input by dimensions in cm, e.g. 29.63 × 19.75, which is equivalent to 3500 × 2333 pixels (constrained by the aspect ratio).

may be less than ideal due to movements of the patient, operator or incorrect equipment positioning. These failings can partially be compensated at the processing stage by cropping extraneous objects to concentrate on the points of interest, as well as aligning the image so that it is standardised according to guidelines for the EDP (essential dental portfolio) and EPP (essential portrait portfolio) discussed in Module 5 and Module 6, respectively (Figures 9.47–9.49).

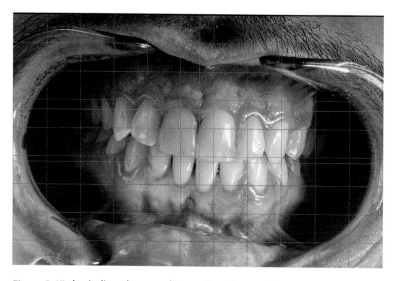

Figure 9.47 A misaligned captured image. In order to realign this image, a vertical grid line (vertical orange line) is placed at the dental midline, and horizontal grid lines (horizontal orange lines) at the cervical and incisal aspects of the maxillary anterior teeth, and the image rotated accordingly to coincide with these orientation lines.

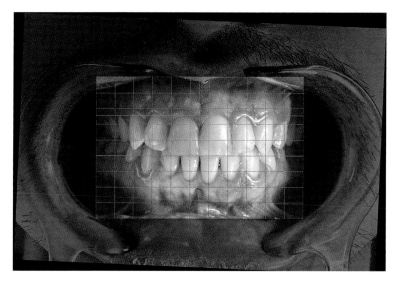

Figure 9.48 Correctly aligned and cropped image to exclude extraneous objects such as cheek retractors and superfluous extra-oral anatomy.

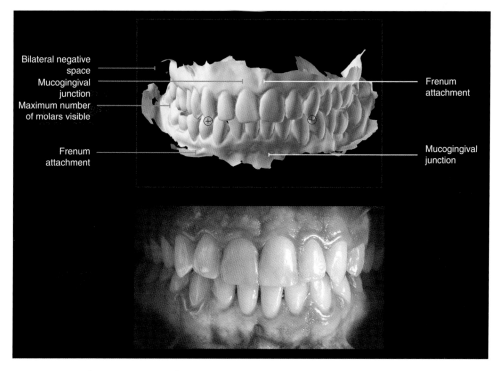

Figure 9.49 Final image corresponding to standardised EDP image #4.

Artefact Removal

One of the most annoying things about digital photography is accumulation of dust or fluff particles that adhere to the camera sensor by static electricity. This is particularly pronounced with cameras that have a mirror, or if lenses are constantly interchanged. Many cameras have built-in sensor cleaning mechanisms to mitigate this phenomena. Also, numerous sensor cleaning kits are available for cleaning sensors consisting of lint-free cloths, mild detergents and mini vacuum cleaners. It is worth emphasising that sensor cleaning is a very delicate and fiddly procedure, and if performed causally, can cause irreparable damage to the sensor. Therefore, it is prudent to delegate this task to a skilled professional who is proficient in this field. Dust particles tenaciously stuck to the sensor appear as tiny white and black dots or blemishes on the image, which are particularly conspicuous on light or white surfaces such as teeth. If the sensor is scratched, the artefacts are larger and even more conspicuous. Most software has spot removal, healing or cloning tools for removing these artefacts, but if dust particles are widespread, the process is onerous and time-consuming (see Figure 1.13 in Module 1).

Another issue is condensation on the glass covering the sensor that occurs with extreme changes in ambient temperatures. This may occur when using the camera at the beginning of the day during the winter months, or taking the camera outside from an air conditioned room. The resultant images are hazy, and the only solution is to allow the camera to acclimatise to the new temperature before starting a photographic session.

Local Adjustments

The editing described above affects the entire image, and the adjustments are termed global. However, in certain circumstances, it may be beneficial to edit only particular parts of an image that perhaps maybe underexposed, or require some form of enhancement for conveying the intended message. This is probably the most gratifying aspect of digital photography for compensating inadvertent photographic mistakes, which can be rectified after taking a picture. In theory, any variables such as colour, exposure, sharpness, cloning, etc., can be adjusted locally. However, local adjustments are highly contention for ethical reasons, and steer into image manipulation territory. For example, changing the colour of inflamed tissues from red to pink in a particular region can fraudulently convey health, and lead to misdiagnosis of an underlying pathology. Therefore, local adjustments should be limited to those variables that are compensating for fallings in photographic technique, rather than surreptitiously masking pathology or deficiencies in treatment for enhancing post-operative outcomes.

An example of a justifiable local adjustment is correcting exposure in part of the image that was poorly illuminated. Furthermore, some pictures cannot be repeated, but nevertheless benefit from minor corrections, e.g. recording treatment sequences or surgical procedures. The image in Figure 9.50 shows surgical crown lengthening of the maxillary anterior teeth using a

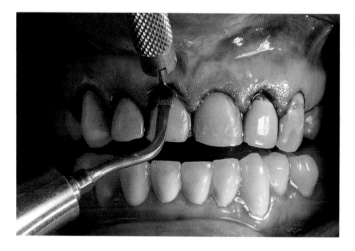

Figure 9.50 Poorly illuminated piezo tip and Zekrya gingival retractor.

piezo surgery tip for performing ostectomy and osteoplasty. Although the picture is correctly exposed, the piezo tip and Zekrya retractor are poorly illuminated and could benefit by increasing brightness to make them more conspicuous to guide the eye to the main point of interest. The local adjustment tool creates a separate layer, consisting of an airbrush (depicted by an airbrush emoji) to draw a mask (green) delineating the parts requiring an increase in exposure. The exposure was increased by 1 *f*-stop and the shadows lifted by a factor of 11 (Figure 9.51). The final image shows the effect of the local adjustment, restricted only to the piezo tip and part of the Zekrya gingival retractor, making them brighter and more visible (Figure 9.52).

Sharpening

The last item to consider in post-image processing is the sharpness of an image. Sharpness is determined by the hardware, the magnification factor and the viewing distance. In addition,

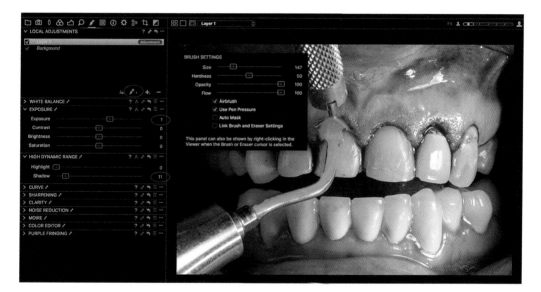

Figure 9.51 Local adjustment limited to piezo tip and Zekrya gingival retractor.

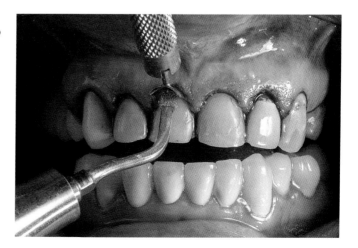

Figure 9.52 Adjusted image with a brighter and clearly visible piezo tip and Zekrya gingival retractor (compare with Figure 9.50).

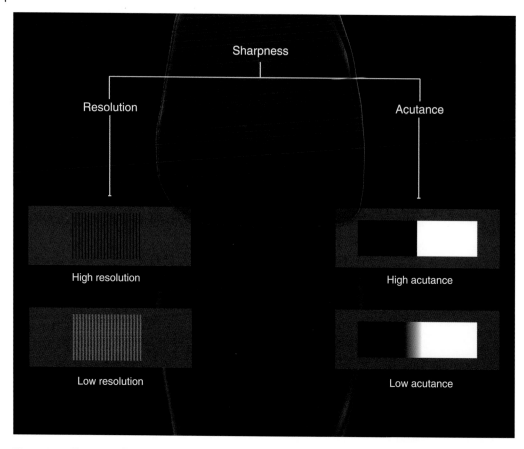

Figure 9.53 Sharpness depends on resolution (property of lens to discriminate fine detail) and acutance (ability to discriminate edges of objects).

proper photographic technique plays a crucial role such as correct focusing, preventing camera shake, and setting an appropriate ISO number for mitigating 'image noise'. The sharpness of an image is highly subjective, varying from individual to individual, and for the same person at different times depending on their state of mind. In objective terms, in order for an image to appear sharp depends on two fundamental parameters: resolution and acutance. Resolution is unchangeable since it is an intrinsic property of the lens and its ability to discriminate detail between closely spaced objects, e.g. the number of lines resolvable per millimetre. Acutance is the ability to clearly discern the edges of objects, i.e. the tonal contrast between two objects, and is the parameter that is adjustable in imaging software[6] (Figure 9.53).

Most images captured by digital cameras are unshaped due to the colour filters covering the pixels for adding colour, usually Bayer or Fovean interpolation filters (see Figure 1.4 in Module 1). There are two methods for compensating this unwanted side-effect, either applying immediate sharpening by in-camera processing, or sharpening in imaging software. The latter method is preferred since it allows greater control for increasing sharpness both globally and locally to only selected parts of an image. However, most cameras, by default, are configured to perform

---

6 http://www.photoreview.com.au/tips/shooting/sharpness,-acutance-and-resolution

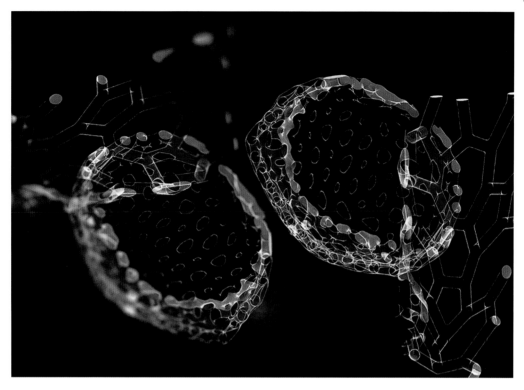

Figure 9.54 The image on the left is out of focus at its periphery, which cannot be sharpening by imaging software, and therefore it is better to take another in-focus image (right).

in-camera sharpening before displaying the image on the LCD screen for previewing. If the intention is to use imaging software, the factory default settings for sharpening in the camera menu should be disabled beforehand. Also, it is important to realise that no amount of processing will render sharpness to blurred or out-of-focus images (Figure 9.54).

The basic principle of sharpening is increasing the relative contrast between the edges of objects by altering three variables, 'amount', 'radius' and 'threshold', thereby giving an illusion that the objects appear sharper. It is advisable to create a separate layer to perform the sharpening so that the original image is left intact in case the results are not as anticipated. Also, the image should be viewed at 100% zoom, and sharpening is always the last step in the imaging (editing) chain. The extent of sharpening depends on the subject of the image (skin tones, gingiva, teeth), intended use of the image (e.g. websites), or the media on which the image will be displayed (monitor, projector screen, or paper). Coated or glossy paper is usually more punchy and sharper as it confines ink 'bleeding', whereas matt paper allows inks to disperse, and therefore the image appears softer.

There are two options for sharpening an image, the easiest is using built-in presets in imaging software that offer numerous choices for the degree of desired sharpening (Figures 9.55 and 9.56).

For experienced photographers, the manual option involves individually adjusting values for the three variables; amount, radius and threshold (Figures 9.57 and 9.58). Some guideline parameters for manually sharpening dental images are summarised in Table 9.2 (Kelby 2003; Benz 2003).

However, these recommendations are broad guidelines, and a little experimentation is necessary for achieving optimal results. Finally, over-zealous sharpening is counterproductive as it

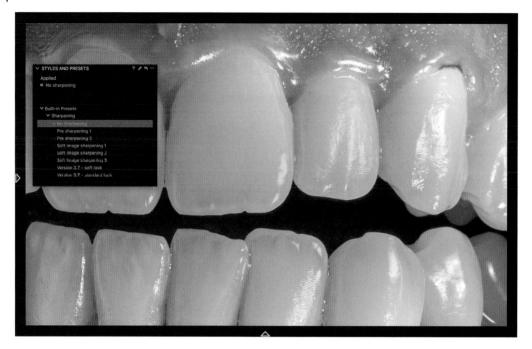

Figure 9.55 The easiest method of sharpening is using built-in software presets, and preview the effect before accepting the changes. Original image before sharpening.

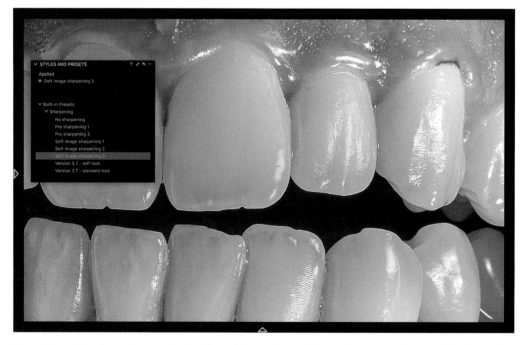

Figure 9.56 After sharpening: notice the effect of sharpening on the perykymata on the enamel surfaces of the maxillary left lateral incisor and canine and the mandibular left lateral incisor. The gingival stippling and incisal edges are also markedly sharper.

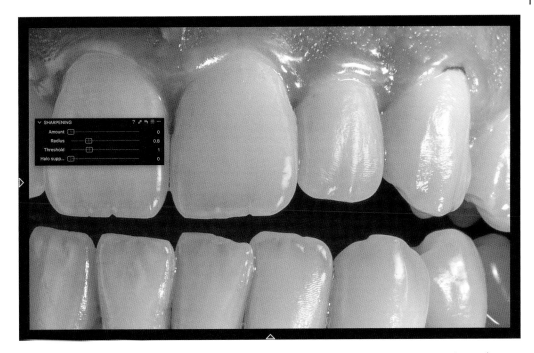

Figure 9.57 Manual sharpening involves inputting values for the three parameters: amount, radius and threshold: Original image before sharpening.

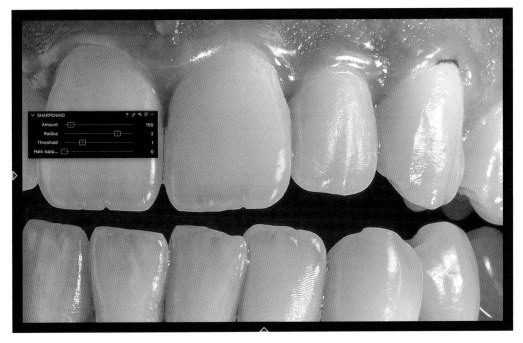

Figure 9.58 After sharpening: notice the effect of sharpening on the perykymata on the enamel surfaces of the maxillary left lateral incisor and canine and the mandibular left lateral incisor. The gingival stippling and incisal edges are also markedly sharper.

Table 9.2 Parameters for manually sharpening dental images.

Type of image	Amount (%)	Radius	Threshold
Intra-oral	100	2	1
Extra-oral/portraits	75	2	3
Bench images	65	4	3
Web use	400	0.3	0

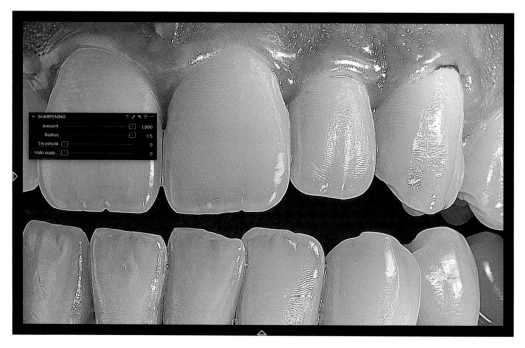

Figure 9.59 Over-zealous sharpening is detrimental to image quality as it introduces image noise, and creates unwanted halos at the edges of objects, e.g. at the incisal edges of teeth. Notice the Halo suppression slider indicated by the red circle.

creates unwanted halos at edges of objects and introduces image noise,[7] which can mimic pathology, especially when applied to intra-oral radiographs (Brettle and Carmichael 2011) (Figure 9.59). Some imaging software have a halo suppression tool for reducing this nuisance, but the results are contentious.

After completing the editing process, the final stage is exporting the images for the intended use, which is the topic of the last module.

---

7 https://helpx.adobe.com/photoshop/atv/cs6-tutorials/sharpening-an-image-with-unsharp-mask.html

References

Ahmad, I. (2009a). Digital dental photography. Part 9: post-image capture processing. *Br. Dent. J.* 207 (5): 203–209.

Ahmad, I. (2009b). Digital dental photography. Part 3: principles of digital photography. *Br. Dent. J.* 206 (10): 517–523.

Badano, A., Revie, C., Casertano, A. et al. (2015). Consistency and standardization of color in medical imaging: a consensus report. *J. Digit. Imaging* 28: 41–52.

Benz, C. (2003). Digital photography: exposures, editing images, and presentation. *Int. J. Comput. Dent.* 6: 249–281.

Brettle, D. and Carmichael, F. (2011). The impact of digital image processing artefacts mimicking pathological features associated with restorations. *Br. Dent. J.* 211: 167–170.

Devigus, A. and Paul, S. (2006). Preparing images for publication: part 1. *Eur. J. Esthet. Dent.* 1: 20–29.

Kelby, S. (2003). *The Photoshop CS Book for Digital Photographers*. Berkeley, CA: New Riders.

Nordberg, J.J. and Sluder, G. (2013). Practical aspects of adjusting digital cameras. *Methods Cell Biol.* 114: 151–162.

Ramsthaler, F., Birngruber, C.G., Kröll, A.K. et al. (2016). True color accuracy in digital forensic photography. *Arch. Kriminol.* 237 (5–6): 190–203.

Sandler, J. and Murray, A. (2002). Manipulation of digital photographs. *J. Orthod.* 29: 189–194.

Sheridan, P. (2013). Practical aspects of clinical photography: part 2 – data management, ethics and quality control. *ANZ J. Surg.* 83: 293–295.

Snow, S.R. (2013). Myths vs reality. *J. Cosmet. Dent.* 29 (1): 62–70.

10

Exporting, Managing and Using Images

The last module of this book deals with exporting, managing and using images for a variety of purposes, and disseminating via various media. This is the final part of the CDP (Capture, Process, Display) imaging chain triad, discussing how images are displayed. After editing images in processing software, the next stage is understanding how and where to export the image files.

Exporting Files

The first priority is deciding the intended use of the images and the requirements of the recipient. These criteria also determines the file format, file size, image dimensions, aspect ratio, naming conventions, and the necessary embedded metadata. The use or recipient of the images have different requirements, and it is better to anticipate these at the outset so that the export process is efficient and productive. Besides archiving, the array of uses include documentation (e.g. dento-legal, treatment planning/monitoring), communication (e.g. e-mail attachments, sharing pictures on mobile devices), marketing (web-publishing, e-marketing, social media, office stationery, treatment portfolios) and education (e.g. lecturing, training) – Figure 10.1. The ensemble of recipients are patients, dental colleagues, dental laboratories, printing houses and publishers. Finally, the images can also be exported externally for manipulation in drawing, image management or practice management software (Figure 10.2).

As explained in the previous module, basic image processing is accomplished with relatively simple and inexpensive software. However, choosing an intermediate or professional level software pays dividends by offering additional features such as bespoke exporting recipes or managing the rich media assets. Rich media assets are any multimedia data, including photographs, annotated images or audio-visual files that are digitally captured, and stored for sharing on various devices such as computers, tablets, smart television, or smartphones.

Output Location

Before exporting files, it is necessary to specify the location where the images are to be stored. The destination can be directly into the patient's named folder and subfolders created by the user, within the editing software (if it offers cataloguing facilities), or alongside dental records of the patient in a dedicated image or practice management software. Also, the files can either be stored on local internal, or peripheral external storage hard drives. In addition, the files may

Essentials of Dental Photography, First Edition. Irfan Ahmad.
© 2020 John Wiley & Sons Ltd. Published 2020 by John Wiley & Sons Ltd.

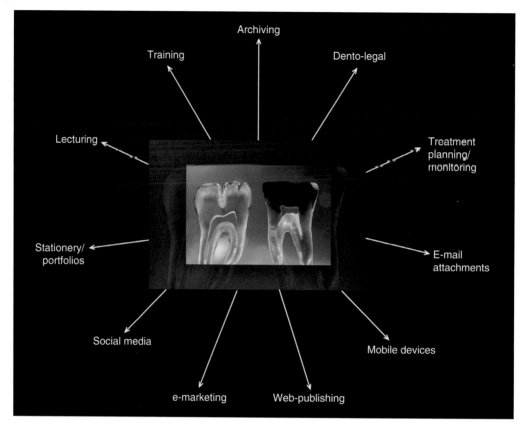

Figure 10.1 Intended uses of dental images.

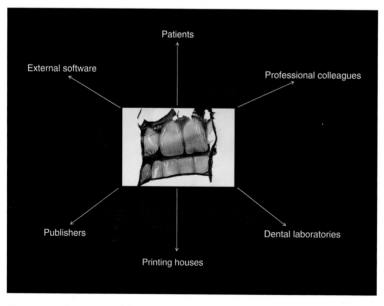

Figure 10.2 Recipients of dental images.

be output to a cloud storage application. Irrespective of the destination, it is advisable to regularly back-up onto remote, preferably off-site, storage devices.

Although digital dental photography offers convenience and accrues possibilities, it also calls for responsibility by safeguarding the integrity of patients, no different to radiographs or dental records. This includes conforming to guidelines according to the HIPAA law (Health Insurance Portability and Accountability Act of 1996). The foremost intention is, of course, to archive and safe keeping of the images. Whichever option is chosen for storing files, the paramount concern is that confidentiality is not compromised, and the medically sensitive data is secure and accessible with stringent security and password protection protocols (Sheridan 2013). The cloud storage option is relatively new, and although it offers benefits by saving local hardware disk space, security may be breached if the server is hacked or fails. Another drawback is that cloud storage requires constant high-speed internet access to retrieve data, and download speeds can be painfully slow for large files. Although no electronic device is foolproof, the hardware storage option is more suited for protecting sensitive data, and offers the benefit of easy and rapid access without having to rely on WiFi connection.

Naming Conventions (Formats)

A naming convention for images is no different to organising a conventional filing system. As an image library expands it soon becomes overwhelming, and trying to find images is a laborious and time-consuming task. The naming convention, or format, can either be custom made by the user, or predefined in dedicated dental asset management programmes. Since dental photography is a niche category, most generic photographic imaging software do not offer a naming convention catering specifically for dentistry. However, it is relatively simple to modify keywords and tokens in any imaging software for dental needs (Figure 10.3). The example shown below is easily saved as user preset, and recalled for future use (Figures 10.4 and 10.5).

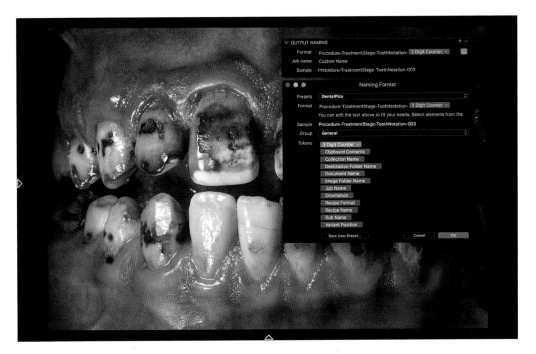

Figure 10.3   A bespoke naming format for dental images.

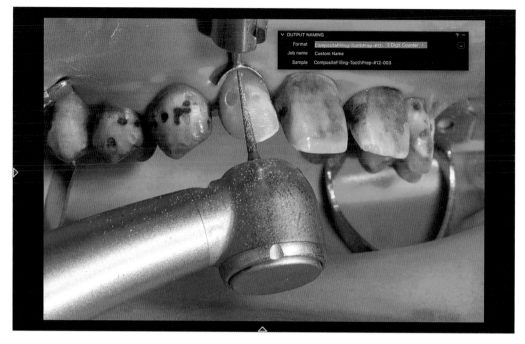

Figure 10.4 Example of a naming convention for CompositeFilling.

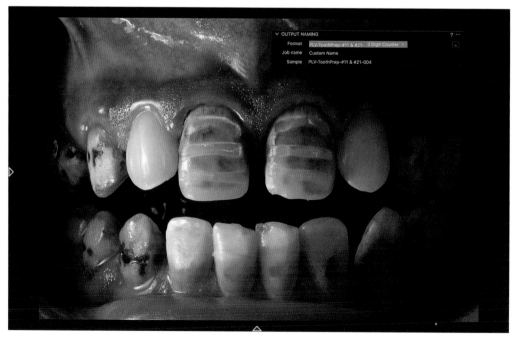

Figure 10.5 Example of a naming convention for PLV.

Export Recipes

An efficient method for exporting images is using export presets, or recipes, which define certain criteria or parameters for specific export requirements. In addition, multiple export recipes can simultaneously be applied to a single or a collection of images for different uses. Most software offers several built-in export recipes containing export settings for helping to export images quickly and efficiently. These recipes can be modified to suit specific needs by changing any parameter, or new ones created and saved for future use. Also, many service or application vendors including printing/publishing houses or website designers have specific requirements for images, and supply export recipes in the form of plug-ins that can be installed in the processing software for exporting the images with the necessary customised settings. Some important ingredients to consider for export recipes are detailed below.

- File properties – It is possible to either export the original files (masters) as captured by the camera, or variants (versions) that have had adjustments applied to them during the editing and manipulation process. However, since the initial captured image always requires some form of modification, in most circumstances it is the edited version of the image that is exported. The file properties include file format, bit depth, compression, resolution, scaling, sharpening for screen or printing, and assigning a default software for viewing the images. Every programme has its unique interface for these items, which are accessed by toolbars, tabs, dialogue boxes and floating or cascading menus.
- Colour spaces – Other useful information to attach when exported files are the ColorSync or ICC (International Color Consortium) profiles (colour spaces), LUTs (Look Up Table) and XMP (Extensible Metadata Platform) sidecar or 'buddy' files. The ColorSync or ICC profiles allow the recipient to match colour profiles on different monitors for ensuring colour consistency, which is essential for diagnosing pathological lesions or shade analysis (Figure 10.6).

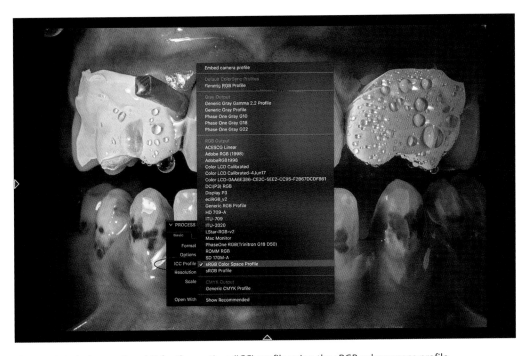

Figure 10.6 An International Color Consortium (ICC) profile using the sRGB colour space profile.

Although there are innumerable colour spaces to choose from, the most frequently used are the sRGB, Adobe° RGB and CMYK (see Figure 9.9 in Module 9). The XMP files contain all processing (developing) changes made while editing the original captured file. This allows the recipient to open the file in another software, or on another computer, and still have access to the original file as well as all data relating to any subsequent developing that was performed. Also, if processing is delegated to an external editing house, after completing the editing, only the XMP file containing the editing changes needs to be returned to the client who can apply them instantly to the original file for reviewing the changes.

- Metadata – In addition to exporting the image file, it is useful to attach technical, administrative and copyright information about an image. These details are termed metadata and are embedded with TIFF or JPEG files. PNG (Portable Network Graphics) files, which are often used for web-publishing, do not support the inclusion of metadata. There are two universally accepted forms of metadata called EXIF (Exchangeable Image File Format)[1] and IPTC (International Press Telecommunications Council) information.[2] The EXIF metadata contains information about the type of camera, lens, flash, camera settings, file format, colour space, date, and GPS location (Figure 10.7). The IPTC information header has three categories of information; administrative, descriptive, and rights. These categories list the creator's name, address, description or content of the image, and can also include patient details and consent, keywords, ratings, colour labels, plus intellectual property and copyright limitations (Figure 10.8). When disseminating images, the metadata can be included or excluded, depending on the intended use or recipient. For example, it is appropriate to include IPTC information containing patient details when liaising with a specialist or professional colleague for co-diagnosis, but inappropriate if the image is intended for web-publishing.

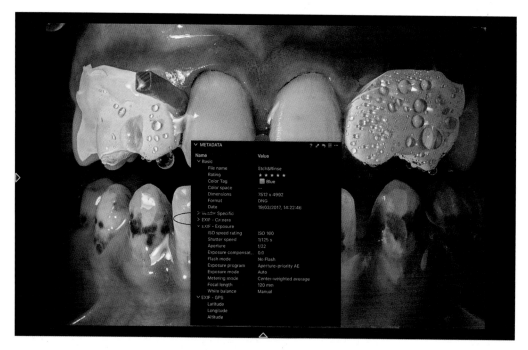

Figure 10.7 An example of Exchangeable Image File Format (EXIF) metadata.

---

1 http://home.jeita.or.jp/tsc/std-pdf/CP3451C.pdf
2 https://iptc.org

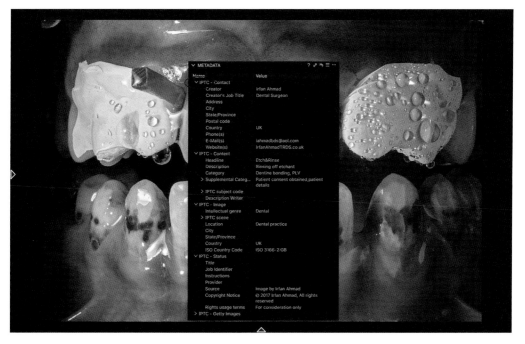

Figure 10.8 An example of International Press Telecommunications Council (IPTC) metadata.

- Watermarks – These are semi-transparent text or logos placed over the image to prevent copyright infringement. It is, of course, easy to save any image from the internet by simply clicking on the right mouse button, but placing an indelible watermark on the image acts as a potential deterrent for unauthorised usage or dissemination (Figure 10.9).
- Parameters – As previously mentioned, most photographic software contain several predefined export recipes for a variety of uses. However, the number of recipes can be reduced to four fundamental types that fulfil almost every requirement. Table 10.1 summarises the recommended parameters for export recipes, which are readily modified to suit individual needs by changing any criteria.

To summarise, there are five easy steps for exporting files (Figures 10.10 and 10.11):

1) Select file(s) to export
2) Select export recipe(s)
3) Select, and/or create, output location folder(s)
4) Type file name(s) according to naming format (convention)
5) Click 'Process' or 'Export'

Image Management

After exporting images, the next stage of the digital dental workflow (Goldstein 2015) is managing the rich media assets. There are several options for image management ensuring security and accessibility of data. Compared to conventional photography, the digital dental workflow presents unique challenges, the most important of which is maintaining confidentially. There are two protocols for organising images, either patient based, or treatment based. The first protocol is sorting according to personal details of the patient, including name, date of birth,

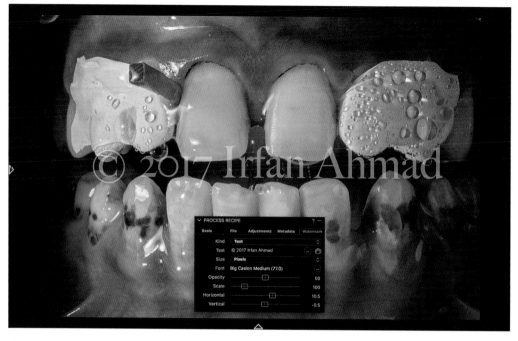

Figure 10.9 A watermark on an image acts as a deterrent for unauthorised usage.

contact information and hospital or practice reference numbers. The second is labelling images according to the types of treatment, and forming a keyword tree that grows over time to include clinical finding, diagnosis, procedures, phases of treatment, outcomes and follow-up (Niamtu 2004). Both options can be combined for filtering and accessing the relevant images for particular needs. Also, images should be processed immediately after a photographic session to facilitate labelling while the memory is fresh to prevent misfiling at a later date.

The first method for storing images is manually creating a hierarchy of folders and subfolders for managing patient images (Nayler 1998). A simple schematic is a main folder titled 'Patient Images' that contains patient name subfolders, followed by date subfolders, which contain consecutively numbered images corresponding to the date folder (Figure 10.12). This manual workflow strategy should be familiarised by members of staff and followed precisely for ensuring consistency. The limitations of the manual option are that the images are not linked with the patient's dental records, and filtering is impossible for retrieving images for specific criteria such as the type of treatment, or stage of treatment.

The second option for storage is purchasing dedicated image management software, which can be a standalone, or integrated within an editing or dental practice management package.[3] Since standalone image management software are catering for many photographic genres, a degree of customisation is necessary for dental use. Examples of the latter include Image Fx, Adobe Lightroom, Capture One, Cumulus, IrfanView and Apple® Photos. These software organise images by systematically cataloguing them in folders, albums, smart albums, etc. This is essentially creating an image database, no different to a patient database for electronically filing dental records (Figure 10.13). The advantage of this method, compared to creating manual folders, is that filters can be applied for retrieving particular images by using keywords such as 'composite fillings', 'implants' and so on. Furthermore, entire folders and albums, which are stored within the software, can be exported to other imaging or dental practice management software.

---

3 http://www.dentalcompare.com/Restorative-Dentistry/4454-Dental-Image-and-Management-Software/

Table 10.1 Recommended parameters for export recipes.

Parameter/principal use	Archiving	Archiving	Web-publishing	Print ready
File format	TIFF	JPEG	JPEG, PNG	TIFF, JPEG
Colour (bit) depth	16-bit or 8-bit/channel	8 bit/channel	8 bit/channel	8 bit/channel
Compression/quality		Maximum or 100% quality	–	Uncompressed TIFF or maximum quality JPEG
International Color Consortium (ICC) profile	sRGB, Adobe RGB[a]	sRGB, Adobe RGB[a]	sRGB, Adobe RGB[a]	sRGB, Adobe RGB, CMYK[a]
Resolution	300 dpi	300 dpi	300 dpi	300 dpi[b]
Scale	100%	100%	Long edge,1600 px[c]	Long edge (never upscale), 4724 px[c]
Sharpening	None	None	Output sharpening for screen[d]	Output sharpening for print[d]
Metadata	Exchangeable Image File Format (EXIF) and International Press Telecommunications Council (IPTC)	EXIF and IPTC	Copyright	EXIF and copyright
Watermarks	None	None	Optional	None
Other uses	Publishing, presentations/lectures	Publishing, presentations/lectures	E-mail attachments, e-brochures, e-marketing, social media	Offset printing, proofing, publishing

dpi: dots (pixels)/inch.
px: pixels.
[a] Recommended colour spaces.
[b] Increase to 600dpi or 800 dpi for line drawings.
[c] Variable, according to requirements of recipient.
[d] Automatic output sharpening by imaging software.

A surfeit of software is available that satisfies dental needs, but each is configured for specific tasks such as image editing, radiographic or cone beam computed tomography (CBCT) imaging, smile design and cosmetic simulations, practice management, accounting and invoicing, payrolls, ordering supplies, and so on. The major advantage of dental management software is the ability to link images with the patient's dental records so that everything is in one place. It is difficult to recommend a particular dental software since every practice and institution is unique, with unique requirements. If a practice already has a dental management software and is looking to incorporate dental imaging into their daily workflow, it is obviously useful to purchase software that can be integrated within the existing programme. Alternately, other practices may prefer software for specific purposes such as digital smile design or simulating aesthetic/cosmetic enhancement procedures for treatment plan acceptance. Furthermore, practices specialising in periodontics may require DICOM (Digital

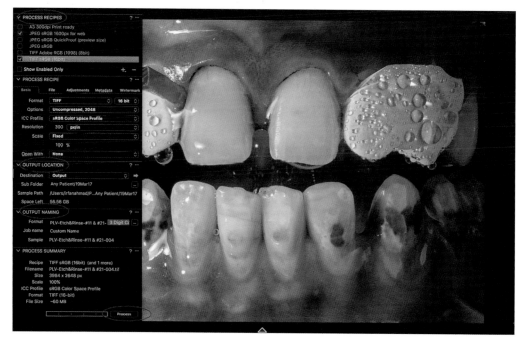

Figure 10.10 Summary of steps for exporting image files.

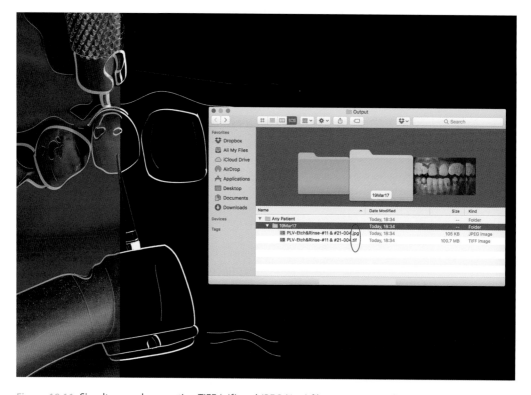

Figure 10.11 Simultaneously exporting TIFF (.tif) and JPEG (.jpg) files to an output folder.

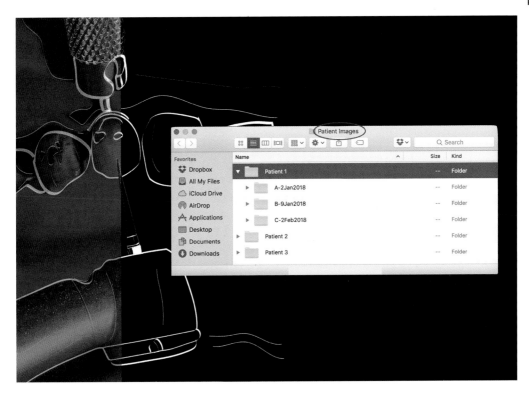

Figure 10.12 Custom hierarchical folders for organising and storing patient images.

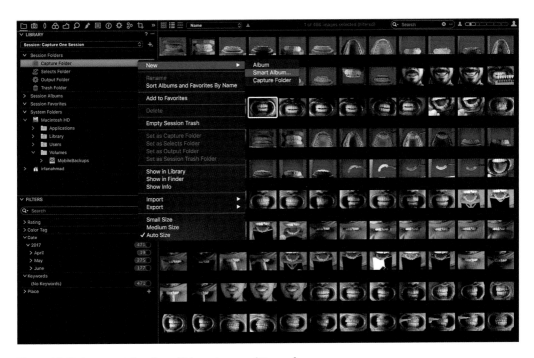

Figure 10.13 Image cataloguing within an image editing software.

Imaging and Communications in Medicine) file format compatibility for viewing CBCT scans for planning implant placement. Examples of popular dedicated dental software include Dentrix, CS Imaging Version 7, MacPractice DDS, Planmeca, Visora and Extensis Portfolio, but many others are available that concentrate on specific tasks. In addition, training and technical assistance from the vendor are indispensable for realising the maximum potential of these programmes, especially the dental digital assets management (DAM) varieties.

Whichever software is chosen, either standalone or integrated programme, each has specific images requirements. This is especially relevant for dental imaging or management software, which require particular file formats, sizes, and dimensions, etc. Therefore, it is advisable to contact the software house to enquire about plug ins, or image parameters, so that export recipes are tailored for exporting images.

Using Images

Having exported and securely stored the image files, the last item to consider is how and when to use them (Ahmad 2009; Wander and Gordon 1987). Besides recording the clinical manifestations of the oral cavity, there is a host of applications for dental imagery, which is broadly categorised into documentation, communication, marketing and education (Christensen 2005) (see Figures 10.1 and 10.2). However, the lines between these categories are nebulous, and the same image if often used for several purposes at different times.

Documentation

The first and foremost usage is dento-legal documentation before starting any therapy, and for subsequent monitoring, progress and outcome of treatment. A collection of pre-operative and treatment progress images form an invaluable record, which should be incorporated into a code of good practice, for defending against litigation of negligence or malpractice.

The second use is for the provision of dental care including clinical findings, diagnosis, treatment planning, outcomes, anticipating complications, and rectifying mistakes. A photographic record is a diagnostic tool, similar to radiographs, study casts or CBCT scans for analysing the clinical status and devising treatment options. Furthermore, any overlooked conditions during an intra-oral examination may be scrutinised at leisure so that a comprehensive plan is devised encompassing all oral lesions and predicaments. Several studies have concluded the importance of photographic documentation for facilitating diagnosis of conditions such as caries (Boye et al. 2013), developmental defects of enamel (DDE) (Chen et al. 2013) and acute trauma (Pinto et al. 2015; Casaglia et al. 2015). Another topical issue is safeguarding vulnerable adults and children; and having a photographic record is irrefutable evidence if abuse is suspected. In addition, dental records, including photographs, are one of the main forms of forensic identification of body remains (Bernstein 1983; Pinto et al. 2015), and for criminal investigations involving matching victims' bite marks to potential suspects (Levine 1977; Golden 2011).

Monitoring is not limited to treatment progress, but also reviewing pathological lesions that fail to heal over a period of time, or following the success or failure of a prescribed modality. In these circumstances, early referral, or intervention, is essential to halt local progression and systemic spread, especially for pre-cancerous lesions such as leukoplakia or suspected squamous cell carcinoma. With the rising demand for elective medical procedures, particularly esthetic dentistry, a series of images showing the initial, during and after status is imperative. Aesthetic dental procedures are highly subjective, and a clinically acceptable outcomes may be greeted with ambivalence and dissatisfaction by the patient. Although any form of treatment is a potential legal nightmare, particular attention is warranted for documenting aesthetic and surgical procedures.

Communication

Every picture not only tells a story, but is also worth a thousand words, especially when faced with the task of typing them. It is far easier to show something rather than explain something; words can be misconstrued or forgotten, but a visual record is unambiguous and indelible. In addition, a photographic depiction compensates for inaccuracies resulting from variations in descriptive ability. The mode of communicating with pictures is either electronic or paper-based. Nowadays, the former is the preferred method, provided stringent security measures are in place such as encrypted e-mails and adhering to HIPAA 1996 guidelines. The main parties to communicate with are patients, dental technicians, professional colleagues or specialist and healthcare providers. Furthermore, the type of image varies according to the intended recipient.

Most patients are unfamiliar with dental modalities, or oblivious to the latest advances in dental therapies. However, other patients are extremely tuned in; a Google search displays a plethora of information about any dental procedure. Therefore, the type of image that is suitable, or demanded by a given individual, varies considerably. Some patients are indifferent to seeing harsh clinical reality, while others only wish to see the before and after shots, without the intermediary stages of how the outcome was achieved. This is particularly the case for treatment involving surgical procedures showing graphical depiction of bone or soft tissue augmentation. At the other end of the spectrum, some patients are pedantic about every single detail, and insist on seeing every stage of a procedure, irrespective of how gory this may seem. Therefore, clinical case studies should be tailored for each patient, respecting his or her wishes regarding the content of the presentation. As well as gaining informed consent for treatment after showing various treatment options, together with their advantages and limitations, case studies are also motivational by emphasising the long-term benefits of achieving and maintaining good oral health (Figure 10.14). Another issue patients may be unaware of is the importance of oral health on their general well-being. For example, the mounting evidence linking periodontitis with cardiovascular diseases, or the mutually destructive nature of diabetes and periodontal health.

Figure 10.14 Pre and post-operative split mouth images are invaluable for showing the importance of good oral health.

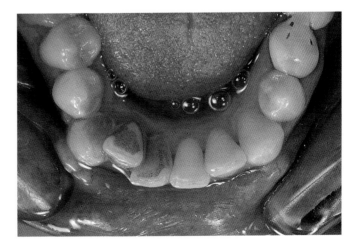

There is currently a burgeoning trend for digital smile design using various simulation soft-ware (Figure 10.15). This involves using a pre-operative intra-oral image that is imported into a smile design software, and using various drawing and manipulation tools, a simulation is created for smile enhancement (McLaren et al. 2013) (Figures 10.16 and 10.17). While these programmes are useful for communicating treatment possibilities, their limitation is that what is achievable on a screen monitor may not be reproducible in the mouth. Therefore, a prag-matic approach is advised; making extravagant claims that may not, or cannot be substantiated

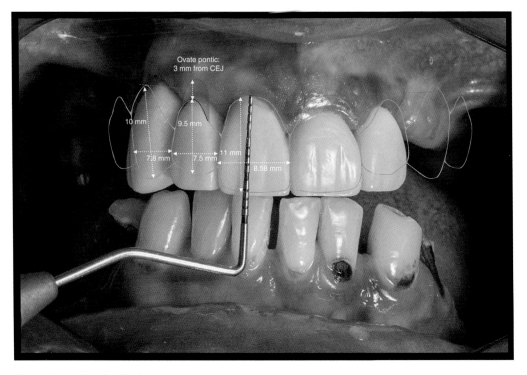

Figure 10.15 Digital smile design.

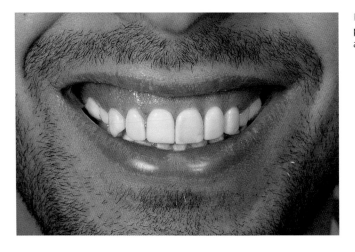

Figure 10.16 Software simulation: pre-operative image of patient with a 'gummy smile'.

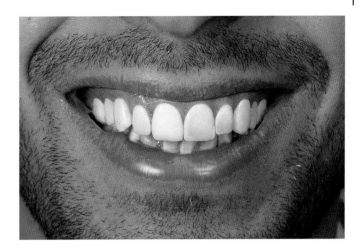

Figure 10.17 Software simulation: digital simulation showing aesthetic enhancement of the smile.

in the clinical environment is committing hara-kiri. On an optimistic note, most treatment is successful and immensely satisfying for both the clinician and patient, and offering patients an electronic slide show or printed portfolio of before and after results does wonders for the reputation of a practice or clinician.

An effective method for communicating with the dental laboratory is with images. This includes visual prescriptions for diagnostic wax-ups, articulating study casts, indirect restorations, orthodontic appliances, surgical guides, removable denture frameworks, etc. (Terry et al. 1999; Mahn 2013) A laboratory prescription can incorporate shade analysis, as well as detailed annotations showing chromatic and characterisation maps for helping the ceramist recreate these effects in the definitive restoration(s). If the ceramist does not have access to the patient, a series of images act as a guide for every stage of treatment such as pre-operative analysis, intra-oral mock-ups, temporarie and try-in stages, which are invaluable for anticipating and correcting problems before delivery of the final prostheses (Figures 10.18–10.25). This methodology is also crucial for involving patients with treatment, and gaining their approval before proceeding with subsequent stages of therapy. All images used for laboratory communication should faithfully reproduce the clinical environment with fidelity, especially colour rendition for consistency of shade matching.

In many instances a second option is advisable for pathological lesions (Riley et al. 2004), or for a collaborative interdisciplinary treatment plan. In these circumstances, standardised images are mandatory, i.e. colour space profiles and metadata should be included for calibration and identification, respectively. This prevents misdiagnosis, which is essential for arriving at a correct prescription for the prevailing condition. In addition, images showing pathology should always include some form of reference for scaling and orientation. This could involve framing the picture so that adjacent teeth or surrounding oral anatomy are in the field of view, or reference markers such as periodontal measuring probes or graduated rulers placed next to suspected lesions for accessing scale. Lastly, annotations and grid lines are useful adjuncts for orientation (Figures 10.26 and 10.27).

A further use of dental images is liaising with government or insurance-based healthcare providers. In some instances, a proposed treatment may require pre-authorisation, and the insurance company or health authority may request pre-operative images for assessing the validity of the proposed therapy. Also, claims-processing or disputes are facilitated by forwarding pre and post-operative images regarding a particular item or course of treatment.

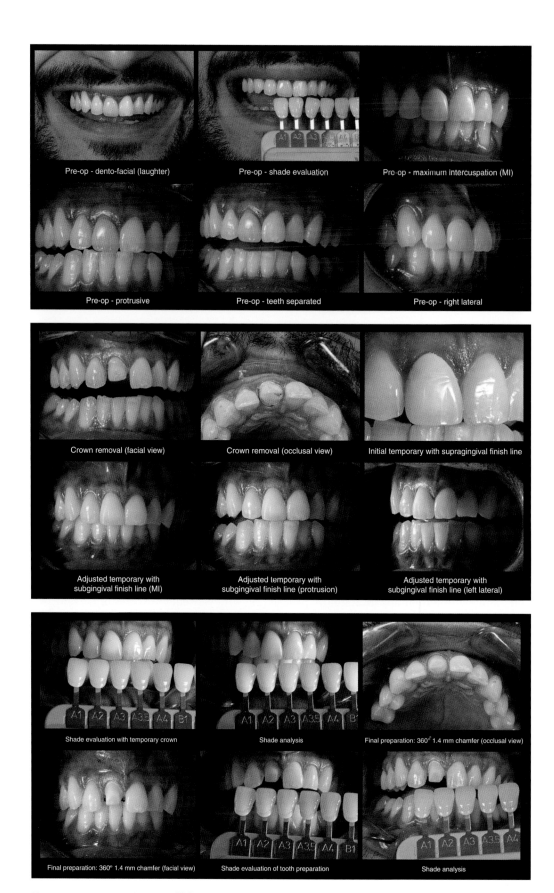

Figures 10.18–10.23 Annotated laboratory prescription for replacing a defective crown on the maxillary right central incisor.

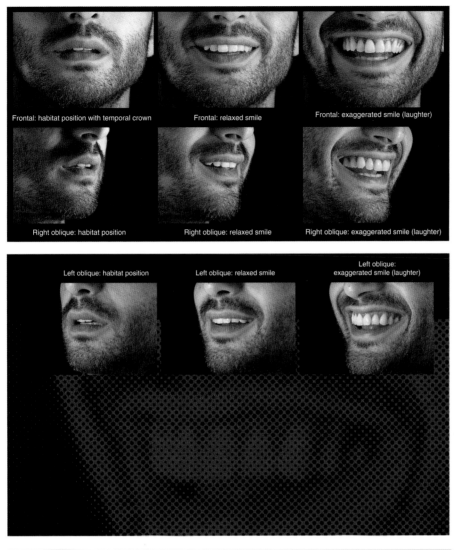

Frontal: habitat position with temporal crown

Frontal: relaxed smile

Frontal: exaggerated smile (laughter)

Right oblique: habitat position

Right oblique: relaxed smile

Right oblique: exaggerated smile (laughter)

Left oblique: habitat position

Left oblique: relaxed smile

Left oblique: exaggerated smile (laughter)

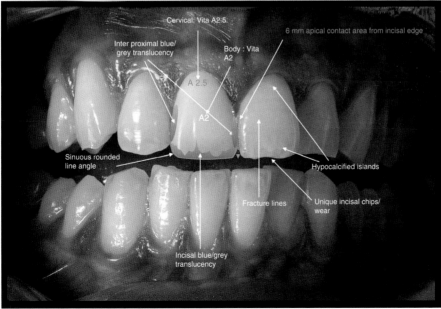

Cervical: Vita A2.5

Inter proximal blue/ grey translucency

Body : Vita A2

6 mm apical contact area from incisal edge

A 2.5

A2

Sinuous rounded line angle

Hypocalcified islands

Fracture lines

Unique incisal chips/ wear

Incisal blue/grey translucency

Figures 10.18–10.23 (Continued)

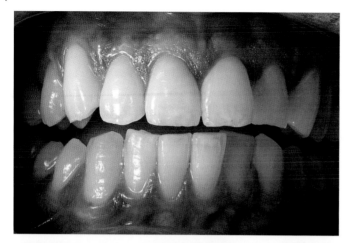

Figures 10.24 and 10.25 show the post-operative result after replacing the defective crown on the maxillary right central incisor with an all-ceramic e-max™ crown.

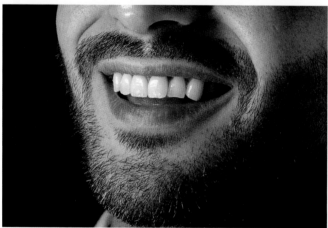

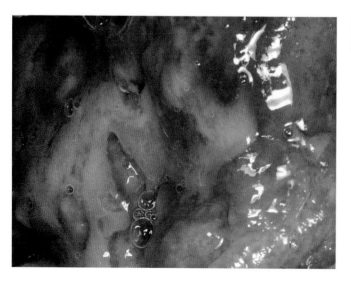

Figure 10.26 A potentially malignant lesion without surrounding anatomical landmarks.

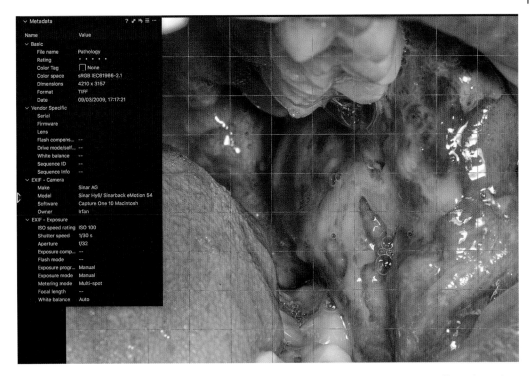

Name	Value
∨ Basic	
File name	Pathology
Rating	• • • • •
Color Tag	☐ None
Color space	sRGB IEC61966-2.1
Dimensions	4210 x 3157
Format	TIFF
Date	09/03/2009, 17:17:21
∨ Vendor Specific	
Serial	
Firmware	
Lens	
Flash compens...	--
Drive mode/self...	--
White balance	--
Sequence ID	--
Sequence Info	--
∨ EXIF - Camera	
Make	Sinar AG
Model	Sinar Hy6/ Sinarback eMotion 54
Software	Capture One 10 Macintosh
Owner	Irfan
∨ EXIF - Exposure	
ISO speed rating	ISO 100
Shutter speed	1/30 s
Aperture	f/32
Exposure comp...	--
Flash mode	--
Exposure progr...	Manual
Exposure mode	Manual
Metering mode	Multi-spot
Focal length	--
White balance	Auto

Figure 10.27 The same image as Figure 10.26, but framed to show surrounding anatomy, grid lines for scaling, and colour space metadata for colour calibration (blue circle).

Marketing

There is a thin line between marketing and coercion. Ethical marketing is laudable since it offers a service that the populous may be unaware of, or for seeking a clinician proficient in a particular treatment modality. However, the distinction between ethical and non-ethical marketing is often blurred, and unfortunately, transgression into hyperbole is common. What constitutes ethical marketing is difficult to define, but blatant statements claiming miracles or exaggerating treatment outcomes are encroaching on an abyss that is unsurmountable. Therefore, it is left to the individual or practice to seek guidelines from governing bodies and indemnity organisations before embarking on a potentially costly and vain marketing campaign.

The images used for marketing purposes are usually sanitised to show the best 'view' or emphasise positive outcomes of dental treatment. In this respect, they may be construed as contrived and not clinically 'honest', but because their intended use is for promotion and moti-vation, and hence, a certain degree of latitude or artistic licence is permissible (Figure 10.28). This should not translate to carte blanche for disguising poor outcomes or hiding defects and mistakes by flagrant manipulation. Instead, the images should covey an aura, or highlight a beautiful veneer or composite fillings with appropriate lighting – or, put another way, showing results in the 'best possible light'. However, some take a dim view of this form of portrayal as being deceptive. On the flip side of the coin, the argument is that the purpose of these stylised images is motivational, and therefore differs from standardised clinical images that serve an entirely different purpose (Figures 10.29–10.31).

There are two types of marketing, internal (within the practice or institution) and external (online or print). However, with the advent of mobile devices such as smartphone and tablets,

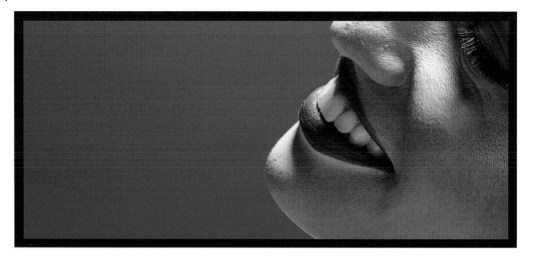

Figure 10.28 Marketing images are not always clinically honest, since their purpose is to entice and allure.

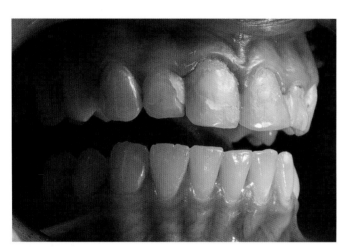

Figure 10.29 Images used for marketing and presentations are motivational and alluring. The pre-operative image shows defective composite restorations in the maxillary anterior sextant.

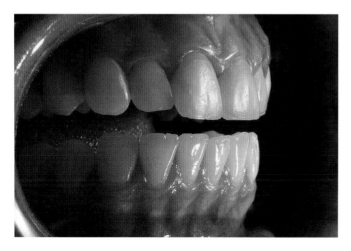

Figure 10.30 Replacement fillings after contouring, but before polishing.

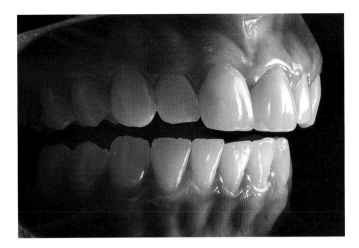

Figure 10.31 Post-operative image after polishing the composite restorations. The key light was positioned on the left side of the patient to encourage specular reflections for conveying vitality, and showing the fillings in their 'best possible light'.

this distinction is somewhat obsolete. The traditional choice of media is printed stationery, branded gifts, brochures and leaflets. The electronic media are digital picture frames, laptop or tablet presentations, e-brochures, e-mails, social media, websites and blogs. Hence, even compared to a few decades ago, the scope for dissemination is immense.

Although the conventional printed methods are somewhat antiquated, a well-designed practice brochure showing high-quality before and after shots still carries weight; tactile sense hasn't totally surrendered to the virtual era. Nevertheless, the order of the day is embracing new technology. All the information compiled in a brochure is converted into a digital form as an e-brochure PDF file, and attached to targeted e-mails to existing or potential new patients. There are several marketing companies offering e-mail addresses of specific socio-economic groups in any given locality. Also, the marketing material can be uploaded to various hosting domains such as Facebook, Twitter, Instagram, Flickr, Google, WhatsApp, LinkedIn, Viber, Baidu Tieba and so on.

Whereas in the past building a website involved engaging a web designing agency at considerable cost and time, now even a novice can build a professional-looking and interactive site in a few days at almost no cost (Figure 10.32). Online web designing companies such as WordPress have revolutionised and simplified building websites. Most of these companies offer a free starter pack, plus the option to upgrade by purchasing specific templates, 24/7 online help and hosting services for ensuring the integrity of the site for a relatively modest fee. Besides listing practice details, a website is probably the best way of showcasing treatment outcomes, practice or clinician(s) achievements, which can regularly be updated with blogs and posts. Another feature of interactive websites is allowing visitors to respond to the content of the site. This instant feedback is ideal for gauging the 'thumbs-up' or 'thumbs-down', and making changes in order to increase web traffic. Finally, the password-protected statistical analysis is useful for tracking visitor numbers and for assessing the success (or failure) of a website.

Education

The last use of dental images is the education realm that expounds self, patient, staff and professional learning. The protagonist on this list is the clinician, who benefits the most by learning from failures and critiquing his or her own work. This is essential since without clinical self-deprecation there is little possibility for improving clinical skills and foreseeing and mitigating mistakes.

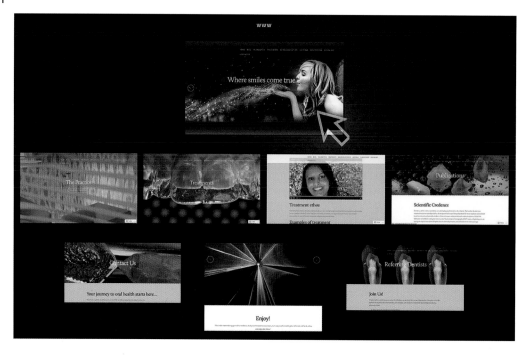

Figure 10.32 An interactive and professional looking website can be created within days, with little or no cost.

The images for educational purposes should 'talk to the audience' by effusing vitality and spark. Furthermore, they should inspire and motivate the delegates rather than causing tedium and boredom. This is not to say that the images should be frivolously altered with pyrotechnic effects that neither add to the understanding of a particular technique, nor enhance the message being delivered. Instead, the photographer should concentrate on using photographic techniques for producing pictures that captivate the audience and secure their attention. There are several methods for achieving these objectives. For example, composing pictures using the rule of thirds, converging lines, or thinking outside the box for capturing views that are unusual and interesting (Figures 10.33 and 10.34). Other methods include unidirectional lighting for enhancing texture and depth, lighting from various angles to create specular reflections

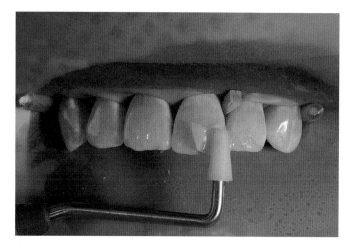

Figure 10.33 Unusual images captivate the audience and enhance the learning process, such as this image showing placement of the last incremental enamel layer of composite for restoring a Class IV cavity.

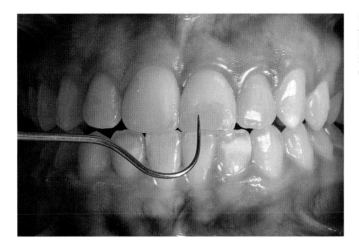

Figure 10.34 Remnants of cement following removal of orthodontic brackets can be detected by scratching the labial surface with a dental probe.

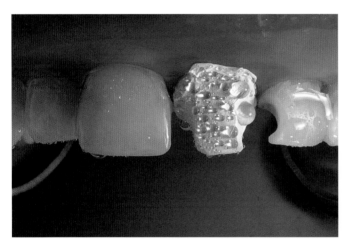

Figure 10.35 Unidirectional lighting creates shadows that convey depth, while specular reflections confer vitality.

(Figure 10.35), and illuminating only a few teeth or a particular part of the oral cavity. Also, the picture should be framed to include only relevant items, extreme magnification for highlighting a particular anatomical feature (Figures 10.36–10.41), adding annotations (Figures 10.42–10.45), or selective focusing on items of interest and blurring the background. If a series of images are showing a particular technique, a simple approach is association, i.e. placing instruments or materials adjacent to the teeth or soft tissues to add relevance (Figures 10.46 and 10.47), especially if these are an integral part of the procedure (Figures 10.48–10.60). To add credence to a lecture, it is always beneficial to show the longevity of a particular restoration or procedure (Signori 2018) (Figures 10.61–10.63). Finally, a striking effect is using colour for visual impact, e.g. selectively isolating a coloured item for emphasis, while making the remainder of the picture black and white (Figure 10.64).

Staff training and education conveys a sense of belonging and unity, making everyone feel that they are part of a team. It also informs staff members about dental procedures so they are fully conversant with various treatment modalities, and can relay this information to patients who may be apprehensive about the therapy they are about to embark upon. Another benefit is updating colleagues with the latest clinical techniques and legislative changes for smooth running of a practice or institution. Also, clinical appraisal is particularly relevant if an office has a dedicated treatment coordinator who is responsible for discussing treatment options

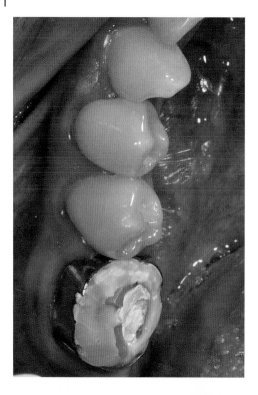

Figure 10.36 Framing only a few teeth allows the viewer to concentrate on the relevant technique being shown. Pre-operative view of a failing mandibular left first molar.

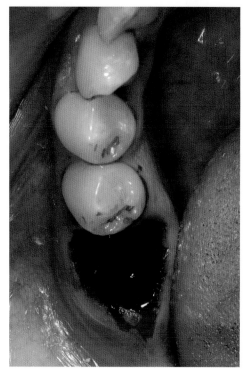

Figure 10.37 Atraumatic extraction with intact buccal and lingual alveolar plates.

Figure 10.38 Immediate implant placement and simultaneous augmentation with bovine xenograft.

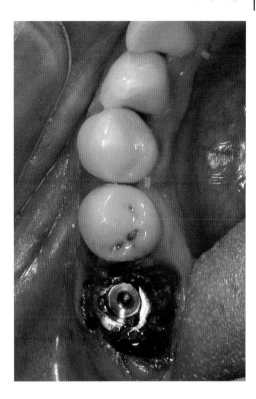

Figure 10.39 Immediate screw retained acrylic crown.

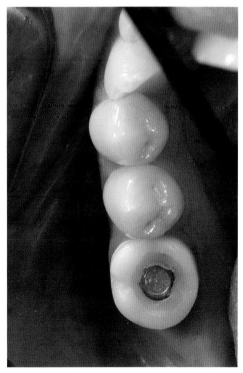

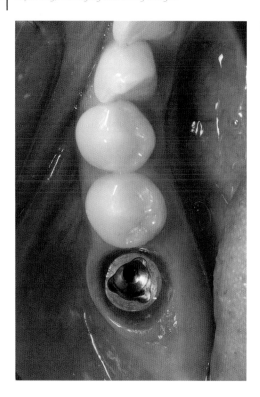

Figure 10.40 Osseointegration after six month healing.

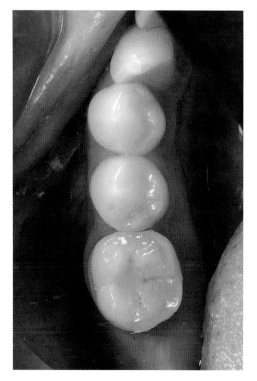

Figure 10.41 Definitive porcelain fused to metal screw retained crown.

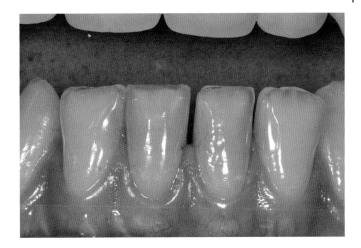

Figure 10.42 Adding annotations is extremely useful for teaching, such as a chromatic map for these complex composite restorations in the mandibular central incisors: pre-operative status showing defective and stained restorations with a median diastema.

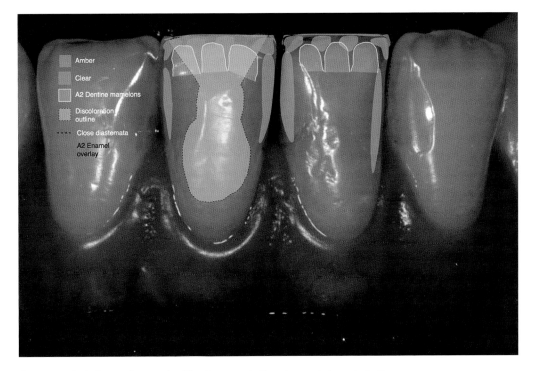

Amber
Clear
A2 Dentine mamelons
Discoloration outline
Close diastemata
A2 Enamel overlay

Figure 10.43 A chromatic map detailing incremental layering and characterisations.

with patients, and counselling them about the importance of diet and home oral hygiene procedures.

The next education endeavour involves clinical research, lecturing, publishing and presenting at dental conferences. Besides the obvious egotistical self-gratification of having your name in print, the spin-off is adding kudos for a clinician or practice that reassures patients they are receiving state-of-the-art dentistry. Although academia is not for everyone, it is still worthwhile meticulously documenting clinical cases for sharing with colleagues on an informal basis.

In an academic environment, use of dental photography can inspire creativity for both undergraduate and postgraduate students (Siegle 2012). Furthermore, many prospective and

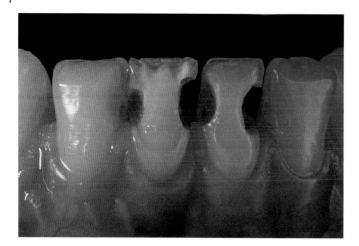

Figure 10.44 Tooth preparation.

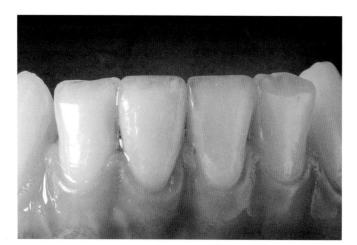

Figure 10.45 Post-operative result.

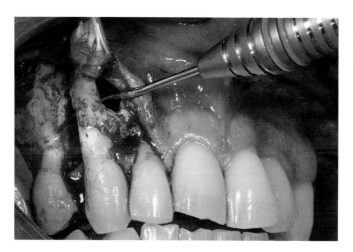

Figure 10.46 Placing a probe in this photograph shows the extent of bone loss encircling the root of the maxillary right canine.

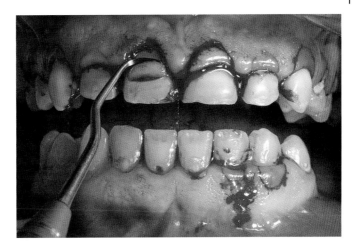

Figure 10.47 A curette being used to remove excised soft tissue after gingivectomy during an aesthetic crown lengthening procedure.

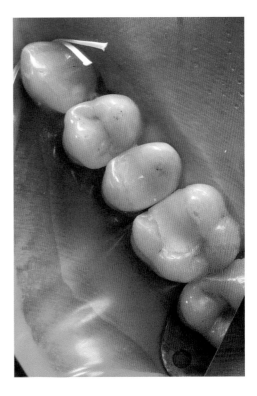

Figure 10.48 Incorporating instruments and materials in a series of images showing a clinical technique aids the learning process: pre-operative defective filling in the maxillary right first molar.

retrospective studies rely on photographic documentation for monitoring changes in treatment outcomes over time, and ascertaining survival and success rates. The use of simulation software for intentionally altering images is useful for epidemiological survey studies, especially relating to aesthetic dentistry (Ker et al. 2008). If images are to be sent to publishing houses, it is prudent to read the author guidelines for ensuring the correct file format, size and dimensions. Also, if large TIFF files are required by the publishers, it is better to use applications such as Dropbox for transmitting the files, rather than waiting hours for e-mail attachments to upload.

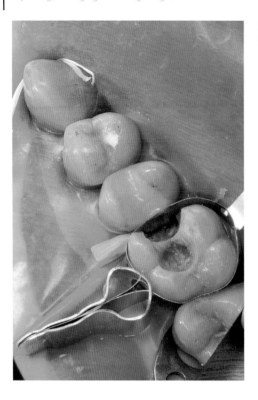

Figure 10.49 After removing the filling, a matrix band is secured with an interdental wooden wedge.

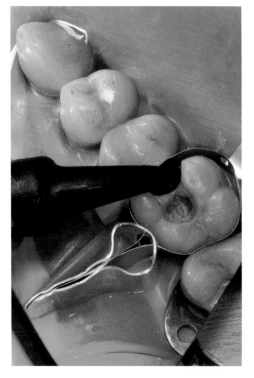

Figure 10.50 Bulk-fill composite being introduced into the cavity following etching and application of a dentine bonding agent.

Figure 10.51 A craving instrument for sculpting the composite.

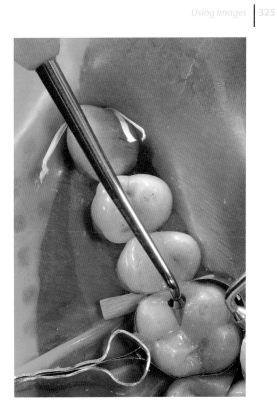

Figure 10.52 Post-operative result.

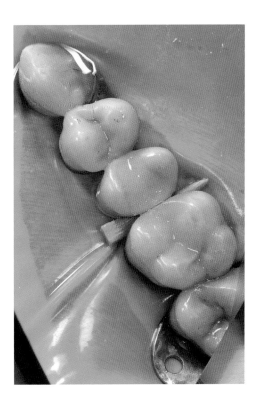

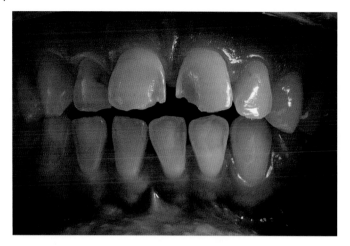

Figure 10.53 Incorporating instruments and materials in a series of images showing a clinical technique aids the learning process: pre-operative status showing profound tooth surface loss associated with both the maxillary and mandibular teeth (intra-oral fontal view).

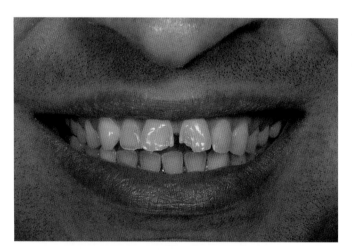

Figure 10.54 Pre-operative dento-facial frontal view showing compromised anterior dental aesthetics.

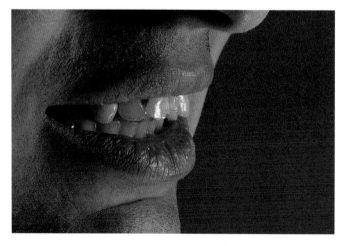

Figure 10.55 Pre-operative dento-facial right oblique view showing compromised anterior dental aesthetics. Notice that the patient's left cheek and background are out of focus to concentrate on the anterior teeth.

Figure 10.56 Intra-oral acrylic mock-ups for the maxillary incisors fabricated from a diagnostic wax-up.

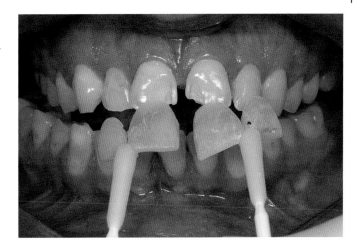

Figure 10.57 Intra-oral acrylic mock-ups 'luted' with a glycerine water soluble try-in paste.

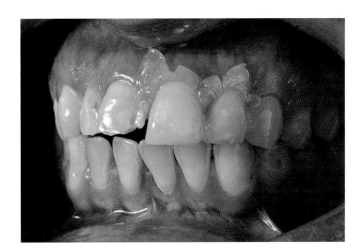

Figure 10.58 Intra-oral frontal view of mock-ups in-situ after removing excess try-in paste.

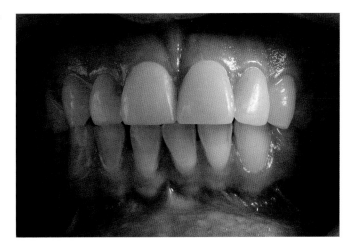

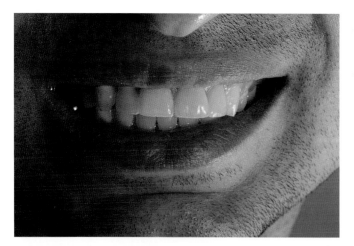

Figure 10.59 Dento-facial frontal view of mock-ups in-situ photographed with unidirectional lighting to emphasise highlights and shadows.

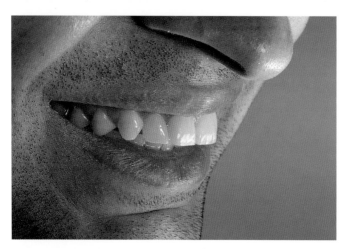

Figure 10.60 Dento-facial right oblique view of mock-ups in-situ. Notice that the patient's left cheek and background are out of focus to concentrate on the anterior teeth (similar to Figure 10.55).

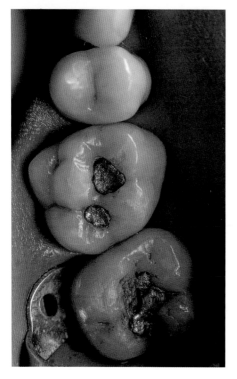

Figure 10.61 Monitoring the longevity of restorations adds credence to a presentation: pre-operative defective amalgam restorations in the maxillary left first and second molars.

Figure 10.62 Immediate post-operative replacement of amalgams with resin-based composite (RBC) restorations.

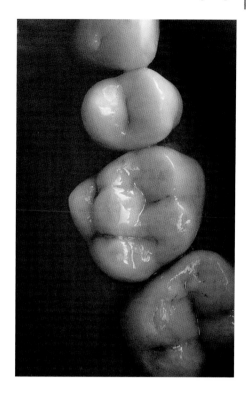

Figure 10.63 Resin-based composite (RBC) 14 years later.

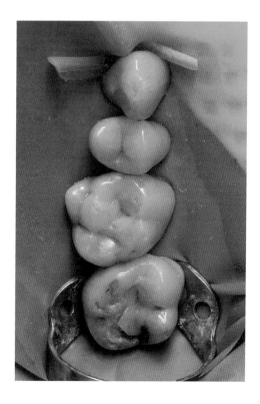

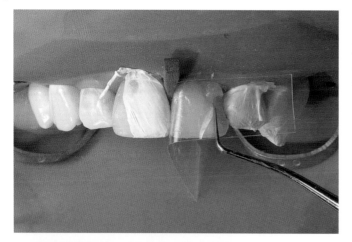

Figure 10.64 Selective colour isolation for emphasising the use of a wooden [pink] wedge for transiently separating the teeth during a composite build-up for ensuring a tight contact area between the maxillary central incisors.

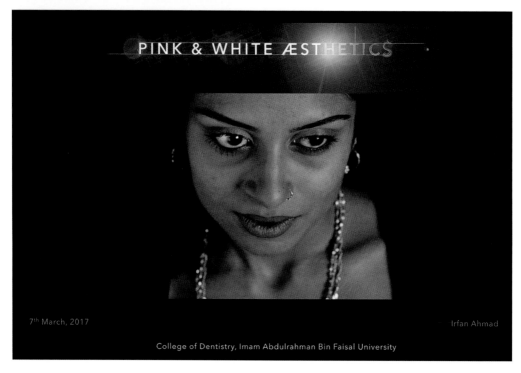

Figure 10.65 The most popular presentation programmes are PowerPoint and Keynote.

Preparing a lecture for conferences requires using presentation software. The most widely used applications are PowerPoint™ or Keynote™, which are both relatively easy to use and require minimum or no training for basic features (Figure 10.65). An important issue before starting is setting the correct aspect ratio of the presentation, which should correspond with the projector at the venue. Also, the aspect ratio determines whether the images require cropping to accommodate the chosen ratio. For example, some popular aspect ratios are 4 : 3, or widescreen 16 : 9, but some conferences or projectors require different ratios, and it is worth checking beforehand to ensure that the presentation is compatible with a particular projector. Besides the aspect ratio, the native resolution of the auditorium projector, e.g. 720p, 1080p or 4K, also influences the dimensions of the presentation. The second issue is using relatively small files,

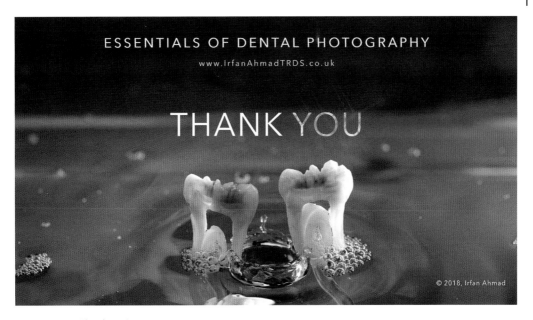

Figure 10.66 *Thank you!*

preferably JPEGs rather than TIFFs, so that the upload and transition time between slides is quicker. Preparing a presentation is time-consuming depending on the vision of the lecturer. However, images supplemented by line drawings and synoptic text are accomplished relatively easily. On the other hand, if the intention is incorporating videos, audio, sophisticated transitions and animation effects, the task is far more demanding, and some training, as well as patience, is necessary for creating memorable visual impact – *Thank you!* (Figure 10.66).

References

Ahmad, I. (2009). Digital dental photography. Part 2: purposes and uses. *Br. Dent. J.* 206: 459–464.

Bernstein, M.L. (1983). The application of photography in forensic dentistry. *Dent. Clin. North Am.* 27: 151–170.

Boye, U., Pretty, I.A., Tickle, M. et al. (2013). Comparison of caries detection methods using varying numbers of intra-oral digital photographs with visual examination for epidemiology in children. *BMC Oral Health* 13: 6.

Casaglia, A., DeDominics, P., Arcuri, L. et al. (2015). Dental photography today. Part 1: basic concepts. *Oral Implantol.* 8 (4): 122–129.

Chen, Y., Lee, W., Ferretti, G.A. et al. (2013). Agreement between photographic and clinical examinations in detecting developmental defects of enamel in infants. *J. Public Health Dent.* 73 (3): 204–209.

Christensen, G.J. (2005). Important clinical uses for digital photography. *J. Am. Dent. Assoc.* 136: 77–79.

Golden, G.S. (2011). Standards and practices for bite mark photography. *J. Forensic Odontostomatol.* 29 (2): 29–37.

Goldstein, S.H. (2015). Adobe Photoshop Lightroom and its application in dentistry – An overview of digital dental workflow. http://www.stevenhgoldsteindds.com/for-doctors/dental-workshops-scottsdale-az-coming-2015/.

Ker, A.J., Chan, R., Fields, H.W. et al. (2008). Esthetics and smile characteristics from the layperson's perspective. *J. Am. Dent. Assoc.* 139 (10): 1318–1327.

Levine, L.J. (1977). Bite mark evidence. *Dent. Clin. North Am.* 21: 145–158.

Mahn, E. (2013). Dental photography. Part II. Protocol for shade taking and communication with the lab. *Intern. Dent. Australas. Ed.* 8 (2).

McLaren, E.A., Garber, D.A., and Figueira, J. (2013). The Photoshop Smile Design technique (part 1): digital dental photography. *Compend. Contin. Educ. Dent.* 34 (10): 772. 774, 776 passim.

Nayler, J. (1998). A clinical image library using photo CD. *J. Audiov. Media Med.* 21: 99–103.

Niamtu, J. (2004). Image is everything: pearls and pitfalls of digital photography and PowerPoint presentations for the cosmetic surgeon. *Dermatol. Surg.* 30: 81–91.

Pinto, G.D., Goettems, M.L., Brancher, L.C. et al. (2015). Validation of the digital photographic assessment to diagnose traumatic dental injuries. *Dent. Traumatol.* 32 (1): 37–42.

Riley, R.S., Ben-Ezra, J.M., Massey, D. et al. (2004). Digital photography: a primer for pathologists. *J. Clin. Lab Anal.* 18 (2): 91–128.

Sheridan, P. (2013). Practical aspects of clinical photography: Part 2 – Data management, ethics and quality control. *ANZ J. Surg.* 83: 293–295.

Siegle, D. (2012). Using digital photography to enhance student creativity. *Gifted Child Today* 35 (4): 285–289.

Signori, C. (2018). *Journal of Dentistry* 71: 54–60.

Terry, D.A., Moreno, C., Geller, W. et al. (1999). The importance of laboratory communication in modern dental practice: stone models without faces. *Pract. Periodont. Aesthet. Dent.* 11: 1125–1132.

Wander, P. and Gordon, P. (1987). Specific applications of dental photography. *Br. Dent. J.* 162 (10): 393–403.

Index

Note: **Bold** page numbers indicate Figures and *Italic* page numbers indicate Tables.

Essentials of Dental Photography, First Edition. Irfan Ahmad.
© 2020 John Wiley & Sons Ltd. Published 2020 by John Wiley & Sons Ltd.